SAGE was founded in 1965 by Sara Miller McCune to support the dissemination of usable knowledge by publishing innovative and high-quality research and teaching content. Today, we publish over 900 journals, including those of more than 400 learned societies, more than 800 new books per year, and a growing range of library products including archives, data, case studies, reports, and video. SAGE remains majority-owned by our founder, and after Sara's lifetime will become owned by a charitable trust that secures our continued independence.

Los Angeles | London | New Delhi | Singapore | Washington DC | Melbourne

PSYCHO-SOCIAL HEALTH ISSUES
in Indian Youth

Thank you for choosing a SAGE product!
If you have any comment, observation or feedback,
I would like to personally hear from you.

Please write to me at **contactceo@sagepub.in**

Vivek Mehra, Managing Director and CEO, SAGE India.

Bulk Sales

SAGE India offers special discounts
for purchase of books in bulk.
We also make available special imprints
and excerpts from our books on demand.

For orders and enquiries, write to us at

Marketing Department
SAGE Publications India Pvt Ltd
B1/I-1, Mohan Cooperative Industrial Area
Mathura Road, Post Bag 7
New Delhi 110044, India

E-mail us at **marketing@sagepub.in**

Subscribe to our mailing list
Write to **marketing@sagepub.in**

This book is also available as an e-book.

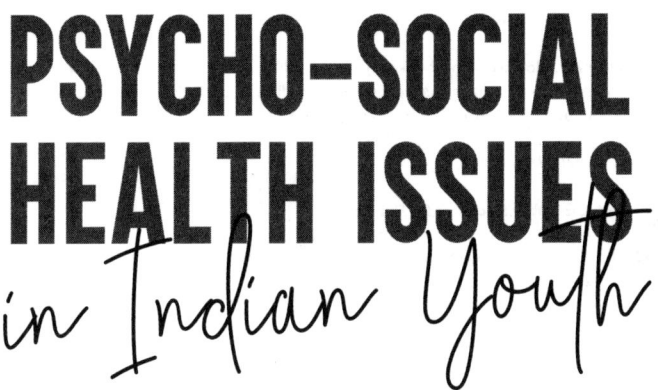

PSYCHO-SOCIAL HEALTH ISSUES
in Indian Youth

Emerging Trends
and Intervention

ALKA WADKAR

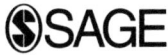

Los Angeles | London | New Delhi
Singapore | Washington DC | Melbourne

First published in 2022 by

SAGE Publications India Pvt Ltd
B1/I-1 Mohan Cooperative Industrial Area
Mathura Road, New Delhi 110 044, India
www.sagepub.in

SAGE Publications Inc
2455 Teller Road
Thousand Oaks, California 91320, USA

SAGE Publications Ltd
1 Oliver's Yard, 55 City Road
London EC1Y 1SP, United Kingdom

SAGE Publications Asia-Pacific Pte Ltd
18 Cross Street #10-10/11/12
China Square Central
Singapore 048423

Published by Vivek Mehra for SAGE Publications India Pvt Ltd and typeset in 10.5/13 pt Berkeley by AG Infographics, Delhi.

Library of Congress Cataloging-in-Publication Data

Names: Wadkar, A. J., author.
Title: Psycho-social health issues in Indian youth : emerging trends and intervention / Alka Wadkar.
Description: Thousand Oaks : SAGE, 2021. | Includes bibliographical references and index. |
Identifiers: LCCN 2021042986 (print) | LCCN 2021042987 (ebook) |
    ISBN 9789354791055 (hardback) | ISBN 9789354791062 (epub) | ISBN 9789354791130 (ebook)
Subjects: LCSH: Youth—Mental health—India.
Classification: LCC RJ502.I4 W33 2021 (print) | LCC RJ502.I4 (ebook) | DDC 618.92/8900954—dc23
LC record available at https://lccn.loc.gov/2021042986
LC ebook record available at https://lccn.loc.gov/2021042987

ISBN: 978-93-5479-105-5 (HB)

SAGE Team: Rajesh Dey, Syed Husain Naqvi, Aishna Bhatt and Rajinder Kaur

CONTENTS

PREFACE

This book is written with a unique approach. It is a blend of scientific knowledge, factual information of daily life and application orientation. It is a brief and informal communication with the readers. Salient features of the book are lucid language and an account of relevant research done abroad and in India. Every phenomenon is explained with reference to Indian culture and the Indian situation. Indian incidence, peculiar Indian problems, psychological and logical flaws in thinking, feeling and behaviour of the Indian community are discussed in depth. This book is focused on challenges to psycho-social problems of Indian adolescents and youth.

Youth are the future of the family, society and the nation. Adolescence and youth are the golden periods of human life. On the one hand, an individual is increasingly becoming more capable of handling various responsibilities in day-to-day life, and on the other, they have to resist various temptations and maintain a balanced view. Due to global impact, new individualistic values are emerging. A substantial number of adolescents and youth are attracted to some socially unacceptable and individually damaging behavioural practices. This results in various risks: physiological and psychological. This book is about strengthening awareness about the same. It is an attempt to enhance understanding of the risk and ways to regain psycho-social health. The present book also suggests ways to deal with the problem situation and intervention necessary for that.

The aim of this book is to discuss contemporary common issues related to psycho-social health from different perspectives:

psychological, social, cultural and biological. It will be useful not only for psychology students and counsellors but also for other students, parents and teachers and even for laypeople. To give some examples, it includes the impact of sex addiction and pornography addiction, along with drug and alcohol addiction. The book explores the psychological impact of hidden and neglected issues, such as emotional abuse and marital rape with sexual abuse, harassment and rape. It deals with serious psychological clinical disorders and discusses suicide among youth. Effects of trauma and chronic and terminal diseases are considered at length. Most common behavioural problems, such as aggression and violence among youth, are depicted in detail. The most recent issue in human life—corona—is also explained with reference to its psychological impact.

A modest attempt to suggest ways to deal with these life challenges is also incorporated in the book. Some things that can be taken care of by the family and professional help that needs to be provided are recommended.

The book includes incidence, box comments and real case studies for in-depth understanding. The author sincerely hopes that it will be beneficial to enhance the well-being of the next generation.

ACKNOWLEDGEMENTS

It gives me immense pleasure to write an acknowledgement for this book. First of all, I would like to express my heartfelt gratitude to SAGE authorities for accepting this book for publication. This gives me an invaluable opportunity to continue association with one of the most prestigious publishing houses. I am deeply indebted to them for publishing *Life Skills for Success* in English, Hindi and Marathi. I am grateful to my readers for giving positive feedback and motivating me.

I deeply appreciate the generous support given by Mr Amit Kumar, the Executive Editor, and express gratitude for his suggestions and directions. Ms Indrani Dutta, the Commissioning Editor, invested a lot of efforts in making the book both more interesting and scientific. I would like to thank her sincerely for her guidance. Mr Rajesh Dey, the Managing Editor, guided me for essential modifications and motivated me to complete the work without further delay. I am indebted to him for enhancing clarity regarding the work. Without the kind cooperation and able guidance of these three mentors, this book would not have been possible. I feel obliged by their favour. Mr Syed Husain Mendhdi Naqvi, production editor reviewed every minor detail of the book. His enthusiasm for perfection is highly appreciated. I thank him wholeheartedly for the same.

The basic idea regarding the book emerged during brainstorming discussions with my daughter, Dr Prachiti. Without her academic and technical support, this book would not have been completed. As she has a multidisciplinary perspective and in-depth understanding of neurology, genetics, clinical psychology, psychiatry, forensic psychology and the like, her guidance was especially valuable in understanding the multidisciplinary nature and implications of various psycho-social health issues discussed in the book. I owe a great deal to her.

I express a sense of gratitude to all the known and unknown experts and colleagues from SAGE Publications. Their hard work and efforts to maintain quality will always be remembered.

I am proud to be a part of the SAGE family.

Psycho-social Health during Adolescence and Youth

1.1. INTRODUCTION

Mental health is the ability to adjust satisfactorily to various strains. It is that state of well-being in which an individual realizes their own potential, can cope with the normal stresses of life, can work productively and fruitfully and is capable of contributing to their community. Mental illness is defined in terms of deviant behaviour from socially approved standards of interpersonal behaviour or as an inability to perform one's social roles. It is dysfunctional behaviour judged to be so with reference to norms and values held by the observer. (Wolman, 1977).

Psycho-social health may be treated as a hypothetical construct. No one in this world may be perfectly psycho-socially healthy from all perspectives: mental, emotional, social, cultural, behavioural and so on. What is considered as healthy in one situation in a specific environment and in a particular culture may not be considered so in other situations, environment and culture. An individual's age, gender, education, socio-economic status and background, everything should be considered before labelling their behaviour as healthy or otherwise.

According to the World Health Organization (WHO), 90 million Indians suffer from some form of mental disorder.[1] It is suggested that half of the world's population may be affected by psycho-social illness, more or less serious, which affects their self-esteem, relationships and ability to function in everyday life.

There is a space between normal and abnormal, and many people are in that space. If we consider psycho-social health as a continuum, the differences in characteristics of the two ends are well documented, but the middle portion is not well understood. Every individual

[1] bmcpsychiatry.bioedcentral.com 16 November 2020

experiences distress, failure and difficulty coping with situations at some time. Hence, one's psycho-social health may not always be equally good. It may vary or even deteriorate to a substantial degree. There is hardly any awareness about how that person should be helped in such a temporarily unhealthy condition. The person may or may not be aware that they should seek some help and help themselves.

If one is able to understand the exact status of one's own psycho-social health and the psychological status of near and dear ones, it will be easy to objectively accept it. It is essential to evaluate various mental health problems, symptoms and their severity. One should try to analyse, synthesize and arrive at a conclusion about what should be done. Self-understanding, self-acceptance, self-help and systematic attempts to improve psycho-social health should be the outcome.

According to the WHO, half of the mental health conditions start during teen age. If not treated, these conditions extend to adulthood.[2] India tops the list of countries with the highest proportion of mental and behavioural disorders. It is reported by researchers that 12 per cent of Indian students suffer from psychiatric disorders.[3]

Adolescence and youth are the most crucial periods in human life as these stages decide the whole future of an individual. Indian youth represent the largest youth population in the world. So it is essential to generate maximum opportunities for utilizing their potential, better education and employment, as well as satisfaction and effectiveness.

According to recent estimate, 27 per cent of the total Indian population comprises youth.[4] In global population, it is about 16 per cent.[5]

In a country, like India, many social traditions, customs, rituals, attitudes and styles of interaction are very stereotypical and unfair. Still, one has to choose conformity as it is the only important condition for achieving social acceptance. This may ruin individual's psychological health. Considering this fact, who should be considered as

---

[2] who.int 28 September 2020

[3] lawctopus.com 12 July 2019

[4] www.outlookindia.com>story 12 August 2020

[5] www.un>sites>2019/08

psychologically healthy in India? One who is leading individually satisfying life or one who is leading socially effective life? Both these criteria should be simultaneously applied. If happiness is accepted as a major contributor to mental health, an Indian housewife is supposed to get happiness in enhancing others' happiness and sacrificing her whole life for the family. She may be leading a socially effective life that may not be individually satisfying. Psychological health is optimal living. It is a subjective viewpoint when one defines optimal living. It may be interpreted as personal well-being without considering anything about others. This is difficult to accept as social interactions play a major role in psychological health. Hence, it is the capacity to adjust and function well in a given community.

The concept of positive mental health has attracted attention of researchers for last several decades. WHO's definition of mental health includes physical, psychological and social well-being. Self-actualization, sense of mastery over environment and autonomy are three basic aspects of mental health. Autonomy includes freedom to identify own problems and to deal with it. Psycho-social health can be defined as a state of mental, emotional, social and spiritual well-being. All these aspects of health are interdependent as shown in Figure 1.1. They are overlapping as well.

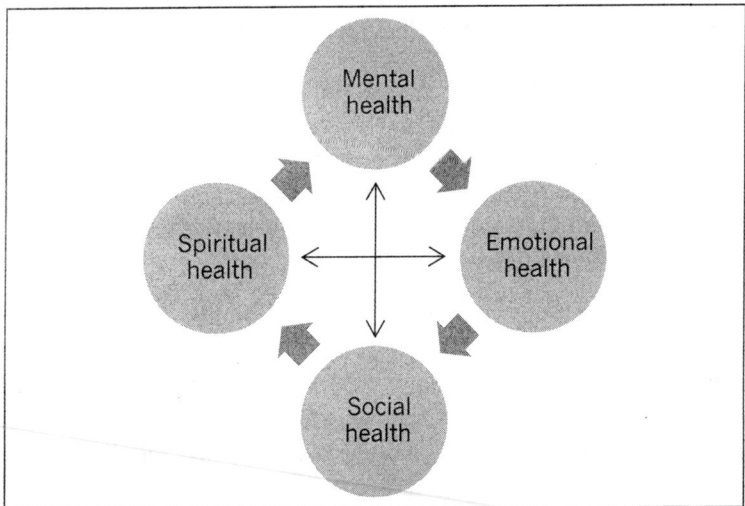

Figure 1.1 *Interdependence of Different Spheres of Psycho-social Health*

The exact nature of psychological health includes not only absence of disease or negative viewpoint but also understanding self, others and environment, balancing demands and resilience, stress and coping and achieving homeostasis. It is spontaneous happiness, curiosity, motivation, freshness of affect, capacity to enjoy life to an optimum level, giving every opportunity to self for enhancing potential. Social health means optimum interpersonal relations and playing various social roles effectively. Researchers have given different perspectives such as personal values, self-reliance, sense of direction, sense of responsibility, individuality and cultural and religious considerations.

There are different models of mental illness. Biological models are based on genetics, neurobiology and neuroimaging. Psychological models include psychodynamic model, behavioural model, cognitive behavioural model, and existential and humanistic model. The behavioural model stresses the importance of learned behaviour. Cognitive processes like thoughts may take a distorted form and affect behaviour. This leads to mental disorder, according to the cognitive behavioural model. The humanistic model is interested in self-actualization and all-sided growth of an individual. Failure of that results in mental illness. According to the social model, social interactions and restrictions may result in mental problems. Interaction between psychological and social aspects is held responsible for mental illness as per the psycho-social model. Inadequate peer relations, early deprivation, trauma, inappropriate parenting style, marital discord and divorce are some factors responsible for that. The biopsycho-social model puts forth that interaction between these three types of factors, that is, biological, psychological and social, may result in abnormal functioning. Figure 1.2 depicts some important factors affecting mental health.

Adverse conditions responsible for poor psycho-social health are given by researchers. Lack of basic trust in childhood regarding the availability of parental unconditional love, and poor attachment are major contributors. Unfair or traumatic experiences in childhood, like accidents or chronic disease, disability, sexual abuse, deprivation of parental love, learned helplessness, are some glaring examples.

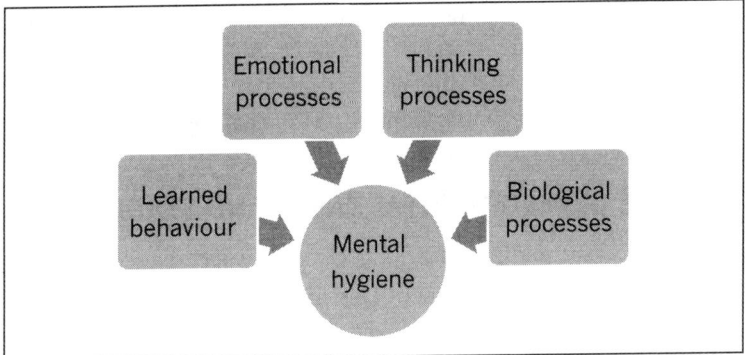

Figure 1.2 *Factors Affecting Mental Hygiene*

Characteristics of psycho-socially healthy persons specifically indicate the following features.

- **Like themselves:** Self-understanding and self-acceptance lead to liking self as a worthy human being. Unconditional acceptance of self is the most essential basic requirement of psycho-social health.
- **Accept their mistakes:** Self-development and improvement requires objective perspective and accepting limitations and mistakes of self.
- **Take care of themselves:** Instead of being over dependent on someone else, psycho-socially healthy individuals take care of their own health and psychological conditions.
- **Have empathy for others:** Empathy leads to better understanding of others' conditions and better interpersonal relations.
- **Can control negative emotions:** Such as anger, hate, tension, hostility and anxiety.
- **Are optimistic:** To keep one's mood fresh and spontaneously enjoying positive moments, being optimistic helps.
- Can work alone and with others equally well.

Those who are mentally healthy are optimistic, have better coping styles and have better contacts with reality. They are more oriented to personal growth. In short, it is the capacity to experience spontaneous happiness in everyday life. It is well documented that recovery from various diseases and traumatic situations depends on psycho-social health. As there are many demands and challenges that adolescents and youth are facing, it is difficult for them to achieve psycho-social health without special efforts. Some common challenges are as follows.

1.2. DEVELOPMENTAL TASKS AND STAGES

Developmental tasks are guidelines for individuals and families to understand social expectations. The members get motivation out of it. Due to its hierarchical nature, one can get an idea of what to expect next. However, if a normal individual skips a stage because of not mastering the developmental tasks, it may be detrimental to their future adjustment. Although the developmental tasks are in accordance with age and developmental stage, shifting from a stage to the next becomes challenging. Sometimes, it is not less than a crisis. This affects an individual's attitude towards self and behaviour as well as others' attitudes and behaviour. Unfavourable labels leading to stigma are generally seen. This is associated with negative self-worth and illness, feeling of inadequacy, negative thinking, poor self-efficacy and disturbed interpersonal relations. Physical defects, psychological disorders, poor health, lack of motivation, low mental abilities, retarded development, lack of opportunities and lack of guidance are important causative issues.

Accepting one's role in the social world is the most crucial task during adolescence. In Indian culture, gender differences are essentially linked to social acceptance and roles. Acceptance of one's sex role and physique are important stepping stones to maturity as one has to shoulder many responsibilities, learn appropriate behavioural patterns and develop one's identity with reference to that. It not only affects an individual's social self but real self and ideal self also. These things depend on culture and the margin it gives for various expressions and interactions. Achieving emotional independence is a difficult but essential job. Mostly in India, boys exaggerate and girls can't achieve it completely.

As far as appearance is concerned, adolescents become more conscious about it, and if it is not as per their ideal image, they become unhappy. Material pleasure available is related to their life satisfaction.

Accepting reality as it stands and maintaining motivation to go ahead are even more difficult tasks. Selecting and preparing for occupation is a major area having controversial issues. Parental expectations about son's achievements are too high and about girls are too low. Their intellectual capacities, aspirations and interests are generally not considered. Hence, it is unfair for both. This may lead to perception of discrimination by parents, sibling hostility, frustration and helplessness among offspring. Motivated intelligent girls and guys not interested in a typical masculine career may face many problems.

Youth's developmental tasks also include developing intellectual skills for civic competence, socially acceptable behaviour patterns, preparing for marriage and family life and achieving economic independence. In India, male members, especially, are supposed to be economically independent as they are perceived to be the main source of income of the family.

Indian child-rearing practices are such that the parents want their children to be dependent on their parents in case of cognitive, emotional and economic matters as they want to control the lives of their children. Everything significant or insignificant, parents want to decide about their children's lives, may it be hairstyle or education, occupation or marriage. Typical Indian parents don't want their children to earn while they are studying.

Career and marriage are the most significant decisions in life, and an individual's self-understanding plays an important role in them. Family and social support enhances an individual's well-being. Selecting a marriage partner, adjusting to the marriage partner, managing home, starting a family, bearing and rearing children are related developmental tasks and roles.

Adolescence is a period of very high unrealistic aspirations and dreams. Emotionally, the individual becomes too sensitive. Influence of peers is one more important characteristic. Changing lifestyles and values are also seen during this period. Family frictions are common due to different perspectives about parental discipline, criticism, standards of behaviour and family rules. Positive self-illusion is a fake or unrealistically favourable attitude towards self. In a way, it is self-deception. Taylor and Brown coined this term in 1988. Although, in the short term, the individual feels more comfortable and is capable of stress reduction due to positive self-illusion, the disadvantages in the long run are well documented.

Due to substantial changes in every area of life, it becomes difficult for adolescents and youth to maintain appropriate psycho-social health.

1.3. PERIOD OF RAPID CHANGE

1.3.1. Physiological and Psychological Changes

External physical changes during adolescence are an increase in height, weight, general body proportion and sex-related changes regarding primary and secondary sex characteristics. Internal changes are regarding the endocrine system and development of various systems, such as respiratory and circulatory.

Among psychological changes, the most important are heightened emotionality, self-doubt, instability, inferiority and inadequacy. Generally, these feelings are not openly accepted but are kept as secret and overcompensated by superficial self-assurance (Hurlock, 1979). Unrealistic aspirations and heightened emotionality are related to each other. As unrealistic aspirations increase, intense feelings of being disappointed, hurt, angry and not capable of fulfilling self and parents' aspirations increase. Youth become gradually capable of accepting the reality of life and the limitations of self. The transition from dependent adolescent to an independent young adult is the major expected achievement. If the parents are supportive, the environment is conducive and enough opportunities are available, then an individual may develop self-confidence, motivation and appropriate aspirations. Unconditional acceptance by parents and understanding and proper guidance lead to psycho-social development of individuals.

1.3.2. Relation with Family and Friends

Due to the stereotypical image, adults perceive adolescents as irresponsible and immature. As adolescents are aware of this, they become defensive. During these years, individuals become more involved with friends, interact with them and are accepted by them. Happiness, sense of well-being and satisfaction depend on interaction with friends. If an individual has to go against parental wish to please friends, they are willing to do it. If parents are too inconsistent, show favouritism, insult and underestimate children, are authoritarian, keep a lot of psychological distance from children, adolescents will just be fed up with their parents and want to get rid of them. In such a case, not communicating anything with the parents may be a general trend. If parents are democratic, understanding, supportive, share things with children, respect their opinion, consistent and fair, then the relationship between parents and children will be satisfactory.

1.3.3. Conflicts and Other Interpersonal Problems

Due to a lot of confusion about one's exact role in the family and society, an individual may experience a lack of self-understanding and understanding others. If the intention of parents and other significant adults is not understood, an individual may develop a distorted interpretation. This may lead to a number of conflicting situations and generation gaps. Avoidance of shouldering responsibilities of household, different expectations about life and human relations and ideas about freedom cause serious disharmony in relations with family. Things are taken for granted and every facility is expected as a right without fulfilling the duties properly. Care and concern about safety expressed by parents are interpreted as botheration.

Young adults accounted for 69.3 per cent of victims of road accidents in India.[6] Rash driving, not wearing seat belts and driving under intoxication are common practices among youth. Hence, road accidents are a leading cause of death of young male members in India (*The Indian Express*, 23 December 2019).

Insulting others, disrespectful behaviour and not caring for them are common behavioural patterns. Selfish motives, underestimating others' needs and exaggerating the importance of self, immature verbal and non-verbal communication increase conflict with family. In general, anger and aggression are very commonly seen among adolescents and

[6] www.deccanherald.com>youth

young adults, which may be irrational, indicating immaturity. During adolescence, there are unrealistic attitudes and hedonistic values.

1.3.4. Sibling Rivalry

A well-known leader, Pramod Mahajan, was shot dead by his own brother on 3 May 2006.[7] Sibling rivalry is one of the major issues which starts in childhood and may continue for the whole life. Levy in 1939 introduced the term sibling rivalry.[8] According to researchers, sibling rivalry can be reduced but can't be completely eliminated.

It generates from sharing of attention and love of parents. According to Adler, siblings are striving for significance. Birth order is also considered as an important issue. Age and gender play an important role. However, parental interaction is of top most importance. Undue comparison between siblings, partiality while providing facilities to children, praising one and blaming the other child continuously, withdrawing expressions of love and affection, declaring rejection are some parental practices which are proved to be the basic causes of sibling rivalry. It leads to hostility, aggression and negative attitudes towards siblings and parents also. A twenty year old killed his father, mother, sister and grand mother as the father declared that the property will be given to his sister (*Hindustan Times*, 2 Sept. 2021). As children grow older, sibling rivalry becomes intense, its expression becomes more harmful to siblings and to themselves also if proper care is not taken by parents. In such intense rebellious activities, the person is confirming their own negative self-image and reminding others of their nuisance value. That is equally harmful to the individual and their siblings. It may lead to inadequate intraindividual relations, poor interpersonal relations, depression, frustration, low self-esteem, anxiety, low self-efficacy, rebellious attitudes, self-harm, attention seeking and intense hostility.

Even it affects educational achievement, as one's thoughts are revolving around how to prove one's superiority and make one's sibling feel awkward. One can't concentrate on studies.

[7] https://en.wikipedia.org/wiki/Pramod_Mahajan

[8] www.jstor.org>stable>pdf

To reduce sibling rivalry, parents should avoid favouritism and treat all offspring in a fair and just manner. Teaching children emotional intelligence, problem-solving negotiation skills, conflict resolution and practising win-win proactively is recommended.

1.4. IDENTITY AND SELF-WORTH

An appropriate and strong sense of identity gives a lot of confidence to adolescents to face youth and adulthood. They develop self-efficacy and trust that they are worthy. Self-worth is a value assigned to self and one's abilities. According to Rosenberg, 'Self-esteem is favourable or unfavourable attitude towards self. It is the extent to which an individual values or appreciates self.' Low self-esteem means the individual does not realize their potential fully. Their self-perception is they are unworthy, incapable and have low self-efficacy. Their self-esteem is low. Those who have high self-esteem have a fair image of their abilities, and such individuals appreciate self. They are happy, well-adjusted and confident. They are extrovert and encourage and support others. Such individuals learn from their mistakes.

Self-esteem develops from the forth grade, and there are additions and enhancements during adolescence. If the environment is conducive and the individual gets enough opportunities to take new challenges, confidence is enhanced during adolescence. Experience of success increases one's confidence and generates more confidence so that one will be able to succeed in other areas also. Self-esteem is relatively stable and is related to the general behaviour of the individual. Self-esteem boosts one's belief that one will be able to face the challenges of life and lead a happy life. Emotional warmth expressed by parents, unconditional positive regard and acceptance by parents lead to high self-esteem of adolescents and youth. Fake confidence and unrealistically high self-worth may develop due to overindulgence by parents. Such inappropriate self-esteem is expressed in terms of arrogance, underestimating others while overestimating one's abilities and self-glorification.

Self-respect, self-love and self-efficacy contribute to self-esteem (as shown in Figure 1.3). Self-esteem decides one's perception of the

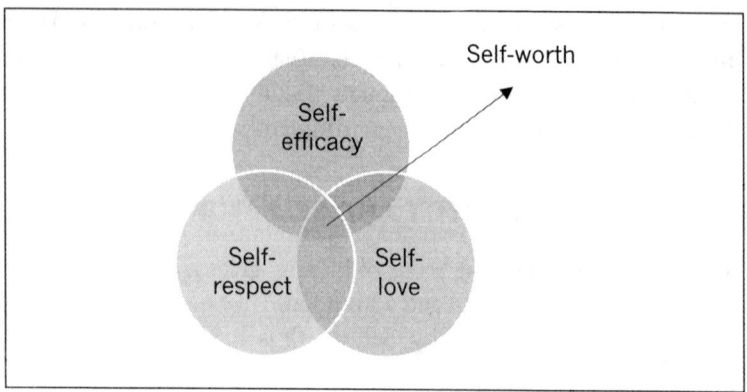

Figure 1.3 *Factors Contributing to Self-worth*

world and one's role in it. This indirectly affects how others perceive the individual and how they treat them. It is essential to accept reality as it is about self, limitations and potential of self. One should have the courage to make up for shortcomings. Encouragement and support given by others increase frustration tolerance. That results in a tendency to take healthy risks and feeling proud of one's achievements.

Experts have given some important correlates of self-esteem and identity. The most preliminary source is material belongings, which is a superficial compensation for insecurity and self-doubt. The second type of borrowing self-identity and self-worth is educational and professional achievements as a completion of the highest degree in a specific field, member of some prestigious university or association with a company. In India, it is reported that women and girls have low self-esteem as compared to men and boys.

1.4.1. Unrealistic Self-perception and Confusion regarding Various Roles

As a consequence of rapid growth, an individual experiences new emotions, new challenges and new relationships. They want to try various excitements. They perceive themselves as being capable of doing anything anyway. There is heightened vulnerability as a consequence of different and incongruent time frames of physical, cognitive, emotional and social maturity. There is increased sensitivity to criticism, an increased need to belong and heightened self-consciousness. Due to the decreased possibility of parental control, they enjoy freedom to behave in a different self-oriented way. This may be socially unacceptable, troublesome to others and detrimental to the self-image of the individual. The lack of experience and less concern about health leads to defensive optimism. This leads to more serious consequences.

Inaccurate or negative self-esteem may lead to fear of rejection and abandonment, over protection of self, unwillingness to take risks, inability to fulfil one's needs. In severe distortion of self-esteem, even thoughts and tendencies of self-destruction develop. In this case, the individual is not capable of making appropriate decisions, developing close personal relations and friendship and maintaining good interpersonal relations even with family members.

1.4.2. Identity Crisis

A sense of basic trust regarding mother's love in infancy, autonomy in toddler hood, ability to play during preschool years and developing work ethics in elementary school days are the pillars of identity. Adolescence is a period when individuals are confused about their destination, what is the goal of their life, who are their own people and groups and where they belong to. Hence, an individual becomes detached, withdrawn, apathetic and indecisive. There is less involvement in studies and work, as well as in interpersonal relations. Although identity crisis is not experienced by each and every individual, it is the most common problem in adolescence. It is worth noting that some individuals remain in an identity crisis for the whole of their lives. Commitment results in a firm sense of who the person is. This leads to strong feelings regarding choices. Low identity commitment is associated with an uncertain sense of self.

An identity crisis is a failure to achieve an appropriate ego identity during adolescence. Famous psychologist Erikson has given this concept. During adolescence, there is a tug of war between identity cohesion and confusion regarding various roles. This is associated with an imbalance between self-image and what others think about the individual. This leads to a crisis of basic ego identity. The role of an individual in the social world, gender roles, careers and value orientation are the major concerns. Sudden change in career or unexpected role change may lead to identity crisis. Divorce, parental divorce of an adolescent, change in sexual orientation may lead to identity crisis. If an adolescent is forced to get involved in homosexuality while ragging, he will feel completely shattered and may face severe problems regarding identity crisis. Marcia developed a framework having achievement, moratorium, foreclosure, and diffusion as the basis for identity. Achievement is possible with the help of both exploration and commitment. A moratorium takes place when there is exploration without commitment. If commitment is developed without considering the various alternatives, without choice, it is identity foreclosure. Many a time, it is some outer influence like parental pressure that results in it. Parental perceptions, ideas and beliefs are accepted without analysis and evaluation. Identity foreclosure leads to an identity crisis. Diffusion is the condition where there is no exploration and no commitment. If there is a fixed stereotypical identity which is distorted due to some environmental changes, it leads to an identity crisis. Those adolescents who have to suddenly change their role, educational stream, nature of work or basic things, like religion, may face an identity crisis. Identity diffusion, which means lack of identity structure, is a major issue in some serious mental diseases, such as schizophrenia and depression. It is an apathetic state where there is no commitment and no exploration.

According to experts, the development of fidelity is essential during adolescence. The individual develops a sense of duty while interacting with others and becomes genuine and sincere.

Resolving identity crisis and identity achievement are salient stages in adolescence. Firm self-image, self-confidence and self-efficacy depend on that. Major decisions in life are based on it. Identity achievement prepares the individual for developmental tasks in the future. Conducive environment giving appropriate emotional support, guidance and counselling and, in severe crisis, therapy may be useful to resolve identity crisis in adolescence.

1.4.3. Youth in Indian Context

Youth culture and values are directly affected by global impact, advancement of science and technology, and changing social scenario. Today's youth are much more advanced and over civilized as compared to the last generations. According to social psychologists and sociologists, the younger generation has both better and worse characteristics. They have courage and determination and are capable of meeting challenges. In the contemporary world, there are better opportunities for girls and ladies and for disadvantaged groups.

Negative characteristics are related to over socialization from a self-oriented perspective. It results in deterioration of interpersonal relations and a change in the impetus of personality. Relations with family become less important, and an individual is less involved in family matters. There is less respect, love and compassion expressed for family members, such as parents and siblings. Sexual pleasure is justified as a physiological need even when it is not accepted by cultural norms, such as premarital and extramarital sex. Sex is considered just as a game without considering the psychological and physiological ill effects and risks. More importance is given to material pleasure and physical pleasure.

Uncontrolled road rage and aggression, in general, and lack of patience are common. More violence and crimes are reported. Terrorism is also attracting a substantial number of youth. The present young generation is over dependent on technology. They are self-obsessed and want to show off and pretend that they are enjoying every moment of life. Superficial relations and frenemy type interaction having all sorts of negative hidden emotions are very common in the younger generation. There is a deterioration of moral values and humanitarian attitude. The younger generation is becoming egoist and self-centred, has less empathy, is more practical and is more interested in seeking pleasure.

The younger generation is also lonely and isolated. Although there are thousands of friends on Facebook, in real life, nobody is bothered about each other. Everyone wants to pretend that they do not need anyone to support their life and can manage independently.

Self-orientation is so influential that no one is bothered about even their own brother or sister. Due to abandoned premarital and extra-marital sex, the family system is collapsing. The rate of divorce is increasing, and the younger generation is less ready to compromise. As a consequence, there is more loneliness, more depression and alcohol and drug abuse, more HIV patients and patients of sexually transmitted diseases. The importance of a stable family for psycho-social health has been accepted by psychologists right from the beginning. No support and no near and dear ones lead to helplessness, frustration and a reckless lifestyle.

The activities and things which were once considered as tabooed for generations in India are now commonly practised. Barriers are breaking down, and immediate gratification orientation is becoming more popular. Young ladies are getting exploited due to patriarchal culture, on the one hand, and the so-called advancement of youth culture, on the other. All said and done, the girls and ladies who are involved in premarital and extramarital sex pay more as compared to guys. In India, premarital pregnancy and problems of unwed mothers are increasing every year as is reported by researchers.

Social psychologists and sociologists view it as a paradoxical culture. On the one hand, due to the changing value system, there are no limits to pleasure and enjoyment of all sorts; on the other, there is pretension of being with the age-old cultural ethos and traditions. The male member who has been enjoying sex for a number of years and with a number of partners wants to marry exactly as per cultural expectations. Only 4 per cent expressed that they may marry against their parents' wish. He will obey his parents, wants his wife to be a virgin, accepts dowry and other gifts and wants the father-in-law to spend a huge amount for celebration. This is a combination of self and convenience orientation. It may be labelled as consequence-oriented behaviour. One may label it as pretension culture as values, like honesty, are rapidly disappearing. In every relations and every communication, many of the youth are becoming superficial, fake and exploitative (*The Hindu*, 2017).

In Indian families, male teenagers are given more freedom, and many of them can't manage their impulses. Comparatively, less freedom is given to girls and young ladies, and they are supervised as far as possible.

Although this is the general scenario of the majority of adolescents and youth, it is not applicable to everyone. There are more responsible, motivated, stable and psychologically healthy individuals who are coming from a more conducive environment.

Recently, on 6 March 2021, it was reported that 55 per cent of married people in India who responded to the survey accepted that they have extramarital relations.[9] Gleeden, an extramarital dating app, has published a survey of Indian users, and the percentage is 48.[10] Before the age of 16, 75 per cent of students were found to be involved in physical relationships. A total of 1,240 students participated in this survey (*Maharashtra Times*, 24 February 2021).

1.5. STRESS RELATED TO EDUCATION

Competition for admission to prestigious courses, stringent rules and a huge amount of donations, if one is not capable of getting admission by merit, are crucial issues in the Indian educational system today. Parents want their offspring to understand the intricacies and demands of this situation and decide their priorities. A conducive environment at home, parental acceptance and unconditional love, proper facilities and guidance, appropriate and achievable goals and sensible decisions all play an important role in it.

Failure in academics has detrimental effects on self-esteem, self-worth, confidence and general educational adjustment. It disturbs interpersonal relations with family members, especially with parents. Parental rejection and punishment affects the self-image of the individual. The individual feels detached, lonely and frustrated. Every year, many such pressurized students either run away, threaten that they will commit suicide or some actually do it.

Every hour, one student commits suicide in India,[11] like a 24-year management student, Arjun, who killed himself due to depression about failure in an examination. He was also facing problems with drug addiction. Lack of frustration tolerance and inability to deal with failure are the most crucial issues.

[9] news18.com

[10] tv9marathi

[11] www.hindustantimes.com>08 May 2017

In March 2018, a 19-year-old student killed his teacher as the male teacher scolded him for misbehaving in the class in Sonipat, Haryana. Just two months ago, in Haryana, an 18-year-old student killed his female principal. In both these incidences, a revolver was used by students. Many such incidences are reported by the media (*The Times of India*, 2019).

This is the time when the individual faces ultimate rejection and actually needs acceptance, understanding and support, especially by parents. Punishment, rejection and insults everywhere lead to even more frustration, depression, isolation and self-hatred.

Underachievement and drop out are major problems in the Indian formal education system. Underachievement is achieving below the level expected on the basis of intellectual powers. Lack of motivation, lack of necessary facilities, value system not supporting education, hedonistic tendencies, gratification orientation, wrong company are some common causes. Dropping out, in turn, affects the complete life of the student. This may result in antisocial gang-type behaviour as a pass time. Girls generally contribute to household duties after they drop out.

Truancy is intentionally staying away from school or college without substantial reason. It is unjustified absenteeism. Some other students run away from home and never return. School phobia and school refusal are the most common causes. There are some psychiatric problems which are associated with truancy. This leads to multiple problems in school work and even more problems regarding school adjustment. This ultimately results in dropping out. The increasing incidence of crime committed during adolescence indicates the severity of the problem. The percentage of girls dropping out is and has been always greater from the beginning of the formal education system. This is directly related to the traditional perspective about the stereotypical gender role of women.

According to government reports, 20 per cent of the total students are out of school in India. Only 70 per cent among those, who are enrolled, complete even 10th. Millions of youth are dropouts from high school and college.[12]

[12] thehindu.com 4th Jan 2019

Comparison and negative feedback should be avoided. Changing self-talk, controlling negative thoughts and enhancing concentration are the methods useful for helping them. Counselling, relaxation, meditation and self-management are also essential.

1.5.1. Test Anxiety

Performance depends on not only learning but many more psychological and physiological experiences such as stress, anxiety, fatigue, illness, alertness of cognitive processes and motivation. As is well understood, the relation between anxiety and performance is like an inverted U. When there is hardly any anxiety and stress, the performance of the student is also substantially low. If the anxiety level is moderate, the performance is highest, and when it is too high, performance again deteriorates. It is a very common condition during adolescence and early adulthood.

Approximately, 10–41 per cent of school children and 15–20 per cent of college students suffer due to test anxiety.[13] Prevalence is 78 per cent among women medical students.[14] Due to extreme competition and very high parental expectations, fear of failure increases.

The four types of symptoms are as follows:

- **Physiological:** Physiological changes are increased heart rate, dry mouth, headaches, stomach upset, nausea, changes in body temperature, difficulty in breathing, catastrophe, feeling of restlessness, stress hormone secretion, hyperventilation, sweating and light headedness.
- **Cognitive:** Cognitive block, racing thoughts, lack of concentration, loss or partial loss of memory, difficulty in organizing thoughts and lower performance are some cognitive symptoms of test anxiety. The individual can't comprehend things properly, and as a consequence, learning deteriorates.

---

[13] dusunenadamdergisi.org > pdf2020
[14] bmcmededuc.biomedcentrl.com 2019

- **Emotional:** Excessive fear, disappointment, tension, stress, worry, anxiety, negative thinking, lack of self-confidence, depression, negative self-talk, devaluation of self and comparing oneself with others, feeling of dread, feeling of helplessness, uncontrolled weeping or sometimes laughing, extreme discomfort and over arousal are emotional symptoms of test anxiety. In such a situation, students feel helpless, nervous and cold. Too much dependence of self-esteem on academic performance is always detrimental. A panic reaction is experienced.

  Low self-esteem, depression, feeling of hopelessness, anger, agitation, disturbed interpersonal relations, frustration, guilt and shame are some correlates of test anxiety.

- **Behavioural:** Pretension, avoidance of examination, fidgeting, pacing, smoking and substance or alcohol abuse are behavioural symptoms of test anxiety.

Relaxation, understanding the relative importance of examinations in human life, simulation exercises and practising writing in an atmosphere similar to an examination, proactive and positive thinking, emotional support by parents and teachers are most useful for reducing test anxiety. Therapies and counselling have also proved to be effective. Intervention includes parental counselling and family therapy.

Examination phobia is much more intense than test anxiety. The student experiences all sorts of disturbances described in test anxiety and, at any cost, wants to avoid the situation. Examination phobia is an extreme form of irrational fear of examination. It is a mental disorder.

Indian researchers proved that there is a negative correlation between test anxiety and democratic parenting style, and acceptance of the parents by children. It was also found that Indian children of housewives have more test anxiety than that of working mothers. Excessive involvement and interference in studies of children may be the cause behind it.

It is reported that Indian students experience and express more physical symptoms, while American students have more cognitive symptoms.

In March 2018, as 10th examinations were going on, a student suffered from a heart attack in Mumbai.[15] This is an indicator of the uncontrolled and overwhelming stress experienced by students. In June 2018, a student who could not reach the examination hall in time and could not appear for a national-level competitive examination committed suicide immediately.[16]

Generally, more stress is reported by girls and young ladies as compared to boys and young men. Girls are more sensitive to relationship issues in the family and outside the family. Self-destructive and aggressive coping is more among boys. The most frequently mentioned life event by adolescents is regarding interpersonal relations.

1.6. EMPLOYMENT AND UNEMPLOYMENT

During early adulthood, getting adjusted to the world of work and developing an image of self as a worker or employee are significant developmental tasks.

Vocational development is a process which continues for years. Indian youth grossly lack various skills necessary for shouldering different responsibilities and social skills to get along well with colleagues. When they get an opportunity to serve, they interact immaturely with others, can't manage their work and can't express the sincerity expected. Many of them can't tolerate the tension and job stress. Having only theoretical knowledge may not be enough sometimes. One has to develop new skills, face new challenges and shoulder new responsibilities, and it may result in new freedom, new confidence and better self-worth. Happiness and life satisfaction largely depend on securing a good job and adjusting well to it. There are clear gender stereotypes and status stereotypes.

Unemployment is a serious problem in India. According to recent research, 30 per cent of individuals between 18 and 29 years are unemployed. Unemployment results in accepting any lower-level job by well-educated individuals.

---

[15] www.dnaindia.com>education 1 March 2018

[16] www.indiatoday.in>stroy>civ 4 June 2018

Recently, in Uttar Pradesh, over 93,000 candidates, including 3,700 PhD holders, applied for the post of a peon.[17]

In India, there is one more huge class of voluntarily unemployed individuals and that is of housewives. Irrespective of education, due to social pressure and expectations, many women voluntarily choose to be unemployed. This is the ideal role of a housewife that is approved by the culture and community. For example, in Maharashtra, 87 per cent of women are full-time housewives.

> In India, the percentage of housewives is 85 per cent, according to researchers. According to some government reports, in urban areas of India, less than 15 per cent of women work outside home. It is worth noting that the number of working women is decreasing in India. More women in urban areas as compared to rural areas have expressed that they stay back at home out of their own choice. *The New York Times* (23 August 2015) has commented that even in the contemporary world, the Indian community wants to save females from the outer world and other males and wants to ensure the purity of women.

The impact of unemployment on an individual depends on age, socio-economic status, gender, motivation and general perspective towards self-esteem. Substantial frustration, and unhappiness results due to unemployment. The unemployed may experience mental health issues, feel isolated, inferior, and worthless. Such individuals face social rejection, insults and unpleasant atmosphere where ever they go. Unwanted dependency, frustration, depression, hostility, and intense anger are the outcomes.

1.7. POSITIVE YOUTH DEVELOPMENT

In a developing country like India, concentrating on youth should be the prime focus of not only parents and family but also educational institutes and the government. They should be helped to lead a socially effective and individually satisfying life. Regular programmes for those who need special help for adjusting to educational and occupational world may be given these facilities. Parallel programmes for skills

---

[17] economic times..indiatimes.com 30 August 2018

development, guidance and counselling and special opportunities for improving self-worth and self-confidence may help them at least in some areas. Assertiveness, resilience, hardiness and proactive thinking need to be introduced during the developmental period.

Self-actualization is a very significant concept introduced by well-known psychologist Maslow. Every individual should understand that they are the only person who can improve their life after a particular age. Hence, adolescents and youth should be guided to self-understanding, self-acceptance and self-development. Utilizing potential results in intrinsic satisfaction and motivation to go ahead. Once the individual gets insight into self, their psychological health improves a lot.

1.7.1. Self-help and Intervention

Most of the time, we forget that though we can't control everything, we can control many important things, such as our own thinking process, behaviour and feelings. All these can be used to promote psycho-social health.

Various strategies for maintaining good psycho-social health are as follows:

- **Understanding self:** It includes understanding one's potential and limitations. It is essential to improve one's style of interaction considering its effects on others.
- **Accepting self, others and the environment:** Accepting one as one is with all the things that can't be changed saves a lot of psychological energy and defensive reactions. Accepting others as they are reduces negativity in interaction and that, in turn, improves psycho-social health.
- **Respecting self and appreciating self as a worthy person:** One should respect oneself, value oneself, be kind to oneself, give margin to err to oneself, get involved in hobbies and value activities.

Developing realistic and achievable goals, proper communication skills, life skills like assertiveness enhances psycho-social health.

1.8. SUMMARY

Psycho-social health is a multidimensional concept. Everyone may face some psycho-social problems and need to enhance one's coping strategies. In particular, adolescents and youth are vulnerable due to various challenges. Adolescence and youth are two unstable stages of human life. Due to rapid physiological and biochemical changes, the person is confused. There are substantial demands from the family and society regarding academic, job related and domestic responsibilities. The individual has to be competent and prove that they are capable of leading their life independently. It is a challenge to select a career, a life partner and get settled in the social and work-related world. As the severity, nature and frequency of these problems depend on environmental and intraindividual variables, solutions and guidance also may be adjusted accordingly.

Impact of Gender

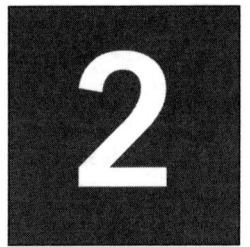

2.1. INTRODUCTION

Sex is the most significant single issue in human life. The term 'sex' indicates biological status as being male or female. 'Gender' means an individual's characteristics that are believed to be learned by an individual as a result of social interactions. Gender is more relevant and significant to understand psychological perspective. Gender identity is the extent to which an individual perceives themselves as being masculine or feminine (Bem, 1974). All over the world, gender and gender-related impact play a very critical role in an individual's psycho-social health, life in general, social as well as legal issues. Various aspects of human life are coloured by traditional or modern perspectives of family and community, customs, expectations and stereotypical gender roles. An individual's potential experiences, direction of development and motivation depend upon gender. Masculinity is demonstrated by possession of crucial traits, such as independence and leadership. Femininity is the presence of expressive traits, such as compassion, sensitivity and cheerfulness. Being androgynous is having high levels of both masculinity and femininity or undifferentiated with low levels of both. Masculine males and feminine females are gender schematic and perceive the world and themselves through a gender bias. Others may not have such a strong gender bias.

> Androgyny is the ideal state. In this case, both boys and girls, men and women are treated on par, and both of them are encouraged to develop all good qualities irrespective of gender. As a consequence, they can utilize their potential and develop a combination of positive traits from both stereotypical gender roles.

The controversy about whether gender differences are innate or acquired is an important issue which has attracted the attention of numerous researchers. Now, it is well accepted that the gender differences reported by researchers are due to complex and complicated interaction of innate endowment and socialization. Gender decides the complete future, social expectations, aspirations, achievements, opportunities, self-worth and interpersonal and intrapersonal relations of an individual. Socialization may be oriented towards systematic ways of passing a particular culture to next generations; however, it may not be appropriate and just for an individual's development, happiness and self-actualization.

In a developing country like India, the scenario is changing gradually; however, the change is negligible. Concepts like women's empowerment are hardly accepted, and practising them in day-to-day life is extremely rare. There is a lot of rigidity about most of the issues among the majority of Indian families. All sorts of international discrimination indices and gender inequality reports unanimously accept the fact that gender discrimination and inequality are very severe problems in India. The correlates are the values, attitudes, behavioural patterns and socialization practices of Indian masses.

2.2. GENDER DIFFERENCES IN SOCIALIZATION

Gender socialization is a lifelong process. It has a significant impact on an individual's cognitive, affective and behavioural spheres throughout life. Traditionally, the role of a homemaker is perceived as a woman's role, and the role of a bread winner is associated with being a male. The Indian cultural and social set-up is mostly patriarchal where men are considered as the supreme power. They colour the whole life of both the sexes. Since birth, significant adults start influencing their lives in a specific way. It is well accepted that there is a substantial difference in social expectations regarding gender-specific behavioural patterns in any given community.

By the age of three, children have formed their gender identity. Even in make believe plays, they pretend to play a gender-specific role of adult in a specific culture. During the age range of 5–7, their ideas about what boys and girls can and can't do are very rigid. Afterwards, these ideas become flexible. Some experts think that there are two sexes and different genders. Gender is decided on the basis of various combinations of traits irrespective of sex.

Researchers have given three types of theories for understanding gender development: biological, social learning related to socialization and cognitive theories. One more perspective is to integrate elements of biological, social learning and cognitive theories and study their interaction to find out its effects. Biological theories assume that biological factors, such as genes and hormones, are the basis of male–female differences in behaviour. Social learning theories focus on the impact of socialization on developing gender related personality and behaviour. Early social learning approaches highlighted the roles of observation, modelling, imitation and reinforcement in the emergence of gender differences. The contribution of significant others such as parents, teachers, peers, siblings and the mass media provide models for gender-specific behaviour.

Some social cognitive theories of gender development give triadic causations of gender development. They include personal, behavioural and environmental influences. Personal are related to cognitive, affective, motivational and self-regulatory aspects. Behavioural are activities that are gender-linked, and environmental influences are social influences in day-to-day life. These factors interact and influence each other. Self also plays an important role as an agent. An individual is actively processing and interpreting gender-related information and makes decisions regarding one's conduct throughout life.

In the cognitive approach, Kohlberg (1966) proposed that, from childhood, an individual is an active processor of information. The child categorizes individuals according to gender. Since then, gender identity and gender stability have been seen. This leads to understanding appropriate behaviours for males and females to behave accordingly and to achieving consistency between the self and the environment. Bem (1981) gave the concept of gender schema, through which an individual perceives the world and self. They are cognitions, ideas and beliefs related to male–female differences and masculinity and femininity. These schema can influence and bias behaviour (Martin, 2000).

Socialization identification and self-induced socialization are essentially important forces that determine the future of an individual. The whole socialization process depends on principles of conditioning. Parents and significant adults give rewards and reinforcement to an individual child according to gender-specific expectations and sex stereotypical roles in the future. Sexism in socialization acts in two ways, first, by encouraging gender-specific characteristics and, second, by discouraging or suppressing other traits. Punishment for gender-atypical activities and reward for gender-typical activities is the most common style. Hence, an individual repeats activities for which they get reward and reinforcement and avoids doing things which are not rewarded. Girls are over socialized and given hot house treatment in almost all cultures. They are protected and are under constant supervision. In 110 cultures, females are socialized for nurturance. Their exposure to the world is limited. Researchers have reported that social sex roles are more important for girls than for boys.

Gender stereotypes consist of beliefs about psychological traits and characteristics as well as activities appropriate for men and women. These are attitudes and opinions regarding the abilities, aptitudes and worth of an individual just on the basis of gender.

Gender role conformity is a very decisive issue in socialization for generations almost all over the world. Its roots are in strong belief in sex differences with reference to all physiological and psychological traits also. In almost all subcultures of India, most parents, in laws and other social agents want the woman to be meek, docile, subjugated, cultured, obedient, sacrificing and serving type. They expect the male members to be confident, self-directed, more logical, tough-minded and strong.

Double standards of morality are practised for girls and boys, which result in enlarged super ego of women. They are aware of others' expectations, feelings and reactions. They are socialized to be more kind, considerate and conservative. Men are encouraged to have goal-oriented, self-directing qualities such as assertiveness, decisiveness and independence of thought and behaviour. These qualities exactly match their sex role and social expectations. Even boys perceive themselves as strong, powerful, dominant and potent. They have less need for affiliation. Males establish their identity by separation and by being different than females. They want to show that they are not influenced by females. Women are conditioned to possess emotive qualities which are oriented towards interpersonal relations. According to research findings, women's need for affiliation is so strong that they put others' needs first. They have empathy, are sensitive and emotionally responsive. They are less achievement oriented, hence play domestic roles exactly as per social expectations. Internalization of social values leads to development of personality as is expected by the community. The most difficult but important task for women is to separate self from others psychologically and be autonomous. Division of labour and division of authority are two salient features of socialization of the genders. These two things are diagonally opposite for two genders in India. Right from childhood, such bifurcation is highlighted every now and then. For example, a girl or a woman is not supposed to make her own decisions and must serve others, while a boy or a man is expected to know how to deal with difficult situations and should never be emotional. Various theories are proposed by psychologists to explain gender differences.

Eagly's (1987) social role theory explains that the physical differences between men and women lead to division labour. The fact that men have more physical strength as compared to women results in different gender roles from men and women. Gender roles are the behaviour patterns expected of men and women. They are the origins of gender stereotypes. According to this theory, gender-specific careers are also linked to inborn proficiencies of a particular gender in that particular field. If one's behaviour does not match with the perceived gender role, it may lead to substantial confusion and stress. This may lead to limited opportunities for that individual, a lot of social criticism and awkwardness.

As is depicted in Figure 2.1, gender influences every sphere of human life. Individuals' self-respect, self-worth and self-expectations depend on biological sex, on the one hand, and culture and socialization, on the other. What the individual will be doing for the whole of their life depends on these aspects.

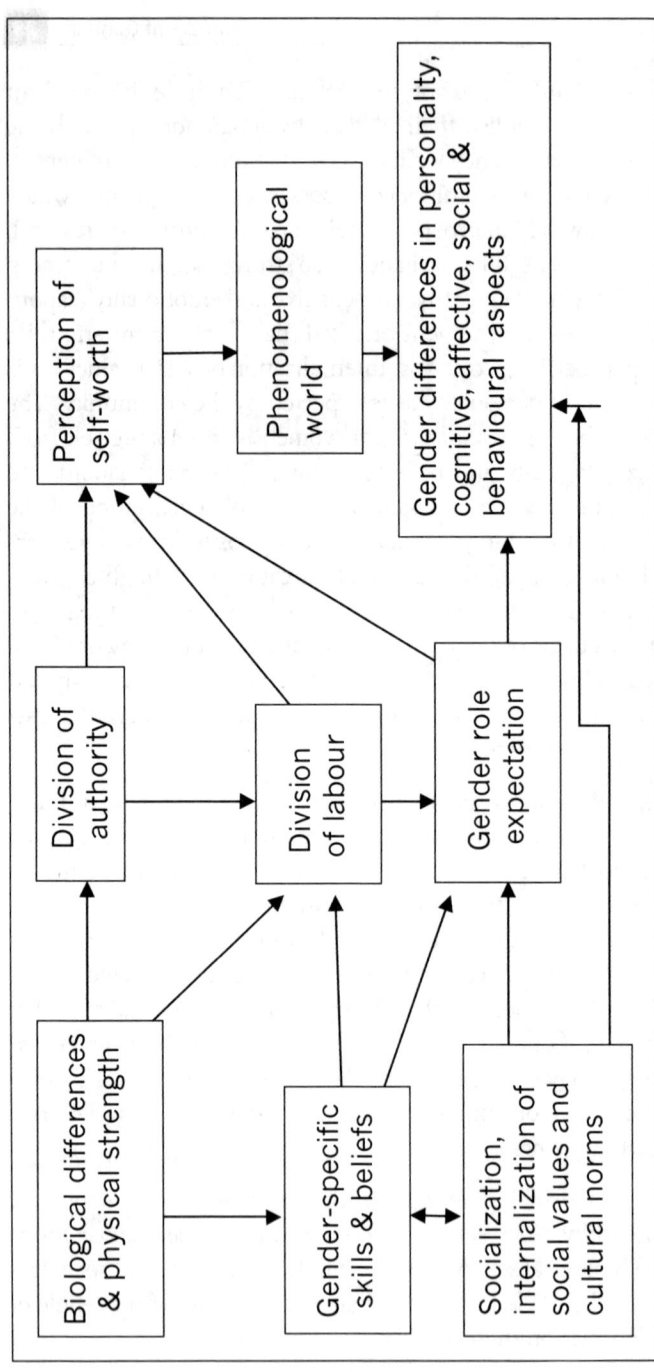

Figure 2.1 *Basic Constructs Resulting in Gender Differences in Every Sphere of Life: An Indian Model*

Source: Proposed by the present author.

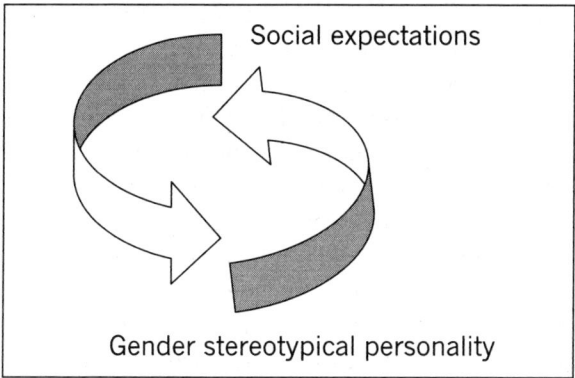

Figure 2.2 *Relation between Social Expectations and Gender Stereotypical Personality*

Over-generalization of gender-specific psychological make-up may lead to injustice to both male and female members. It may be detrimental to their adjustment, self-actualization and social effectiveness.

It is a vicious circle. Society expects women to be submissive and less capable, and they are treated in the same way. As a consequence, women become less confident and less oriented towards self-development. One depends on the other (Figure 2.2).

Cultural impact is obviously seen in these constructs. Even in developed countries, like America, males are expected to be independent, confident, objective and logical, active and less emotional. However, African-Americans believe that they have both masculine and feminine traits irrespective of their gender. They are less gender role specific while socializing their children. Capability is explained and associated with age and competency (Redway & Miville, 2013).

In India, there are many traditional ideas, customs and ideologies, assuming and indicating that a woman is not supposed to be an independent and competent human being who is free to develop her potential and lead a self-fulfilling life. Old religious Hindi and Sanskrit literature clearly indicates that a woman does not deserve freedom and should be physically beaten and controlled. Generally, the socialization of girls is oriented towards virtue and acceptance rather than power and competence. Opportunity, respect and power are difficult to acquire for a common Indian woman. Most of them are conditioned to accept subordinate status, underestimate their abilities and be overwhelmingly dependent and vulnerable. In traditional Indian families, a married lady has to take permission of her in-laws if she wants to meet her own parents, friends or attend a social function. Restricted field of activities is a critical and common character of socialization of an Indian girl. She is supposed to be at home, play nearby and should be under constant supervision. She is not encouraged to participate in social activities other than family functions. This, in turn, leads to a lack of sufficient social skills. Both boys and girls are not only encouraged but forced to be ready to accept a sex stereotypical role.

The basic differences in socialization of a male and female offspring are as follows:

Male child	Female child
More freedom	Less freedom
More social exposure	Less social exposure
More pampering	Less or no pampering
More outdoor group play	Indoor isolated play
More mobility granted	Hot house treatment
Physically demanding activity	Less physically demanding activity
Aggressiveness tolerated	Submissiveness expected
More opportunities for new experiences	Less opportunity for new experiences
Special attention, better food and facilities	Less attention, poor food, facilities
Less household jobs	More household jobs
No emotional expressions granted	Emotional expression expected
Major decisions to be made	No independent decisions
Responsibilities as head of the family	Responsibility of household work

Hence, the whole socialization process is totally dependent on gender-specific roles and cultural norms regarding the same.

2.3. GENDER DIFFERENCES: PHYSIOLOGICAL AND BIOCHEMICAL APPROACH

Gender differences originate from sex-determining chromosomes and differences in hormones. Obvious differences seen and scientifically reported are in body building, anatomical characteristics, physiological functioning and biochemical compositions. Males generally have more height, weight, muscular strength, vigour, vital capacity or consumption of air.

Females mature early and are capable of surviving even in the case of adverse conditions before and after birth. They are more viable. It is reported that male members are biologically more vulnerable, susceptible to infections and are more affected by various diseases, defects and disorders. During the past 250 years, in epidemics, hardship or famine, women have consistently overlived men (*The Guardian*, 2018). Men are more vulnerable to life's hazards, illness and trauma.

One very important quality in a woman's personality is endurance. They are capable of surviving even in the case of shock, disease and exhaustion. As we all know, thousands of farmers from various states of India commit suicide every year due to extreme poverty, unfair atmospheric conditions, such as lack of sufficient rain and wastage of invested money. However, their wives don't give up. They struggle for the whole of their lives and take care of their children. Men give up in such a situation as they can't fulfil social expectations and may not be able to share their worries with anyone, as a man is not supposed to do that. The range of bodily functions considered for homeostasis is narrow in the case of males. Their functions are more stable.

Substantial research indicates that there are gender differences in basic things, such as weight, size, volume, composition and functional

Do You Know?

It is scientifically proved that though there are differences in excellence in specific activities and cognitive processes, there are no sex differences in general intellectual powers. Women's brains are more integrated. They utilize greater neural efficiency and both the hemispheres. Multi-tasking is better among women.

differences of the brain. Overall brain size of females is smaller; they have more grey matter. Male members have more overall white matter. They have higher percentage of grey matter in the left hemisphere.

Sex-related differences originate from sex-linked genes and hormones, like testosterone. That, in turn, affects brain development before and after birth. Men and women utilize different parts of the brain while identifying and processing information regarding emotions, making decisions and storing as well as retrieving memories. Men have more lateralized speech functions. Women demonstrate bilateral or right representation of speech. It is reported that men have a larger hypothalamus, and the part of the brain that contributes to regulating sexual behaviour, called the amygdale. The male brain has a thicker right hemisphere which is associated with spatial skills. Women have a larger hippocampus which is associated with retrieval of emotional memories, more volume in cortex for decision-making as well as emotional regulation. Even the neurotransmitter system is different, such as serotonin, gamma aminobutyric acid (GABA) and dopamine. Fine motor coordination is better represented in the female brain, and navigational skills are better represented in men. Females show superiority in language abilities. Males demonstrate more proficiency in visuo-spatial skills and mental rotation.

While processing emotional information, males process the sensory aspect with regard to action. Women are more interested in the subjective experience of emotion and show a greater overt response to emotions. This is because females show involvement in the left region surrounding the amygdale. In the case of males, the right-sided region near the hippocampus is activated.

Socialization practices and experiences enhance these effects (Hines, 2011).

2.4. PSYCHOLOGICAL EFFECTS OF GENDER-SPECIFIC SOCIALIZATION ON MEN AND WOMEN

Gender-specific socialization is accepted to be the most influential aspect of the environment which directs individuals to specific goals, behavioural patterns, values, perceptions, meaning of life and achievements. Right from birth, a specially privileged treatment is given to male children. A male child becomes a matter of pride and social prestige in India. Achievement motivation is more among boys and men. They have enough confidence, better social skills and high self-worth. They work for themselves and their goals and aspirations are higher than their achievements. Roothman et al. (2003) have demonstrated that men score higher on physical self-concept, positive thinking, cognitive flexibility, constructive thinking and fortitude. Women scored higher on religious well-being and expression of affect and somatic symptoms.

As per traditional ideology, a man is considered as a super being. He is never supposed to be timid, weak and dependent. Even at a young age, he is supposed to hide his pain, failure and insults. Right from the beginning, he has to pretend that he can bear and deal with different stressful situations and does not need any help. Self-esteem of an individual depends on being positively valued by others and a sense of mastery of the environment. However, if a woman wants to achieve a sense of mastery, she is rarely valued by others. Women with high self-esteem hold less traditional attitudes than those with low self-esteem. Androgynous men and women are found to have better self-esteem and tend to hold less traditional values. Due to gender-biased socialization, girls think that their life, their achievements and their health are not important. They don't consider themselves as a worthy person and don't work for themselves. Women work to please others. They are reinforced to please others from childhood. Even in adulthood, women work hard so that their boss is pleased to see their achievements.

The responsibility of household jobs restricts their other activities, hobbies and interests. It results in stereotypical life routines and a lack of out-of-the-way achievements. They are taken for granted by others and by themselves also and are convinced that it is their responsibility. Women's sense of competence, self-respect and self-evaluation is poor. All these things depend upon success, power to control others, virtue adherence to moral and affection, attention and acceptance from others. Girls and women give more importance to acceptance over performance. Men are interested in personal achievements: They are goal oriented. Women, on the other hand, are more interested in social affiliation and interpersonal communication.

Although they are capable of academic excellence, they can't be successful as an adult. Although they are sincere, hard-working and obedient, they lack confidence, self-efficacy and independent thinking. Women's achievements and goals are similar. Their aspirations are not much higher than their present achievements. Boys are encouraged, and girls are discouraged to be dominant, independent, competent, rational, analytical, strong, active, ambitious, brave, insensitive, sexually aggressive and achievement oriented. This itself may affect an individual's self-concept.

> In the traditional view, male members learn to manipulate their physical and social environment through physical strength, while girls learn to present themselves as objects to be viewed (Cahill, 1986).

All over the world, most women are more interested in their appearance and they devote a lot of time, energy and money to maintain their beautiful and youthful looks. Women are conditioned for that. They have internalized the values and social expectations to such an extent that they think it is their natural tendency. To be more objective, it must be related to being pleasant for the opposite gender. In a way, knowingly or unknowingly, they are conforming to the role of a sex object. Comparatively, men are less involved in such activities, though the trend is changing in the case of youth.

Interpersonal relations in Indian culture are also largely influenced by gender. By conditioning, women learn to be cooperative rather than competitive. Even in the workplace, they are more interested in harmony and good interpersonal relations than hierarchy and power. Qualities like leadership, self-reliance, and independence are very rarely seen among women. On the contrary, nurturance, gentleness, consideration for others are very common traits of women. Socialization of girls is and has been oriented towards virtue and acceptance and not towards power and competence. Any society admires those who are powerful and competent and only superficially praises those who are loved and ethical. Those women who seek power and competence often lose virtue and acceptance. Men like to compete. They are assertive or aggressive, independent, confident, and are motivated to get power. Men work as per their own ideas and aspirations. They are less interested in maintaining good interpersonal relations. Mostly they are self-oriented.

Emotional experiences and their relation to gender have been a very fertile field of research. Research in this area has shown that though there is no gender difference in infants in the case of stressful situations, women freeze during such experiences. As far as school-going children are concerned, teachers perceive girls and girls perceive themselves as anxious and timid. Self-imposed fearfulness and self-attribution of fearfulness reduce openness to new experiences and adventurous activities.

Girls and women lack confidence as they can't get appropriate social experiences to develop it. They become less creative due to all these. All sorts of discrimination, less wages and discouragement by family and employers, economic dependency irrespective of having a paid job, subordinate status, no opportunity to make important decisions and insecurity in every sphere of life result in overwhelming stress. Sexual exploitation, marital rape, sexual harassment and similar unpleasant experiences add to the difficulties. Women are socialized to being dependent, emotional, kind and helpful, empathetic, oriented towards conformity and accepting subordinate status. As a consequence, women mostly internalize their conflicts, which results in eating disorders, anxiety and depression.

Mental health, personality and adjustment of working women attracted attention of researchers. Multiple roles enrich women's lives and it leads to enhanced satisfaction, better health, and decreased frustration. It is the coordination of various roles and the quality of experience that plays an important role in deciding the exact nature of these feelings. It is found that working mothers are less depressed than non-working mothers.

The network of social relations is reported to be useful for managing stress. However, social relations may lead to various negative consequences, such as criticism, unnecessary waste of time and thankless efforts. If an individual has enough money, physical strength, education and internal locus of control, only then social relations result in gain or advantage. However, Indian women are just taken for granted, and they are expected to put in a lot of energy and effort into social relations without any substantial benefit out of it. Sometimes, social relations result in a negative impact on their lives.

In social relations, men also depict self-reliance. They avoid self-expression. Women, on the other hand, are involved in self-expression. They depend on others socially, cognitively and emotionally. They are generally interested in developing close emotional relations with others.

As far as the parental role is concerned, behaviour of the father changes due to economic status and things happening outside home, but the mother rarely changes her behaviour; she continues to fulfil her duties for the whole of her life. Indian women lack assertiveness. If someone attacks a woman, she may not retaliate. In case of any threat or challenge, it is difficult for her to manage stress. She either asks for help or is extremely dependent on someone. There is hardly any active problem-solving. Women are taught right from childhood that they are safe in the company of others. So even grown-up ladies feel secure when they are with others. Hence, women are more interested in maintaining social relations. They are socialized in such a way that they seek social approval in every activity. They need more social reinforcement and social stimulation. As a consequence, they are not interested in working independently. Due to all these, a young woman becomes timid, docile and vulnerable. She can be easily frightened by others. In the case of difficulty, she passively waits for help and depends on others. If the environment is not conducive, she will not go ahead and easily give up.

Gender differences in adjustment and coping are proved to be significant and substantial. As men and women perceive any problem from different perspectives, their reaction and coping have to be different. According to social expectations and customs, the appropriateness of a particular coping style may be unequal for men and women. Boys and men do not accept their anxieties and fears. They don't openly discuss their problems with anyone else and keep pretending that they can manage on their own. There is no emotional catharsis due to which a lot of pent up emotional energy disturbs them. Male members act out due to frustration. They can't manage their emotional outbursts. They are mostly oriented towards an active coping style. They are less organized. As men generally act out and externalize, they are involved in drug and alcohol abuse. Vivid gender differences regarding experience of stress are reported by psychologists. Men want to achieve self-reliance in social relations. Even when under stress, men don't express their emotions openly. They don't want to ask for help. Women generally focus on self-expression and maintaining good interpersonal relations. While under stress, they immediately ask for help. It is in a way essential for them at some time in life. For example, a lady needs someone's help during pregnancy and delivery. Women's stress increases because of negative evaluation of self, poor expectations and negative thoughts. Due to depression and frustration, women lose hopes regarding what can be achieved after delay of gratification. They internalize their emotional reactions and face problems regarding mental health. They don't expect anything. Women's self-control is much more than men's self-control.

2.4.1. Emotional Management

Women	Men
Emotion-based problem-solving	Solution-focused problem-solving
More impulse control	Less impulse control: Anger
More positive emotions expressed	More negative emotions expressed
Feedback when performance is good	Feedback when poor performance
Communication is ambiguous	Clear communication
Submissiveness	Aggressiveness
Inner direction of negative thoughts	Outer expression, addictions
Accept insults	Hide insults
No mask, more real expression	Mask, pretensions
Empathy and sensitivity to self and others	Less empathy and sensitivity even about self
Ask for help	Do not ask for help
Low self-esteem	High self-esteem
Depression and frustration	Less depression and frustration
Hopelessness	Less hopelessness
Leaned helplessness	No learned helplessness
Dependent emotionally and cognitively	Independent cognitively and emotionally

Coping is of three types: emotion-focused, problem-focused and appraisal-focused. Women are more prone to emotion-focused coping. They experience a lot of emotional ups and downs when they face crises. Men may not express emotions and start solving the problem. However, their coping is more emotional in the long run. Conduct disorders are seen more among boys as they can't understand that such behaviour may lead to failure in the long run.

Seventeen types of substance-related abuses and alcohol abuses are more common among men than women. In this way, male members are using an indirect emotional coping style. Such abuses may decrease the intensity of emotional problems only temporarily. So even if they pretend to be tough, they are vulnerable and easily fall prey to abuse.

Actually, more women suffer from fatigue and similar problems, but still more men consume alcohol, cigarettes, weed and cocaine regularly to overcome fatigue. Social sanction is generally given to men for various abuses. It becomes a part and parcel of their pride, male ego and social status. They perceive it as an essential activity for relaxation, especially with friends. More women are taking help of professionals for their psychological problems. This fact can be interpreted from different perspectives. Women feel free to express their ideas, feelings and problems: They openly accept that they have a problem. Men are reluctant to accept it, and they do not take the help of professionals. All over the world, it is proven that more women are suffering from depression than men. This gender difference is not seen among girls and boys. Hence, it may be the effect of social influences.

As far as attribution style is concerned, women accept the responsibility of their failure and attribute it to their lack of abilities and efforts. They generalize the possibility of failure. However, men do not accept the responsibility of failure and blame it on some environmental issues. If a male student fails in an examination, he explains it by blaming the teacher and saying that the question paper was very difficult and unexpected. He thinks that, next time, he will get good grades. So he continues working even after failure. This is because men externalize their emotional problems after experiencing frustration. They seek satisfaction by immediate gratification of needs and desires. Women, on the other hand, think that it is impossible to achieve success and become helpless. This results in even more deteriorated performance and finally they leave the job or education.

Girls underestimate their abilities and potential and concentrate on limitations. Hence, they feel more helpless and emotionally more vulnerable. Next time, when they start studying, they can't concentrate on studies because of emotional disturbances due to fear of failure. Many researchers have reported that they have fear of success also as it is associated with social rejection and loss of femininity. It is a controversial issue in the changing value system. Most women internalize the belief that competence and achievement are incompatible with femininity and the socially desirable role of women. According to this belief, the achievement-oriented female is supposed to be less attractive as a woman (Hyde, 1985). This directly affects their aspirations and motivation. Negative thinking, underestimating self, generalization of failure, distorted cognition and information processing leading to false beliefs enhances stress of women.

Due to the subordinate status for generations, ladies even today are reluctant to make any important decisions on their own. If no opportunity to learn decision-making is given, an individual will lag behind in it. Social expectations, norms and traditions, following previous generation or ideals, identifications with mother figures, lack of logical thinking result in passively accepting decisions made by others. Self-worth, courage and power necessary for making decisions, are not allowed to develop in girls' and women's personalities. Women are conditioned to be dependent cognitively and emotionally. Even when women earn on their own, they are not allowed to and they don't feel confident enough to spend any major amount. Even when mothers spend their life rearing children, they don't make any decisions about their children.

If an individual gets appropriate opportunities for self-development, it may lead to hope, and if not, it leads to hopelessness. Self-respect results from respect given by others. Power generates both opportunity and respect. The lack of power may lead to dependence and vulnerability. These three things, namely power, opportunity and respect, are rarely seen in women's lives. If they want opportunities, they will not be respected. Love and acceptance accompanies respect. Opportunity

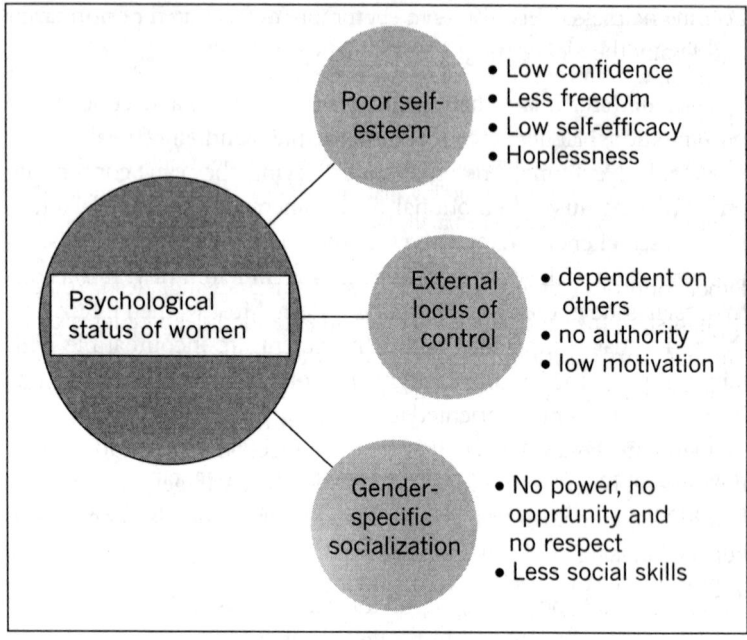

Figure 2.3 *Correlates of Psychological Status of Women*

results in opposition, criticism and conflict. One critical issue is the restricted field of activities (Figure 2.3).

There are so many restrictions and limitations and perceived inabilities due to which women generally prefer to forget about opportunities and stay back at home for routine responsibilities. Due to over socialization, women's achievement motivation remains low for the whole of their lives. As they don't have enough freedom of thought also, they are less creative.

Male members are generally given maximum opportunities by family. They are respected right from birth as the future head of the family, and power is essentially a way of life for males. Expectations about education and career are different for girls and boys (Basu et al., 2017). Indian researchers have proved that, in general, motivation for education and vocational aspiration depends on gender. Vocational aspiration of girls is, in general, low irrespective of their cognitive abilities and availability in the family.

In a research done recently in 2017 by the International Labour Organization Gallup Survey conducted in 142 countries, it is reported that 70 per cent of Indian women neither work nor are interested in it. Around 26 per cent of women work, and most of them are part-time workers. Only 30 per cent of women in India expressed that they would like to or prefer to work, as compared to 41 per cent of women who clearly said that they would prefer staying back at home. It is worth noting that more Indian women, as compared to men, think that other women in the family also should not work outside home.

Other countries giving similar results are Pakistan, Bangladesh, Yemen, Afghanistan, Iraq and Algeria. This is an extended deep belief regarding male superiority internalized by women in Indian culture. Many young women can't work because their in-laws do not accept the idea.

Time management is also totally different among men and women. If we accept the division of activities based on two dimensions, namely important and urgent, then there are four types of activities: urgent and important, urgent but not important, not urgent but important and not important not urgent. A typical Indian woman has to devote a lot of her time to activities that are urgent but not important and, second, not urgent and not important. Women are incharge of household responsibilities, children and old individuals. They have to struggle hard to fulfil family expectations. The activities such as cooking, cleaning and washing are urgent but may not contribute anything to her development. Hence, they can't be accepted as important. The other domain in which women devote their time is not important and not urgent. The traditional lifestyle expects women to devote their free time to decorating homes, embroidery and social interaction, such as kitty parties and non-productive interactions. These activities contribute hardly anything to personal development.

Men, on the other hand, devote time to activities which are urgent and important and not urgent but important. Important decisions regarding family matters, economic transactions, emergency actions and similar other things are related to the basic roles of men. They plan their future and work hard to accomplish their goals. These are important but not urgent activities. As a consequence, in due course of time, they can achieve certain things. Social interactions are also different as men are task oriented: They can manipulate important issues even in a dinner party.

The impact of gender-specific socialization is seen even in academic achievements. Here, gender differences include verbal and mathematical abilities. Many researchers found that verbal abilities are more among girls, and mathematical abilities are more among boys. However, it is a controversial issue if these differences are innate or acquired due to different socialization. Similar controversy prevails regarding the findings that women are people oriented and men are things oriented. Women are reported to be higher in aggreeableness and neuroticism (Lippa, 2010). Hyde (2005) and many others analysed numerous research and concluded that there are very negligible differences among genders, and these are seen in insignificant dimensions. According to them, such differences should not be worth bearing the ill effects.

To sum up, it can be said that gender stereotypical roles play a very decisive role in the personality make-up and self-perception of an individual. For example, very rarely, like in Arapesh culture, females are the head of the family and, hence, entirely different more manly traits are seen in them.

2.5. DEVELOPMENTAL TASKS: MEN AND WOMEN

According to Havighurst (1953), developmental tasks are based on physiological maturation, socio-structural and cultural forces and personal values and aspirations. Developmental psychology has been a fertile field of research for more than 100 years. However, there is hardly any consideration regarding the different expectations related to gender and different ways of evaluating men and women as being acceptable and successful from a social perspective.

During the first few years, developmental tasks for both genders are the same. They are walking, talking, leaning basic skills, language acquisition and so on. As children grow older, academic achievement becomes important. However, as far as the Indian situation is concerned, during adolescence, developmental tasks for two genders start following entirely different orientation. Settling down in a profession and rearing children are mentioned in young adulthood irrespective of gender. If approximately 78 per cent of women do not gainfully work, there is no possibility of settling down. Still, they are leading a socially acceptable life. There are certain responsibilities that nature has assigned to females. In addition, society expects that they should devote a lot of time and effort when they become mothers. For the whole of their lives, they are in charge of child rearing. The same is true in the case of responsibilities regarding family maintenance. The division of labour is a critical issue due to which not only the meaning but also the actual scope of various developmental tasks differ and lead to non-ending demands regarding women's duties necessary for social acceptance. This bifurcation is so vivid that their developmental tasks are also totally different from each other.

In a very interesting research, men and women were asked to enumerate various jobs they do to maintain their family. Men gave a long list of tasks, such as purchasing monthly groceries, payment of light bills, property tax, major shopping and cutting the branches of trees in the garden. The list given by women was comparatively very short, such as cooking, cleaning, washing and looking after children. However, the frequency of the tasks was a number of times a day in the case of women and once a month or even once a year in the case of men.

In a survey, it was found that male members devote on an average 19 minutes to household work in a week. Some researchers were curious to know the exact time the father of a newborn baby spends with it. Data were collected from different countries, and the average time was calculated. It was approximately 2 seconds. It is essential to remember that this depends on culture and socialization.

Developmental tasks have flexibility as per the gender, culture, education and expectations of the individual from self. A woman is still supposed to get a sense of satisfaction and achievement only by keeping the man happy, bearing and rearing children and taking care of his family. These are her developmental tasks according to the traditional Indian perspective. Even today, most Indian ladies are devoting their lives to these goals. If some very well-educated women want to go ahead and think of developmental tasks related to self-development and self-actualization, mostly they are not appreciated by even their own family members. Irrespective of her worth, she is considered only a female and expected to work for others.

A man who is not earning enough to support his family is considered as unworthy and is criticized by the family and community. Even when a man is a great artist and wants to pursue his art further or may be a social worker, he still has to earn. Like that, the developmental tasks are rigid and unfair in the case of both genders.

Genital mutilation and similar other rites are also perceived as essential by some particular communities and are considered as developmental tasks. A young adult female or adolescent girl is not accepted as a member of a specific community until that traumatic procedure is performed. In some other religious groups, similar procedures are performed in the case of male adolescents also.

Hence, it is necessary to reconsider the exact nature of developmental tasks of adolescents and youth with reference to the Indian perspective. If considered in detail with reference to gender, it may lead to a better understanding of the life of both genders.

2.6. DISCRIMINATION AND LIMITATIONS

Female foeticide results in a deteriorating sex ratio all over India. That too, it is seen more in a metro city like Mumbai: There are 777 females as compared to 1,000 males. In the case of comparatively less-advanced communities, like primitive people, this ratio is far better, that is, 1,005 females as compared to 1,000 males. The proportion of girls in a population under 6 years is constantly decreasing. It is 914. Due to the enhanced medical facilities, death rate of adult women has decreased. Various ways have been used for generations to kill female infants in some communities, which indicate society's perspective and attitude towards females. This leads to increased crimes and malpractices as some male members can't get a marriage partner. In 2020, 1 man out of 12 Indian men could not get a marriage partner. The basic human right to life is violated, and a female is denied the status of a human being.

The most critical issue in this case is that the mother herself is eager to get rid of female offspring. If she is not ready to do so, her mother-in-law insists that she must do it and essentially produce only male children. The social pressure is so much that there are incidences of divorce and even killing grown-up daughters for producing male children. Many ladies commit suicide as they can't reproduce a male child and hence are harassed severely by their family. If not direct, there is hidden rejection and subtle negative emotional expressions which a girl child can feel. They are effective in deciding her sense of security and psycho-social health.

In an extensive research by Merdhekar and Wadkar (2012), it was reported that more educated housewives feel hopeless and helpless as compared to working women. Housewives face more frustration and depression. In particular, educated housewives experience more isolation, vulnerability and invasion. They think that they are doing only insignificant and non-productive work. They experience more monotony, restlessness and boredom. More housewives feel that their life is meaningless and vegetative. Some of them think that their future is meaningless. They suffer from more psychological problems.

Crime is another example of extremely inhuman treatment given to girls and women. Every third woman in India suffers from sexual and physical violence at home (News 18, 8 February 2018). According to a recent National Family Health survey released by the Union Health Ministry, 27 per cent of Indian women have experienced physical violence since the age of 15. Most of the perpetrators, that is, 83 per cent, are present and 9 per cent are former husbands. About 5.4 per cent of violence takes place to force sexual intercourse, 4 per cent for other unwanted sexual acts.

It is reported recently in an Indian study that in the case of most of the murders, termination of sexual relations or doubt about a woman's infidelity are the major reasons.

The ideal male member is perceived as being independent and a decision-maker of the family. He may or may not consider others' inconvenience while doing that. Men are taught to underestimate emotions; however, they express emotions like intense anger readily and neglect if their behaviour hurts women. If a man is abused, there is hardly any legal provision for men to get justice, and he does not accept it. As it is not socially acceptable, it hurts their male superiority ego, and they keep mum about it.

Throughout life, more prestigious tasks are assigned to men, and hardly, any prestige and importance is given to what housewives do for the whole of their lives. The worst part is they also do not value their own efforts. It is assumed that there is nothing special and no special skills are required for doing these jobs assigned to women. According to researchers, an Indian housewife works for 99 hours a week to maintain her family.

> The World Economic Forum has done thought-provoking research about the Global Gender Gap Index around the world in 2017. Hierarchically, the rank of India is 108, which is lower than Bangladesh and China. The contribution of women to the economy and wages they get as compared to men are the major indicators. In opportunities that women get, India's rank is 139, and in health and facilities, it is 141. The percentage of women getting education is decreasing. *The Economic Times* (2 March 2021) reported recently that 85 per cent of women in India face strong gender bias and are deprived of raises and promotions only because of their gender. It is the 'LinkedIn Opportunity Index 2021'.

Most young women are forced to stay back when they are carrying and deliver a baby. It is a monotonous and tiring job, and if the mother is doing it alone, she gets frustrated. In the Indian community, a myth has been prevalent for generations that if the mother is working, it may lead to ill effects on the baby's development: psychological, cognitive and even physical. However, it is proved scientifically that it is not necessary for mothers to be with the children for 24 hours. If someone else is playing the role of mother substitute satisfactorily and if the child is safe physically and psychologically, there is absolutely no problem regarding psychological adjustment of the child. There are intense detrimental effects on children if mothers are permanently absent, for example, due to divorce or death. That is deprivation. However, if mothers are going out for a few hours every day and coming back after the work duration is over, that is just separation. Here, children know that mothers will be returning after some time, and they will be able to communicate warmth and love. It is not the quantity of mother–child relations but the quality of mother–child interaction that is more important.

A housewife leads a life where there is very limited scope for cognitive stimulation. It is reported by researchers that if cognitive stimulation is missing for years, cognitive alertness and intelligence quotient may decrease. Her life became boring and frustrating. Due to all these limitations, many adolescent girls in India don't take their career seriously. In a recent Indian doctoral research, it is seen that the vocational aspiration of high-school girls is poor, and there is a lot of ambiguity regarding their future plans. If it is by choice that she is not gainfully employed, she faces comparatively fewer problems. It may be because of internalization of social values that she feels comfortable. In this situation, it is obvious that the lady is not interested in self-development and utilizing her potential. If a woman is not capable of becoming independent, she can't become interdependent for the whole of her life. After a few years of being a full-time housewife, she may lose her confidence and try to justify why she is at home even when children are grown up. She may experience a sense of worthlessness, generalized anxiety, self-pity, devaluation of self, inferiority complex and create a false impression of being satisfied.

Most of the women with psychiatric problems, such as depression, anxiety and sleep disorders, being treated by psychiatrists are housewives. As early as the seventh decade of last century, Friedman found that many women were suffering from depression, being unable to focus on things, feeling tired without substantial reason, sleeping a lot and weeping without substantial reasons. They were unhappy. They had a secure marriage, children, financial security and social network. Most of them were educated and had some college education. There was no substantial biological reason behind it. According to her, it is an identity crisis. After doing feminine duties for years, they felt more and more invalid. 'Who am I?' 'Is it all that is there in my life?' This type of feeling was reported. They wanted to do something more meaningful that would make them happy during middle age. She focused on cognitive dissonance and dissatisfaction of women limited to housewives' life. Many Indian researchers have proved that housewives have low self-esteem and self-respect.

A career woman is exposed to double roles and responsibilities, especially if she is married. She has to complete her household jobs and struggle hard to fulfil the expectations of the job. If this is the first generation of working women, it is difficult to have a role model, and there is more confusion. However, during the last few decades it is proved that the more the roles, the more the possibility of maintaining good psycho-social health. It leads to more life satisfaction and less frustration for ladies. The quality of various experiences is important. Working mothers experience less depression as compared to non-working mothers.

Work is a matter of pride for a man. His status, earning, the time and efforts he devotes to everything is appreciated by his family and community. His convenience, his health, his decisions and everything is respected. However, it is accepted only as a compromise by family in the case of woman. Although she is equally qualified, getting an equal salary and is shouldering similar responsibilities, it is still expected that she should first fulfil her duties related to family, cooking and children. If she is not capable of managing both, it is recommended that she should leave the job. The psychological health of a housewife depends on whether she is willingly staying at home or is forced to do so.

In social life, the political sphere or intellectual achievement, women are seriously lagging behind irrespective of their intellectual capacity. Due to discrimination and social restrictions in most of the important fields, they are hardly represented. They don't utilize their potential to the fullest extent. They contribute hardly anything to the field of civilization. In a list of known contributors to Indian civiliza-tion, at the most, 5 per cent of ladies are represented.

The percentage of female Noble prize winners in physics is 1.4 per cent. Nobel prizes in science, in general, is 3.29 per cent. There are only three female IAS officers per 20 male officers, and 2.5 per cent of the total neurosurgeons are ladies. Out of 431 universities, only 13 universities have women vice chancel-lors. In the 17th Lok Sabha, only 14 per cent of representatives are women. Only 13 per cent of women are represented in the air force, 6 per cent in the navy and 3.85 in the army, as reported in 2018.

2.7. CONDUCIVE ENVIRONMENT AND SUPPORT FOR BOTH THE GENDERS: ANDROGYNY

As the world expects a male member to be a super being and the female member to devote her life to serving others, it is an injustice for both. No one is free to decide; nobody is treated as a human being.

Androgyny is a balance of both masculine and feminine characteristics. Those who perceive themselves as androgynous are more mature in moral judgments. Assertiveness, better self-esteem, and more flexibility in behaviour are correlated to it.

According to Bem (1974), an American psychologist, masculinity and femininity are merely constructions of cultural schema.[1] It is a stereotypical thinking according to which man and woman are perceived as totally different and can be placed at the fag end of the continuum.

According to some researchers, it is a difference of degree. Men are comparatively more oriented towards work, and women are somewhat more expressive.

The impact of culture is so strong that exactly the opposite scenario is seen in different cultures. In Denmark, men are so dependent on their mothers and wives that they commit suicide due to loss of dependency.

Figure 2.4 depicts essential strategies to enhance androgyny and control sexism. Both genders will get benefits out of it.

2.7.1. Modern Youth

India is undergoing rapid social, economic, cultural and technological changes. Its major impact is on youth. A survey of 5,000 youths was conducted. Today's young generation is found to be more ambitious, optimistic, open to change and independent about career decisions. They are eager to face new challenges. Only 19 per cent accepted that they are influenced by families when selecting a field of study. They are more interested in higher education and skills development. About 34 per cent mentioned gender, family background and marital status as a barrier. Around 82 per cent stated that ideal employment would be a full-time job, and very few young ladies wanted to be housewives (World Economic Forum, 2018).

A very popular recent movie, *Kabir Singh* (2019), depicts the life of the new generation and attitudes of the same regarding premarital sex, addictions and extreme aggression in general behaviour. The expression of sexual urge is so exaggerated that it seems to be beyond any control of the hero. Taking

[1] https://en.m.wikipedia.org

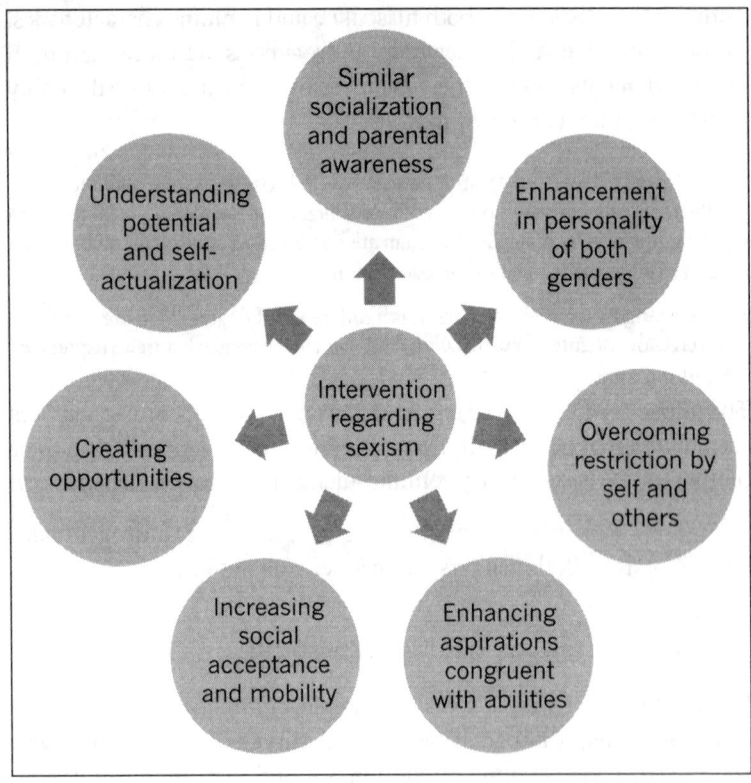

Figure 2.4 *Intervention Regarding Sexism*

drugs, alcohol, smoking, one night stands, no strings relationship, premarital pregnancy, all sorts of anti-traditional behaviour and values are shown as well accepted and dignified patterns of behaviour. At the same time, the heroin is just a sex object, extremely passive and submissive, who without any resistance is ready to surrender sexually (Oddnaari, 21 June 2019).

Mass media, especially movies and series, are very effective in influencing the audience. Some youth are confident and enjoying their premarital and extramarital sex life. There is some cognitive dissonance in all these things. On one hand, there are many psychological problems that women have been facing for generations, including today's youth. They are still sensitive, empathetic, emotionally dependent and perceiving self from others' perspective. Their coping style is emotion based. If they are using the freedom to behave, like male members, it declares that they are still feeling inferior. Their self-worth depends on appreciation and encouragement by others. Most of them still need some support, security and safety to survive in the community.

Crime related to sexual exploitation of women is continuously increasing all over the world. In the work environment, women are commonly perceived as being sexual dolls, easily available by their male colleagues. Women's style and behaviour may contribute to it because of age-old prejudices of male members. New ways, such as premarital sex and live-in relations, are resulting in more problems: sexually transmitted diseases (STDs) and HIV for both. Many of them reproduce during that period and, in spite of legal protection, are outright rejected by the community. Is it that a young lady is now getting more exploited sexually and, that too, willingly? There is still a lot of social stigma about these things. Due to her physiological functions regarding reproduction, it becomes essential for her to be careful about many things. In India, marriage is a strict social norm. It is not considered as a personal matter. The percentage of people who remain unmarried even at the age of 40 is 0.4 in India. It is a social stigma to be single after a particular age.

An intelligent, well-educated, motivated and strong lady is expected to be competing with self, striving hard for self-actualization and more androgyny oriented. For example, she may be more comfortable in dress fashion that never highlights her femininity, is comfortable and declares her self-respect. It is necessary to come out of the burden of femininity and breathe freely as a human being. Stereotypical ideas about being pleasant, attractive and submissive are to be corrected. External locus of control, emotional and cognitive dependence and the need for affiliation are still restricting their lives. They should be able to accept and respect themselves as worthy individuals. They are expected to make their own decisions and face the consequences. They should become self-sufficient in every sense. Only after that, they will be able to think about interdependence.

Both male and female well-educated young adults are free from societal pressure to follow socially acceptable behaviour. It is becoming 'it's my life…. I will do whatever', 'right now, I want to enjoy' and 'so what if they criticize me' type of culture. Young male members are more involved in freely enjoying sex, drugs and alcohol. There is hardly any delay of gratification, and frustration tolerance is low. Showing off one's achievements and happiness with the help of e-communication, like Facebook, has become a common practice. Creating fake impressions and exploiting others are perceived as achievements. Such superficial pretensions and fake impressions even in close relations are generating lack of stability, trust, feeling of security and positive emotions, such as gratitude and compassion. Loneliness and hopelessness are increasing. Fake confidence, unrealistic optimism and hedonism are becoming coping styles. Cybercrime is increasing at an international level. Some women are also involved in such activities (BBC News, 2019; and many other videos on YouTube).

This leads to multiple problems: psychological, social and physiological. It is essential to maintain good interpersonal relations, keep close contact with reality, respect self and manage negative impulses and exaggerated desire for materialistic pleasure. A balanced and mature personality and unconditional positive regard may help the youth to lead a happy and satisfied personal and social life.

Overcoming the ill effects of gender socialization is essential.

Once we accept androgyny, gender-specific roles become less compelling and less rigid. Every individual must get an opportunity for self-development and proper use of potential. Considering the injustice regarding upbringing individuals of both genders in India, it becomes essential to think of carefully avoiding discrimination in every sphere of life. Both genders should be taught to understand and evaluate their own personality, achievements and motivation. Self-respect, understanding self and objective evaluation of self are essential for both genders to develop self-worth.

2.8. SUMMARY

Indian child-rearing practices and social norms heavily depend on a very rigid division of labour and division of authority. As a consequence, the personality of two genders is moulded accordingly. All or none type of conditioning and experiences pressurize both genders to accept a stereotypical sex role, resulting in extremely opposite personality traits of men and women. Their perceptions, their attitudes, understanding, emotional reactions, perceived competence and ideas regarding satisfaction are totally different. Lower expectations, limited opportunities, poor cognitive stimulation and the lack of respect and power make women's life restricted. Male members, especially adolescents and youth, face many problems, such as undue expectations of parents, forced career, compulsion to earn and responsibility of family. A mask of being strong and capable is also difficult to maintain for male members. Extreme internalization of social values and compulsion to perform unwanted duties become essential for both of them.

The Indian situation is such that the majority of both girls and boys, young men and women both are just following a predetermined path and leading life according to someone else's agenda. A lot of injustice and unfair practices are very common in interpersonal relations. The new generation of youth have to utilize their potential and lead an androgynous life which may give them an opportunity for self-development. They should be accepted and treated as a human being rather than just a male and female. Undue comparison between men and women must be avoided.

Emotional Abuse

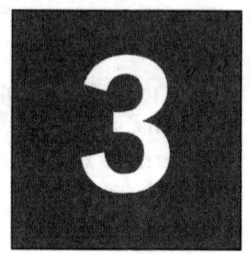

3.1. NATURE AND TYPES OF EMOTIONAL ABUSE

Prashant was never in favour of a second girl child, and he used to abuse his daughter Sanika since her childhood. When she was only 6 years old, Sanika started being threatened by Prashant that she would be sent off to a hostel. Prashant never encouraged her, showed an ounce of affection and used to express rejection. He repeatedly told her that she was an unwanted child. Today, Sanika is 20 years old, and unfortunately, she is suffering from a chronic disorder. Prashant's attitude is still the same; he never enquires about her health or offers any sort of help. He goes to the extent of saying that he won't even attend her funeral.

Emotional abuse is prevalent all over the world, still the most neglected aspect of human interaction. Emotional abuse is a blanket term which encompasses different psychological abuse. It is prevalent not only in parent–child relations but also in every relationship, such as husband–wife, sibling relations, professional relations, relations with friends, teachers and even offspring–parent relationship in old age. There is a difference in degree depending on age, education, personality, self-worth and dependency of the victim on the abuser. Culture also plays an important role in deciding the intensity and ill effects of the same.

There is a lot of ambiguity in the concept and construct of emotional abuse. It is essential to understand that male dominance for genera-tions, cultural expectations about unequal power sharing and socially acceptable roles of men and women depend on religion, race, caste, creed and community, culture, subculture, education, socio-economic status and so on. As a consequence, it is impossible to define it in a universally applicable way. Relationships are labile and keep on changing. The same male may be very kind and caring in the first few years after marriage and may become abusive afterwards. Hence, it is difficult to label a relationship in a particular way permanently.

Emotional abuse is an inherent hidden aspect of any unequal relations where one person wants to control and manipulate the other. It is related to power imbalance. Even in psychological research, it is hardly represented. Until 1996, there was substantial controversy regarding the definition of emotional abuse. Emotional abuse is difficult to identify as it exists with other types of abuse. As its effects are not seen overtly, it is mostly underestimated.

Emotional abuse or psychological abuse means chronic verbal aggression and maltreatment. It is also known as psychological violence or mental abuse. Psychological abuse is included in the International Classification of Diseases, 10th Revision, given by the WHO.

What Is Emotional Abuse?

Emotional abuse can be defined as any interpersonal behaviour that is verbal assault, humiliation, rejecting one's thoughts and ideas, intimidation, treating like an infant, isolation, confinement or any other treatment which may result in a diminished sense of self-worth, identity and dignity of the victim. It also includes manipulating, which may result in self-doubt in a victim's mind.

It includes rejection, exploitation and isolation. Various forms are verbal aggression, yelling, insulting, degradation, terrorizing and deprivation of emotional responsiveness. It may result in psychological trauma which includes anxiety, depression or post-traumatic stress disorder. Emotional abuse produces fear by intimidation and the threat of potential physical harm. This may not only be related to self but to dear ones, like children or parents. Forced separation from family and friends may also be a strategy to emotionally abuse someone. The abuser may constantly insult the victim, practise putting down, nagging and deny that any abuse is taking place. One recent type of emotional abuse is online abuse and cyber bullying.

There are different types of emotional abuse, such as aggression, minimizing and denying. Verbal aggression is shaming, name calling or blaming. Minimizing is covet ambiguous emotional abuse which is difficult to identify. It is underestimating, downplaying the significance of the victim's positive qualities and the abuser's unfair behaviour. It is hidden manipulation. Even the victims can't sometimes understand the reason behind their emotional upset. Denying may take the form of withholding. There is no communication with the victim: no talking and no listening. The abuser may show apathetic behaviour by emotionally withdrawing as disapproval. Some experts insist on the fact that emotional abuse is related to controlling and manipulating a victim's emotions. It means that the emotions of the victim are influenced in such a way that they perceive the issue according to the abuser's perspective.

Emotional abuse is intentionally hurting someone's emotions. Emotional abuse is manipulating emotions and controlling someone through guilt feelings. It is a severe pattern of abuse which is capable of generating a lot of distress. It also includes quarrelling, arguing or giving blunt reactions. Momentary rage, scolding, yelling or expressing disagreement loudly are not examples of emotional abuse. Generally, after that expression of anger, interaction becomes normal, and there is no constant negative interaction repeatedly.

According to a researcher, Romeo (2000), emotional abuse is not just a single event but a continuous behaviour of an abuser for systematic belittlement of the victim so that the victim perceives themselves as unworthy. Only in extreme situations, a single event may be labelled as emotional abuse.

The basic intention of emotional abuse is exactly like physical abuse, which means controlling the other individual's action. Emotions are used as a weapon to harm the other person. Emotional abuse may not accompany physical abuse but is a prerequisite to it. It is seen in scientific studies that if threat, restrictions and damage to the victim's property are used in emotional abuse, the possibility of physical abuse increases.

Sometimes, the victim does not realize that it is emotional abuse. Like in marital emotional abuse, the victim is afraid, confused and somehow wants to cope with the situation.

Hitesh is 24, an engineer, who has been working in a multinational company. Just a few months ago, he got married. He is very particular about food, cleanliness and the neatness of the home. Even if there is a minor change in the taste of food, he starts yelling loudly, throwing things and food and blaming his wife Aashu. Generally, his aggressive gesture is so frightening that she starts weeping and is terribly afraid of physical abuse. After some time, Hitesh again behaves politely, tries to prove that he is a very caring husband and expresses apology. If she is physically hurt, he will apply medicine and behave in a very pleasant way. He tries to convince her that she should not invite such trouble and should behave exactly according to his directions. Again, within a few hours, Hitesh becomes mad with anger, starts blaming her and throwing things.

It is a sort of vicious circle. The abuser emotionally abuses the victim just to show dominance. Then, the abuser feels guilty about the effects of his action. He wants to justify his actions and doesn't want to shoulder any responsibility. Most of the time, the abuser wants to pretend that he is sorry and the abuse never took place or it has taken place due to the victim's mistake. Once he thinks that the victim seems to be convinced, he gets involved in even more serious emotional abuse.

Do You Know?

Gender plays an important role in emotional abuse. In the USA, 80 per cent of abuse is done by men, and in the United Kingdom, approximately 10 per cent of women harass their male partners.

There are gender differences in the perception of abuse, not only by victims but by counsellors also. In most cultures, male members are perceived to be more abusive.

As most of the cases are not reported, the total emotional abuse prevalence rate is estimated to be as high as 80 per cent.[1] Any type of intimate partner violence is related to emotional abuse. Due to the lack of awareness and social acceptance of the subordinate status of women, the percentage of such abuse can't be exactly estimated in Indian culture.

[1] http://www.ncbi.nlm.nih.gov 2013

Equally common all over the world is emotional abuse of children. It hampers their psychological and emotional, social and cognitive development. It results from undue expectations, myths about child rearing and unpleasant childhood experiences of the parents. Sometimes, the paucity of resources and stressful busy life of parents may be the root cause. It is seen that, irrespective of culture or socio-economic status, the lack of empathy and understanding, poor communication and child-rearing skills, and inadequate self-worth of the parents lead to emotional abuse of children. It is reported by researchers that the likelihood of emotional abuse is equal by both the parents. Childhood maltreatment refers to interactions by an adult which endanger the physical or psychological well-being of a child and violate social sanctions regarding proper parenting (Child Welfare Information Gateway, 2018). Childhood abuse can be divided into four basic types: physical abuse, sexual abuse, emotional abuse and neglect. No abuse can exist without emotional abuse.

Researchers have reported that every second a child in India is facing emotional abuse (Bhilwar et al., 2015). The Indian Government's 'Childline India' helpline received 92,000 calls on abuse and violence in 11 days during lockdown due to corona (*The Indian Express*, 8 April 2020). It indicates that there is a 50 per cent increase in these calls. Around 30 per cent of these calls are regarding abuse and violence against children. It obviously means that these children are not safe inside their homes. They are more vulnerable now as they are separated from other people who may support them.

Abusive practices are evaluated on the basis of various dimensions, such as duration, frequency and intensity or deviation from social norms. Of course, extreme expressions do not need any other consideration as it is too intense, when the abuser says, 'go and commit suicide, you are useless, there is no other option.'

Sometimes, the abuser does not have any awareness. However, there is some disturbance in interpersonal relations which is perceived by the victim. For example, a wife may feel insecure and think that her husband does not love her. She is suspicious of his behaviour and ambiguity in sharing information. As a consequence, she may check his whereabouts and details of his plans, which again is irritating. Some of the accusers also expressed the possibility of infidelity and cheating. Here, accusation, blame and repeatedly making sure that the partner is not engaging in affairs are the major ways to abuse.

Generally, emotional abuse in relationships is regarding the following:

- **Sex:** An abuser's stand is that the victim should be able to please him sexually and fulfil all his expectations. If not, he will abuse her.
  - o Shreya is a simple value-based college student. Arman was her Facebook friend. He is trying to convince her that he loves her and wants to marry her. She denied the proposal and stopped talking to him. He, however, consistently calls her until she responds, sometimes even 100 times. He wants her to satisfy him with sex chats and send him her half-nude photographs. He pretends that he will not be able to survive without her love.
- **Emotions:** The abuser openly denies the sincerity of emotional experiences of the victim and says, 'stop your emotional drama'.
- **Threats:** The abuser constantly threatens the victim like 'if you go to your mother, I will drag you back.' This is very common in Indian situations with reference to marital relations.
- **Social issues:** Emotionally abusing with reference to social interactions, like the abuser says to the victim 'my relatives can't stand you'.
- **Finance:** In an Indian situation, especially if a housewife asks for some money, the abuser may deny it outright and may remark that 'such expenditure will result in complete bankruptcy.'
- **Spiritual threat:** An abuser may blame the victim for not accepting a particular thing and may express his anger, like 'God will teach you a lesson'.

3.1.1. Types of Abuse

Researchers have given various types of emotional abuse, which are as follows:

1. **Overt and covert abuse:** Overt means demeaning the victim openly. Covert is subtle, which is equally devastating. Even with the help of visual communication or indirect verbal

communication, this type of abuse can be done. A look with a specific non-verbal communication indicating contempt, hatred, devaluation and mockery can be abusive.

2. **Intentional and unintentional abuse:** Generally, emotional abuse is intentional, but it may take place unintentionally. Especially, when an abuser is just imitating the style of interaction of his parents, he may not notice that it is abusive. Some experts define emotional abuse as 'any behaviour or attitude that emotionally damages another person regardless of whether it is due to conscious intent or not.' Even if the abuser is completely unaware, his behaviour and attitude may be equally damaging and destructive. Many of the abusers were themselves abused in past and repeating the same or re-enacting what was done by the harasser then. This does not decrease the ill effects on the victim.

   Those who had experienced sexual abuse in childhood also have problems interaction with a partner. The abuser may have some stress, anger, feeling that the partner can't fulfil his expectations, feeling rejected, abandoned or betrayed. Insecurity, along with extreme love for a partner, may also lead to abuse. Fear of abandonment and insecurity is more when there is intense love.

3. **Malevolent abuse:** One serious form of intentional abuse is malevolent abuse, which means undermining the victim deliberately. The abuser wants to destroy satisfaction, happiness and health of the victim as he hates the victim, envies her and wants to hurt her.

Fear of intimacy is also responsible for the perception of abuse. In case of sexual harassment, it is not only sexual but emotional also. As it is, sexual harassment is verbal, visual and behavioural. For example, if a boss is harassing a young lady who is his subordinate, he uses all tricks to emotionally abuse her with unwanted sexual advancements and work-related insults.

Some countries have been practising rights regarding relationships. Everyone has a right to have a satisfactory and androgynous relationship. Everyone has a right to have their own perspective and feelings. To get clear and honest answers to one's questions, get respect, to be free from accusation, criticism and blame are the basic expectations. The right to receive encouragement, to be free from threat, hurt and rage are essential for egalitarian interaction. The most significant in marital interaction is to deny sexual contact. The partner is expected to give emotional support and listen politely. If we consider Indian conditions, none of these is seen in the majority of interpersonal relations, may it be husband and wife, parent child or any other.

Various strategies of emotional abuse are as follows:

- Emotional bullying and yelling
- Insult and mockery
- Threats
- Excluding and isolating
- Humiliating and blaming
- Denial of abuse by the abuser
- Not accepting any logical argument
- 'It is so hard to be nice to you' type of pretension

Generally, emotionally abusive interactions are classified into various types. They are as follows:

1. Verbal assaults
2. Abusive expectations
3. Emotional blackmail
4. Gaslighting

Psychological abuse and its impact on human life can't be underestimated at any point of time. Various governments are treating it as part of public health and publishing research regarding the same to develop awareness, for example, the Public Health Agency of Canada.[2]

This report gives various psychologically abusive tactics: neglectful and deliberate. In neglectful tactics, the most common are as follows:

- **Ignoring and rejecting:** No importance given to presence, worth, opinions or any contribution, underestimating victim's thoughts, forgetting promises, communicating that they are inferior, expressing rejection, dislike and treating others more favourably

- **Denying emotional responsiveness:** No sensitive and responsive care, detached and uninvolved minimum interaction, neglecting and ignoring
- **Discounting:** Not taking things seriously, no appreciation or credit, no reciprocation of emotions.
- **Countering:** Claiming that the victim is insane
- **Trivializing:** Denying victim's feeling of being hurt

Some deliberate tactics are as follows:

- **Criticizing behaviour:** Finding faults, unrealistic standards, belittling, diminishing dignity and mimicking
- **Terrorizing:** Creating extreme fear in the mind of the victim by misuse of power, placing them in a threatening environment or threatening to kill family members and destroy property
- **Accusing, blaming and jealous control:** Claiming that the victim is responsible for abuse and is not trustworthy, accusing the victim of affairs, asking for account of every moment, using anger and aggression
- **Degrading:** Insulting, ridiculing and imitating
- **Harassing:** Keeping close watch, sending unwanted messages and gifts
- **Exploiting:** Pressurizing for illegal behaviour, taking undue advantage, forcing to practice sex trade, alcohol or drug use
- **Isolation:** Confined, restricted social interaction, no mobility, limiting freedom, locking, not allowing to use one's money and using someone for controlling the victim

Emotional blackmail is very common in all sorts of relations. An abuser wants to get what they want by controlling the behaviour of the victim and making them feel guilty and upset. If a mother threatens her son, 'I will commit suicide if you marry a girl of your choice', this is a clear example of emotional blackmail. There are many examples of this sort in Indian culture. *Mohabbatein* and *Zakhm* are the two popular Hindi movies very effectively depicting emotional abuse of Indian parents regarding marriage.

Gaslighting is manipulating someone by psychological means by doubting their sanity or reality. All four types may overlap and create a more intense impact.

3.2. PERSONALITY OF VICTIMS AND ABUSERS

Abusers may have some psychological problems, like personality disorders. Some of them can easily impress other significant members and manipulate things in such a way that even the family members, friends and professionals working in the field of law are also convinced that the victim is to be blamed. The personality of abusers is reported to be below normal in the case of psycho-social health. Most of them have one or more problems. They have a desire to control others' lives, have aggressive tendencies, negative self-image, inferiority complex and extreme hostility. If parents are abusive, the victim may develop abusive tendencies while interacting with their own children. The lack of empathy, self-centredness, the wish to manipulate others and get sadistic pleasure, reacting excessively about simple things and extreme views are the commonly seen characteristics. They feel insecure and uncomfortable in social situations. Generally, they exhibit coercive behavioural patterns. Most abusers are involved in substance or alcohol abuse. Many of them have problems, such as antisocial personality, borderline personality disorder, narcissistic personality, obsessive compulsive personality disorder, psychopathic personality and impulse control disorder. In some cases, neurological problems affecting behaviour are reported. They are paranoid about victim's intentions, carefully trying to find out if there are insults or hidden messages.

According to researchers, the abuser, irrespective of gender, has a high incidence of psychological disorders. Approximately, 80 per cent of the abusers have such problems. They don't see any fault in their behaviour, can't accept reality and never seek any treatment. Aggression, jealousy, suspicion, mood swings and poor self-control are very commonly seen.

Avoiding household work and controlling finance are the two main motives of abuse in the case of marital pairs. Abusers may try to convince victims' families also that the victims are to be blamed.

The personality of victims is also a fertile field of research. Generally, the victim over evaluates their need for love and affection. They are ready to bear anything for being loved. That is why even abusive love is also welcome. They are afraid of rejection. Fear of being alone is also seen, as the victim may have dependent personality disorder. The tendency to pretend that the relationship is fine, though it is not, is common. She feels responsible for others' problems. Pessimistic explanatory style and attributing negative events to stable, global and internal causes affect every area of life. Masochistic behaviour and tendencies enhance abuse. Masochism is deriving pleasure or sexual satisfaction from being subjected to humiliation and pain.

The victim has low self-esteem, is depressed and withdrawn. They suffer from anxiety. Some extreme cases have suicidal tendencies. They are timid and always feel threatened. They underestimate self-worth, feel guilty and blame themselves for difficulties in relationships. A strong desire to avoid confrontation is common. Self-doubt results in a tendency to make up and justify the abuser's behaviour. Neglecting the abuser's limitations and finding solace that they were once lovers increases tolerance of abuse. Due to underestimating self after repeatedly experiencing abuse, the victim may think that they deserve the same. They perceive it as their fault that they can't fulfil the expectations of others, they can't stand getting justice. Sarcastic comments, insulting and passing awkward remarks are regular practices of emotional abuse. If the victim is sad, they are criticized for being too sensitive. Whatever happens, it is claimed that it is due to their fault as they force the abuser to act in this way.

In close relationships, there is a combination of emotional, social and financial abuse. Here, the abuser wants to control every significant area of the victim's life. Even today, in most communities in India, traditional practices are in vogue. Due to internalization of social values, women think that it is essential at any cost to adjust to the life partner, and there is no way out. They are emotionally, socially, financially and cognitively dependent on their husbands. Their happiness totally depends on their husbands' mood. They always work hard to please them and underestimate their own capacity to make wise decisions. They are responsive and have no personal boundaries. If their husbands deny it, they can't even meet their own parents. This way, the abuser detaches the victim from the people who may support them if needed. This, in turn, leads to more vulnerability of the victim. The current scenario is such that for control, the abuser wants access to the victim's social media passwords so that they can see every detail of all communications. Sometimes, even women want to do it for their husbands. Women subjected to emotional abuse suffer from gynaecological problems and men get involved in addictions.

3.3. EFFECTS OF EMOTIONAL ABUSE ON NEUROLOGICAL, PSYCHOLOGICAL AND PHYSIOLOGICAL HEALTH

Emotional abuse has a serious impact on the individual's physiological, neurological and psychological health. As the ill effects are not obviously seen, it is neglected by society and mostly by the victim also. Either there is no awareness of abuse, or according to the victim, there is no option other than to tolerate it. However, the effects of emotional abuse are as serious as that of physical abuse.

3.3.1. Neurological and Physiological Effects of Emotional Abuse

Irrespective of age, education, socio-economic status and gender, anyone may face emotional abuse. It results in devastating effects on the individual. Abuse leaves a trace in the brain. This is proved by physiological studies of brain structure and functions. On the basis of memories regarding abuse, it is reported by researchers that emotional abuse results in damage to the hippocampus. According to the research done at Yale University, this, in turn, results in memory deficit. Abuse leads to over secretion of brain hormones, such as cortisol, adrenaline, non-adrenaline and opiates, according to Howard. A number of evidences regarding damage to the brain are available on Google, like brain scans (Downey, 2017). Traumatic childhood abuse may affect thinking, memory and emotions along with the sense of self. If sensory deprivation is a part of neglect and abuse, the child's brain is found to be significantly smaller and has cortical atrophy. There are enlarged ventricles. This is associated with the delay of developmental tasks.

Due to distress, the stress hormone cortisol is over produced. This, in turn, damages hippocampus and generates functional limitations of the same. As a consequence, the individual experiences anxiety, depression, post-traumatic stress disorder and the like. The somatosensory cortex processes intraindividual and interindividual sensations and perceptions. When emotionally abused, an individual wants to block these unpleasant memories. The brain wants to protect them from it. When emotionally abused, the somatosensory cortex is not capable of sending signals for memory recollection. Processing of emotions and self-awareness both deteriorate. Hence, emotional abuse has a negative impact on brain functioning. The basic purpose is to protect the victim from an extremely unpleasant stressful situation. Even after the abuse is over, the brain can't restore its functions.

Abuse leads to psychological symptoms later in life also. The general sense of well-being deteriorates and vulnerability regarding psychological problems increases. Brain scans of people having learning difficulties, relationship or developmental problems and social interaction difficulties indicate similar structural and functional irregularities. Supplements of GABA, vitamins and proper diet may help to overcome some ill effects of abuse.

Research done at the Harvard Medical School has proved that those who have experienced or witnessed domestic violence and sexual trauma and are bullied in their adolescence lack proper connection between the two hemispheres of the brain. This connection is necessary for emotional well-being and proper emotional balance and is responsible for anger, hostility, dissociation, anxiety, depression and even abuse of drugs. Many of the victims suffer from constant severe headaches, stomach aches or other chronic pain in their back, hands and legs.

Verbal abuse is also related to physiological effects such as fatigue, chronic pain, stress-related heart problems. Other problems, such as stammering, gastrointestinal problems, such as diarrhoea, indigestion, ulcers, spastic colon, problems related to eating and sleep, increased blood pressure, headache and migraine are also common. Serious health problems, such as diabetes, hepatitis, stroke and heart disease are reported to be associated with emotional abuse.

3.3.2. Psychological Effects of Emotional Abuse

There is hardly any difference between the effects of physical and emotional abuse (English et al., 2009). Emotional abuse of children affects their personality. Their self-esteem is poor, they lack basic skills, are more involved in acting out, feel insecure and show destructive behaviour. As a consequence of emotional abuse, children suffer from anger, anxiety, dissociation, post-traumatic stress disorder and chronic depression. According to researchers, such adolescents get involved in sexual pleasure at a younger stage to compensate for that. They want to get support and companionship. The feeling of being powerless and unwanted, degrading one's opinion and achievement are the issues affecting every psychological adjustment.

Emotional abuse directly affects emotional well-being negatively. It colours the perception of victims regarding issues utilized by the abuser to harass. Victims sometimes become cognitively dependent on the abuser. Such behaviour is repetitive. Isolation, fear and distrust may result in lifelong difficulties and may result in trouble forming and maintaining relations and academic difficulties.

As far as cognitive problems are concerned, difficulty in concentrating, memory gap disorder and intrusive memories are the most common problems. Intrusive memories are unwelcome and disruptive memories. An individual never intentionally wants to recall these contents.

In the USA, a report of child abuse is registered every 10 seconds. Yearly, 6.6 million children are affected (Huang, 2019).

In addition, immediate or short-term effects of emotional abuse are hypervigilance, shame and guilt, repeated crying, feeling nervous, feeling of being controlled and exploited, learned helplessness, feeling powerless and defeated, becoming passive and submissive overtly.

It is reported that if emotional abuse continues for the long term, the victims think that they can't leave the abuser, and they are not worthy of normal healthy relations. Gradually, they start perceiving self from the abuser's perspective. They get convinced that they are going to become or already have become crazy. Long-term emotional abuse results in long-term detrimental effects on self and integrity.

Johnson (2007) has proved that 24 per cent of total female patients were emotionally abused, and they suffered from higher rates of gynaecological problems. Emotional abuse results in post-traumatic stress disorder, somatization disorders, eating disorders, especially bulimia nervosa, abuse of alcohol, drugs, medicines, boarder line disorders and suicidal thoughts. They have problems with sexual relations. Laurent et al. (2008) have proved that marital dissatisfaction is associated with psychological abuse.

Do you know?

Around 60 per cent of psychiatric parents are emotionally abused. Hence, it is essential to be alert and protect self from abuse before it is too late (Morton, 2014).

Alexithymia or difficulty in identifying and processing one's emotions is seen more in the case of victims of psychological abuse. This may be related to coping or defence mechanisms which may help in tolerating, mastering or minimizing stress or conflict.

'10 Signs of Emotional Abuse in a Relationship (Break the Cycle of Manipulation)' by Barrie Davenport (2019) may enhance our understanding of abuse in relationships and how to get out of it.

As is shown in Figure 3.1, the first is the honeymoon stage where the abuser is perceived as being very attractive and charming to the partner. Others know this, and they also think that they are a nice person. When some problem arises, no one believes it. The abuser impresses

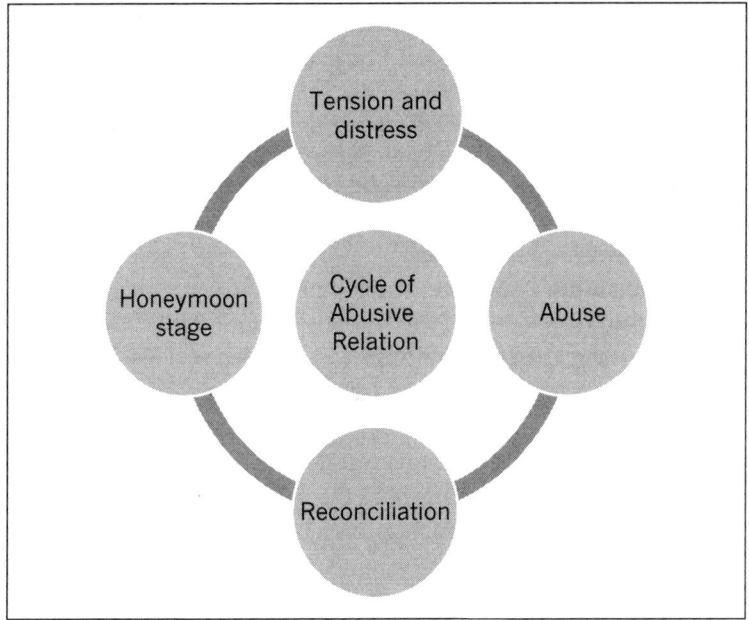

Figure 3.1 *Cycle of Abusive Relation*

the partner with various tricks, and if at all they become angry, they immediately justify and convince that they love the partner. The victim develops an attachment to the abuser and accepts a long-term relationship. At this stage, they never understand that something wrong is going to happen. It is worth noting that when it is the abuse of a partner, it starts after marriage and not before that. In marriage, an abuser wants to continue as they can, exercise power and the victim continues due to social pressure. Most of the time, irreparable damage results from emotional abuse. Some victims develop serious mental disorders and others leave their job or relationship.

In adulthood, victims become helpless, isolated and more vulnerable. They become anxious and depressed. Their self-respect diminishes, and they feel that they are worthless and useless. Panic attacks, post-traumatic stress disorder, reduced sexual desire and nightmares are experienced in the case of severe abuse. Self-harm and suicidal tendencies are reported in very intense cases.

Some specific phenomena related to emotional abuse in couples are as follows:

- **Stockholm syndrome:** Here, for a substantial duration, the victim is afraid of the abuser. Due to those terrifying feelings, they get identified with the abuser to be more safe. There is a binding between the two. Gradually, the victim tries to defend and justify the behaviour of the abuser.
- **Responsibility avoidance:** The abuser would never accept it when the victim tries to hold them responsible for their behaviour. On the contrary, they put the blame on the victim. They claim that if they had been with a better partner, they would have been the most polite person.
- **Extreme jealousy:** The abuser is jealous and hates every person of the opposite gender with whom the victim interacts. In addition to other restrictions, the abuser may ask for passwords for e-mail, Facebook and all the other accounts online to keep a watch. There is no trust, no personal space and no choice.
- **Mask while social interaction:** The abuser may treat the victim very politely in front of others or during any social interaction. No third person will ever know that they are abusing the victim. It becomes difficult to get any support from outside.
- **Loss of credibility:** The abuser may create a fake impression about the victim, especially in the mind of the victim's own family and close friends. Repeatedly, they may try to convince them that it is difficult to deal with the victim, and the victim is crazy.
- **Old discords and memories:** While abusing, past negative interactions and the victim's exact expressions are used again and again.
- **Emotional blackmail:** If the victim wants to get rid of their relationship, the abuser will cry excessively, threaten that they will not be able to live without them and will commit suicide if they leave.
- **Sexual manipulation:** Forcing the victim to do things that they do not appreciate. Manipulating and convincing them that they will enjoy it and if they refuse, blaming them that they are cold and selfish.
- **Physical abuse:** Using physical abuse and creating a fake impression that the abuser is repenting is a usual practice of some abusers.

- **Forced isolation:** Repeatedly, the abuser tries to convince the victim that they should not be so close to some people and should avoid them. Gradually, the trap of emotional abuse becomes even stronger.

3.4. WARNING SIGNS OF EMOTIONAL ABUSE

Due to socialization practices, cultural norms and general submissive personality, the victim may continue tolerating emotional abuse for years. In Indian community especially, ladies accept it as part and parcel of marriage or any other close relations in the family. They just blame their luck, blame themselves as they can't keep the harasser happy, and do not have the capacity to retaliate. Most of the victims, male or female, are confused and can't even label the interaction as abuse.

We can use these behavioural patterns for checking if a particular relation is abusive and, if yes, to what extent (Julia, 2018).

3.4.1. General Experiences of Victims

No communication, excluding an individual or ignoring feelings and priorities, humiliating and embracing remarks and behaviour so that an individual feels ashamed or guilty are very common. Withdrawal of love and affection, refusing to listen, to communicate and emotional withdrawal as punishment, frequent insults, giving fake emotional expression with completely inconsistent intentions and verbal messages are to be noted. Not allowing them to work gainfully and be independent is very common so that an abuser can control everything easily. There are many housewives who are well educated and are motivated to work; however, they are not allowed to do so by their husbands and in-laws. Destroying victim's possessions or threatening them, constant and extreme criticism, use of race, caste, socioeconomic status or even disability to abuse the victim are also seen. Derogatory jokes and put downs regarding any performance of the victim, sarcastic comments, unpleasant voices and unjustified jealousy are observed. Rejection, name calling, like labelling the person as stupid, ugly and useless, spreading false information or private information about the victim, belittling, hostility and outright verbal assault are also some forms of abuse. Manipulation of the victim's emotions, brain washing due to which self-concept and independence diminishes leads to intimidation. Cursing words, control and domination, moodiness, generating guilt in other person's mind are reported very often. Threats to expose private information or blackmailing are one of the serious abuses. In recent years, cybercrimes related to it have increased tremendously. Constantly keeping a watch regarding the whereabouts of the victim by calling or messaging very often, keeping an eye on phone calls, mails and any other communication like WhatsApp, cyber bulling, sending offensive messages or making offensive comments on someone's online profile are recent ways of abuse.

Threatening that if an individual fails to do a particular thing, the abuser will harm self, children, partner or family member of the partner is very common. Forcing one for sex, threatening suicide if the victim leaves or threatening that the abuser will leave the victim, blaming the victim for the unhappiness of the abuser are some disgusting patterns of behaviour. Gaslighting, such as denial of any emotional abuse and justifying one's behaviour, is paradoxical.

3.4.2. Indian Scenario

There is hardly any awareness regarding emotional abuse in the general Indian population, though it is exiting in the majority of relations. There is no legal action that can be taken against emotional abuse in India.

In evaluating emotional abuse, cultural differences must be taken into consideration. General practices of interaction, human rights accepted by that country and general understanding regarding abuse are the basic things. For example, in Western culture, there is more awareness and more legal considerations about emotional abuse. However, a person from Japan or India may label many of their socially accepted behavioural patterns as being abusive. For example, in research, it was reported that a person coming from Japan may perceive the Western practice of leaving infants by themselves at night to sleep as cruel and abusive. Hence, two things make it somewhat ambiguous: the cultural impact on perception of abuse and the actual effect of abuse, which again depends on culture.

Prevention of abuse in intimate relations requires awareness in the first place to recognize it. Even in the case of children, it is difficult to identify emotional abuse. Female victims and young children keep on changing their behaviour patterns to please the abuser, especially in the family.

Emotional abuse is very common in India. In a way, it is accepted as a way to interact and control family members, like children by parents, especially in traditional families. Constant nagging, harsh criticism, controlling every activity and behaviour are general practices. Even in the case of grown-up children, parents still think that they know what is best for their child. Love and affection are conditional. In daily activities, like interacting with others, dress fashion, hairstyle, expression of emotions and everything is expected to be exactly as per parents' wish. Every important decision is obviously tightly controlled by parents. This leads to emotional abuse. In typical Indian families, the concept of privacy to be given to offspring is not acceptable to abusive parents. They keep on checking mail, WhatsApp, etc., and this generates a lot of dissatisfaction, resentment and doubt.

In some communities, extremely coercive practices are prevalent. Along with emotional abuse of various sorts, parents may threaten their own children to prevent inter-caste and inter-religion marriage. Criminal cases where parents have killed their own offspring are known as honour killing. It is worth noting that such parents have intense patronizing gestures: They advocate that as parents they have given birth to children, they can as well kill them for the honour of their family.

Understanding whether one has experienced emotionally abusive parenting helps to avoid similar behaviour with others and own children. These children can't develop trust even in adulthood and can't maintain good interpersonal relationships with others. Low self-esteem results from being subjected to constant criticizing, belittling and verbally harsh punishment. In many traditional Indian families, it is seen that such treatment leads to worthlessness, self-doubt, low self-efficacy, self-hatred and depression with poor capacity to manage emotions. Positive feelings, such as motivation, confidence, hope and pride, are hardly experienced. Even today, a number of parents think that they should never praise their own offspring, others should do that. This leads to pessimism. An ego defence mechanism like repression is used very often to hide true emotions. Due to deprivation of unconditional love, the person is oriented to approval-seeking behaviour. Excessive teasing, humiliation and mockery by parents lead to similar behavioural patterns. Ignoring one's ideas, perceptions and views makes the person feel that they are not okay. Undue comparison with siblings and highlighting negative traits may result in low self-esteem and developing sibling rivalry irrespective of age.

Pressure to achieve something irrespective of an individual's interest, constant critical evaluation, conditional love and affection create a lot of anxiety and insecurity. Abusive parents induce guilt in the minds of offspring for developing close relations with others. This, in turn, is detrimental to the social adjustment of the individual. Disclosing limitations of the individual to relatives and friends and creating a distorted image spoils social relations of the individual and the possibility of getting support diminishes.

In India especially, two roles are perceived to be related to emotional abuse: father and mother-in-law of ladies. According to the stereotypical image, the father is known for his coercive style of disciplining and the mother-in-law is known for her constant nagging and non-ending demands. Emotional abuse is very common in husband–wife relations. Irrespective of age, education and occupation, wives are generally given low status in the family. In particular, as far as decision-making is concerned, her opinion is not considered as worth consideration. Her perspective is neglected, and she is underevaluated and belittled. Practices such as over restrictions and treating her as being her owner, as if she does not have the capacity to behave properly, are very common. She is insulted, exploited, treated as a young child and controlled in every sense. Even when the wife is working and earning equal or more than the husband, he decides how every single rupee will be spent. Economic independence in its true sense is achieved by very few working women also. At least, while making major purchases, she must see to it that her money is utilized as per her convenience. A housewife has to be completely dependent on her husband for every small expenditure. Equally disturbing are the restrictions regarding interaction with any male member outside family. A wife is not supposed to expose her face to any other male in some Indian communities.

Emotional abuse may be seen in every relationship: Husband–wife, mother–child of any age, father–child of any age, sisters, brothers, in-laws or even grandparents may emotionally abuse an individual. It may take the form of bullying in peer relations, body shaming in case of disabled, too strict discipline in schools and hostels add harassment in the workplace. There is no socially accepted and legal way to get rid of it in Indian culture. Even old individuals are emotionally abused, insulted and exploited by their own sons, daughters and grand-children.

Deepak has always been jealous of his sister, who was sincere and obedient and was close to his parents. He always used to compare the facilities his parents gave her and him. Once, when she was selected for republic day pared to be held in Delhi, he was very hostile and lost his balance. He started threatening her that he would burn all her NCC dresses and other materials if she wanted to go to the camp.

There are such other true stories where the books and notebooks of siblings are destroyed just before examination to arrest their progress. A father breaking a guitar of son so that he should study well or killing a pet of his son just to control his behaviour are actually examples of extreme emotional abuse resulting in spoiling their relations forever.

Although both men and women can be the abusers, it is proved in the USA that, in 80 per cent of the cases of heterosexual abuse, men are the abusers. In the United Kingdom, it is 90 per cent. On the basis of these percentages, it is easy to guess the scenario in India. Domestic abuse is not considered as abuse and is never reported. Culturally, men are supposed to be aggressive and dominant and are expected to control family matters. Women are trained to be submissive. Abuse among couples takes place in private, and it is difficult to prove it and that the victim is not responsible for it. Having enough strength to confront the abuser or finding someone who will support the victim are the two possible ways to solve the problem.

Elliott et al. (1997) found that many individuals from Asian cultures assume that family issues are private and should not be discussed with others. In Asian culture, people are of the opinion that parents are free to choose how to rear children. In the same way, it may be found that people think that husband–wife interaction is their private issue, and no third person is supposed to interfere in it. The area that is made a target may be different in the case of every victim.

In advanced countries, workplaces have an open and respectful atmosphere with zero tolerance of abuse. Even then, more females are emotionally abused in the workplace than males. In India, emotional abuse of women has become an inherent part of the job.

Emotional abuse is difficult to prove, especially in the case of children and adolescents. Physical conflict between adults in front of a child, destruction of a child's property, degradation and humiliation, confinement and exclusion result in emotional abuse. It is a very skilful job, even to discuss it with them.

3.4.3. Measuring Emotional Abuse

If one has to measure emotional abuse objectively, one has to use a psychological test for that. By and large, a questionnaire for measuring emotional abuse in a husband and wife relationship may include the following points:

- Feeling that the victim is to be blamed for a partner's problems and problems of interaction.
- Sexual exploitation and unreasonable demands about sex.
- Abuse of alcohol and drugs which results in exploitative behaviour of the abuser and results in put downs, mockery, banter, etc.
- The abuser feels no guilt and never expresses apology for their own mistakes but justifies how others are responsible for it.
- As a victim has to ask for permission even for simple activities, they feel powerless and inferior.

3.5. STRATEGIES FOR OVERCOMING EMOTIONAL ABUSE

If the victim does not do anything to arrest it, emotional abuse increases and becomes worse. Some strategies to overcome it are as follows:

- Make the abusive partner aware of the fact that their behaviour is abusive if they are not aware of it. If the abuser is doing it intentionally, it may make no difference. However, if they are not aware of the victim's feelings and perceptions, it may reduce abuse to some extent.
- The victim has to set personal boundaries which they expect others to be aware of and behave accordingly.
- The victim must be close to their friends, family and well-wishers and share their problems with them as it will create some support.
- If not maintained properly by the abuser, the victim should be ready to leave that relationship. Gradually, they should decrease the interaction with the abuser and limit and avoid harmful relations and interaction. It becomes essential to find out the area where they are dependent on the abuser and try to be independent as soon as possible, like financial.

Many short films are available to guide regarding leaving abusive relationship. Some of these are as follows:
- 'What You Must Do to Leave an Emotionally Abusive Relationship' (Stephanie Lyn Coaching, 2018)
- 'Why I Stayed, Why I Left' (TEDx Talks, 2018)
- 'Why You Can't Leave an Abusive Relationship/Trauma Bonding' (Stephanie Lyn Coaching, 2018)
- 'How to Leave an Abusive Relationship' (Bernardo, 2018)

- Let someone else also know that they are going to leave and the relation is abusive. Close friends and family members may be informed about it.
- Victims should be calm and balanced when the abuser starts abusing them. They may leave the place or keep on doing their routine jobs without being reactive or getting upset. It is essential to train one's mind to be proactive. This reduces the sadistic pleasure the abuser gets. In some cases, this may increase abuse to initiate reactive actions of the victim. However, the victim should have more

patience and pretend that it makes no difference to them. This is the best way to protect self though the abuser may be upset and label them as emotionless.

- Instead of thinking about the abuser's comfort, the victim should think about themselves. She should be able to take care of own self. One has to find ways to maintain one's mental health and happiness.
- Overcoming the pessimistic attribution style enhances confidence to face emotional abuse and to get rid of it. Self-administered optimism training is found to be useful for reducing pessimistic attribution style.
- As no logical argument is accepted and acknowledged by the abuser, any activity like arguing logically with the abuser or losing temper should be avoided. If the victim tries to reason, it will lead to anger and frustration for them.
- When a victim becomes angry and frustrated, abuse becomes easy as they have lost their capacity to reason appropriately. Now, it is only an emotion-based conflict. It is necessary to remember that the victim need not justify one's actions and explain one's perspective. The most upsetting thing is that an abuser has nothing to do with rational thinking. Hence, there is hardly any logical explanation of the relation between how the victim behaved and how and why the abuser is angry. An abuser may argue about worthless things.
- An abuser will compel the victim to do things which are against their wish. Without consulting them, they will make every decision as per their convenience. The victim has to be assertive enough to tell them what they want to happen. This may not change their decision, but the victim's confidence and self-efficacy depends on it.

Nikita got married immediately after her graduation. It was an arranged marriage. Her mother-in-law and husband used to make every decision about her life even without considering her opinion. When she had applied for a job, there was a call for an interview. Her husband told that Nikita was not interested in any job without even informing her.

If the victim keeps quiet, her whole life will be ruined.

- An abuser never respects the victim's privacy. He will try to find out every detail of her whereabouts and phone calls, messages and wants to know everything as to what they are doing, where they are going and with whom they spend time. The victim should be firm and practice self-directed behaviour.

- Possessive behaviour of an abuser indicates that they think they are the owner of the victim. The victim should be alert and try to prove their independent existence.
- The abuser may tell lies even about small things just to make the victim awkward and confused. It is a must to keep a record of significant things with proof.
- Whenever there is abusive interaction, it is necessary to confront rather than withdraw. One should be able to have that much courage and be firm.

If appropriate emotional support and psychotherapy are made available, the human brain can recover some of the traumatic experiences. Diet, exercise and meditation are the basic recommendations to maintain good health. Training one's mind to use various relevant coping styles, maintaining a relaxed atmosphere and spending quality time with family enhance adjustment. It is essential to minimize exposure to negative thoughts and abusive people to improve mental health. Increased self-awareness and regaining sensitivity about self are also equally important.

Let us take an example of a semi-educated housewife in India. Many of these points are essentially applicable for most of them. Without any awareness, without any resistance, for generations, most of them are suffering and take it as an inherent part of married life.

Do You Know?

In a report of a national family and health survey, it is seen that 49 per cent of married ladies have justified even physical abuse in marital relations. They accept that if the wife is not capable of fulfilling all her duties properly regarding her in-laws, does not respect them, does not look after children or rejects sexual relations, he ought to beat the wife. Even today, it is perceived as a natural and inherent part of marital life. So it is obvious that emotional abuse may be justified by most of them (*Maharashtra Times*, 25 January 2019).

3.6. CONDUCIVE ENVIRONMENT, GUIDANCE AND COUNSELLING AND PSYCHO-SOCIAL AIDS

Considering the Indian scenario, it is a must to reconsider child-rearing practices and enhance the development of various skills in individuals while they grow.

The following skills and attitudes are essential for anyone to be relatively free from emotional abuse, at least as a youth. As parents are the most important agents of socialization and contribute a lot to the personality development of an individual, they should also reconsider their interactions with offspring.

The most important thing is that every individual should be able to develop and maintain enough self-respect. Right from the beginning, an individual should be taught to respect self and develop maturity while interacting with others. If parents and other significant adults respect the child as an independent human being, they will develop self-respect. If adolescents are free to decide, their opinion is considered while decision-making and are treated as a responsible person, they will be comfortable and confident. In this case, the individual will be able to combat emotional abuse.

An appropriate sense of self-acceptance, self-worth and self-efficacy, irrespective of gender, education and environmental pressures, are essential for being emotionally strong. There are certain things that no one can change in human life. For example, no one can change one's biological parents, genetic endowment, childhood experiences, permanent disability and gross appearance. If an individual unnecessarily keeps on thinking about it, a lot of psychological energy will be wasted. In addition, negative feelings, like an inferiority complex may emerge. If various opportunities are given to an individual, they may develop a sense of self-efficacy.

Growing children should be encouraged to practice assertive communication style, plan their points, and be firm and calm while confrontation.

Awareness of various options to solve the problem enhances the psychological strength of the victim. If they think that there is no choice, they keep on suffering and negative thoughts dominate their thinking.

Psychological support of family, friends, and significant adults, like teachers or colleagues, helps the victim to develop a sense of security. This enhances the motivation to fight back and get rid of abuse. Knowledge of human rights, tricks to record proof of abuse and the urge to get some help are essential to tackle the situation. Records, if properly kept, are useful as the abuse takes a more severe form.

A professional counsellor may use some of the following therapies:

1. Rational emotive behavioural therapy is the most effective therapy for victims of emotional abuse. Counselling, guidance, techniques to practice changed behaviour are used to help a victim to gain a sense of self-efficacy and psychological security. The importance of identifying and altering thought patterns which increase stress is suggested by Foret et al. (2012). According to Bandura (1997), motivating the victims to develop confidence or self-efficacy in their abilities to complete other tasks successfully helps a lot. It increases competence and decreases generalization of negative attributes.

2. Empathy and unconditional acceptance are the most effective ways to help the victim of emotional abuse. Cochran et al. (2010) have remarked that focusing on empathy and acceptance works very well while helping emotionally abused children. While working with abusers, different cultural images of ideal parenting or an ideal husband may be discussed.

3. Modular cognitive behaviour therapy is useful to help a victim experiencing anxiety. It has 4 stages as given by Chorpita et al. (2004). It includes ranking of fears, psycho education on anxiety, imagining exposure to fears and skill maintenance methods. It is found to be very effective with adolescents and young adults.

4. Relaxation response method is used to manage physiological effects of distress which are generated due to abuse (Benson, 2000). It significantly decreases heart rate, breathing rate, blood pressure and metabolic rate and calms down the systems. It requires an attitude of self-acceptance, being kind to self and focus. Something

like focusing on an external object or using a phrase repeatedly helps. Techniques, such as progressive muscle relaxation and mindfulness meditative exercises, are generally practised for that.

5. Creating a safe environment for both the victim and the abuser by limit setting and structuring helps a lot. Instead of evaluating and criticizing, the abuser, like a parent or partner, should accept and acknowledge the positive side of the personality of the victim (Ginsberg, 2002).

3.7. SUMMARY

Emotional abuse is a hidden abuse which is equally detrimental to the psycho-social health of the victim as physical abuse. As there are cultural variations in expected and accepted ways of interactions with each other, emotional abuse is also perceived in different ways. In India, it is perceived as inherent in close relations, such as husband–wife and parent–child.

Emotional abuse is insulting, belittling, underestimating and taking the individual for granted. Abusing an individual verbally, visually, using non-verbal communication, scolding and completely dehumanizing the individual lead to harmful psychological effects on the victim.

Increasing awareness and giving training to face the situation with the help of various social skills are essential to enhance confidence, self-worth and self-efficacy of the victim.

Aggression and Violence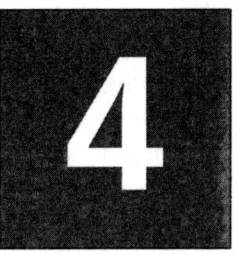

4.1. INTRODUCTION, NATURE, TYPES AND SIGNIFICANCE

According to the WHO (2020), youth violence is a global public health problem. It can range from bullying to physical fighting or more severe sexual and physical assault to homicide. About 200,000 homicides are reported every year, specifically among youth all over the world. Homicide among youth is the fourth leading cause of death in that age group. In a recent research in 40 developing countries, it was found that 42 per cent of males and 37 per cent of females suffer due to bullying. Youth violence has a serious lifelong impact on the psychological, social and physical functioning of the whole generation.

In Buland city, Uttar Pradesh, a 6-year-old girl was killed by her 20-year-old brother because his food fell down due to her negligence. He was extremely angry and lost his mental balance. He punched her continuously till she died (*Maharashtra Times*, June 30 2020). In a two-year survey of five Indian cities, it was found that 80 per cent of Indian youth from the age range of 15–26 are angry and aggressive. According to the National Institute of Mental Health and Neurosciences, the highest percentage is seen in Jammu, which is 92 per cent. The percentage of girls engaged in verbal aggression is higher. Longitudinal studies have proved that physical punishment given to children leads to aggressive behaviour in adolescence and youth (*Bangalore Mirror*, 2 January 2014).

There is a clear link between anger, aggression and violence. It does not mean that anger always leads to aggression, and every aggression leads to violence. People may be aggressive without feeling angry. However, the probability increases. Anger is generated when an individual perceives that there is an injustice, and they can't control it. A wish to hurt someone or self-defence may also generate it. Anger is experienced when an individual feels that they can still influence the situation or cope with it. Anger is related to one's psychological interpretation of having been offended, wronged or denied, and there is a tendency to react through retaliation. Provocation and antagonism are related to it. In 'anger out,' the expressed anger is oriented toward others, and in 'anger in', it is turned inside an individual. Aggressive anger leads to forceful fast action to harm others. Low frustration tolerance is the basic reason behind it. Expression of aggressive anger is abusive, reckless, destructive and harmful. It not only destroys things but interpersonal relations also. In such cases, youth become selfish, do not listen to others, do not consider others' needs and emotions, and are involved in threatening and hurting others physically. Road rage, abuse, even murder and rape are examples of expressions of aggressive anger.

> Naaz is a 20-year-old married lady who stays with her husband and in-laws. Her husband is short-tempered and always wants Naaz to obey each and everything that he tells her to do. Once, she wanted to go to her parents as her father was not well. Her husband became furious and slapped her hard when she asked for permission. Immediately, her ear started bleeding and she fainted. She was admitted to hospital and lost her hearing capacity in that ear forever.

An overwhelming increase in aggression and violence among adolescents and youth has been reported during the last few decades. All over the world, violent crimes are at their maximum during late teenage. It affects the whole society in terms of psychological, social, economic and political problems. Whole socialization, impact of family and peers, personality and self-concept of an individual are the decisive factors. It is not only related to criminal justice but has become an issue related to the psychological health of the whole society. Aggression and violence are fertile fields of research as different disciplines are interested in focusing on the causes and consequences of aggression and violence. Psychology, psychiatry, sociology, law, forensic science, social work, politics and anthropology are some prominent disciplines.

Although there is no title as 'aggressive behaviour' to indicate a disorder in worldwide accepted classification system of abnormal behaviour, there is a mention of intermittent explosive disorder. This is linked to aggression and violence. Aggression can be a sign of hidden mental health disorder, substance use disorders or some physiological problem. Although aggression may result in physical attack, it may be due to defensive or impulsive intentions and sometimes may not be oriented to hurting others. Even violence may be reactive, impulsive, defensive or predatory. The root cause may be environmental distress, psychological problems or biases and prejudices. It may be directed to an individual, a group or even a complete community. Aggression may include physical assaults, verbal threats, tantrum, hostility and property destruction.

A famous movie *My Wife's Murder* is an excellent example of anger outburst and its impact. A man who was extremely angry hits his wife and due to head injury she dies. It is said to be based on a true story. There was no intention to kill. It is impulsive aggression. Similar true stories are reported every day, like on 22 January 2021 in Gualher, Madhya Pradesh, an alcohol addict was so aggressive that he beat his wife who was carrying for 7 months with iron rod. The young lady died in this attack.[1]

The scientific definition of aggression is 'behaviour that is intended to harm someone who is motivated to avoid that harm.' Aggression is observable. Negative feelings and aggressive affect plays a role only as a prerequisite. It has to be intentional. If, in a great hurry, someone hurts an unknown individual while carrying a huge bag, it is not aggression. Aggression must have a clear goal of hurting others. If a laboratory technician pricks a needle in the patient's body to collect blood sample, it can't be labelled as aggression. On the contrary, even if an individual misses an attempt to kill someone, it is labelled as aggression. It means that harm which is for the benefit of the sufferer is not aggression. Actual intention is to be considered. One more obvious thing is that aggression is against a living being. If someone bangs a door, throws a mobile or kicks a pillow, it is not a significant aggression. Finally, the victim should try to and should be motivated to avoid the attack. There are conditions where that pain is welcomed by an individual. Masochism is such a condition that a person achieves sexual pleasure out of pain. In this case, it is not aggression.

[1] https://navbharattimes.indiatimes.com

Three types of aggression are hostile aggression inflicting harm on someone; reactive aggression is a reaction to something or some unpleasant stimulus, and instrumental aggression is related to a specific goal. In sports and games, instrumental aggression is very common (Gaiger, 2016). Reactive aggression is a defensive response to a threat. Instrumental aggression is mostly about getting money, power and control. It results from inadequate social control exerted by the prefrontal cortex.

Violence is considered independent of aggression, but it is a controversial matter. Most experts consider violence as an extreme form of aggression, leading to serious physical damage or the death of a victim. Here again, attempt is considered as violence. Like an attempt to murder is a crime. Hence, it is a difference in degree. On a continuum, one can place anger, aggression and violence at different points depending on severity or degree. Violence is defined by the WHO as the intentional use of physical force or power against self, someone else or against a group or community resulting in psychological harm, deprivation, injury or death. All over the world, millions of people are killed due to violence. Even more are the people who are hospitalized, undergo emergency treatments and suffer for the whole of their lives. The physical, social, psychological and economic ill effects of violence are severe.

There are different categories of violence. It can be self-directed, interpersonal and collective. It can be physical, psychological or sexual. It can be instrumental or reactive and hostile. In interpersonal, family, especially partners, and community are included. Collective violence is social, political and economic. Self-directed violence is regarding self-abuse and suicide attempts. Parasuicide is suicidal thoughts or attempts of suicide and self-mutilation. Interpersonal violence includes physical, emotional and sexual violence, child abuse and abusing elderly individuals. Emotional and physical exploitation of children and teenagers, ill treatment by significant adults and neglect may also be included in it. It may spoil the relationship forever, affecting trust and health: psychological and physiological. Community violence is also interpersonal, which takes place outside the family where the victims are not known. It takes the form of random violence. For example, near railway station, a gang of youths from the slum are generally seen throwing stones at the train that is passing by. The stones injure those who are standing near the door and sitting near open windows. The gang enjoys the situation and counts the number of hits of every member. They are completely unaware of who is getting hurt.

Collective violence is economic violence and structural violence. It depicts the motives of a group or groups. There is a social agenda like casteism, terrorism, and mob violence. Political violence is between two countries or states, and many individuals and groups are involved in it. Some violence is carried out only for economic gain.

Galtung's triangle is an illustration of three types of violence. The first is direct violence, and the second is structural violence, which is invisible, like discrimination, inherent in the structure of society. The third is cultural violence, which is included in the culture and religion of any society. Both justify and support a particular type of violence in a given society (The Peacebuilding Practitioner, 2018). There are overlapping and mixed types of violence. There is non-physical violence which may be in the form of threats, neglect, omission, intimidation, character assassination, insults and indirectly causing loss of opportunity for a specific individual. It can be hidden or latent; however, its effects are seen for years, and it may change one's life to a substantial extent.

Aggression emerges from childhood. There are neurological and psychological diseases and problems associated with it.

Both men and women are equally angry. The difference is in what they do when they are angry. Boys and males get involved in physical fights. Worldwide, it is proven that most violent crimes are committed by boys and men. Much violence takes place between known people and spouses.[2]

Aggression and violence among youths are very commonly seen as fighting, hitting, reckless driving, road rage, truancy and even rape and attempt to murder. Indian researchers have found that approximately 17 per cent of individuals between 16 and 19 years of age more

[2] https://pubmed.ncbi.nlm.nih.gov.2018

frequently experience aggression. Male members were more aggressive than females. They perceive work pressure, alcohol abuse, violent activities, violence in the family and media violence as associated with it. About 34 per cent reported that they were involved in fights, 20 per cent physical violence, 12 per cent used weapons in aggression, and 13 per cent stated that they were injured. It is worth noting that 37 per cent were injured physically or emotionally by parents. Kashmir also has high rates of violence.

There are different types of aggression seen among youth. Some more are as follows. A few of them are somewhat overlapping.

1. **Verbal aggression:** It is a very harsh and abusive language with scary and threatening non-verbal communication. It is a reactive interaction with life partners, siblings, peers, parents, teachers, neighbours or even unknown persons. It is so common in India, for example, in parent–child and husband–wife relations, that it is a socially accepted interaction pattern.
2. **Physical aggression:** Physical aggression includes bullying, hitting, throwing, fighting, kicking, pushing, biting or any harm to the opponent. Mostly, it is seen while interacting with a life partner, siblings, peers or younger children. Generally, illiterate or semi-literate parents and husbands use it to control others' behaviour. This is also known as overt aggression.
3. **Aggression against animals:** When there is a lot of suppressed anger and no other outlet, adolescents and youth direct their physical aggression against animals, such as cats and dogs. Animals are soft targets, and they can't understand the cruel intentions behind human acts. Recently, two elephants were killed. A pregnant female was killed by a coconut bomb in Kerala.[3] In Tamil Nadu, a wild elephant was killed by a burning tyre attack.[4] Many videos depicting it are available on YouTube. Aggression against objects: throwing, kicking, tearing, misusing objects if they are used to hurt someone.

[3] indian express.com>india 6 June 2020

[4] www.news 18.com>india 23 January 2021

4. **Covert aggression:** It includes vandalism and stealing.
5. **Direct and indirect:** Direct is open and face-to-face, like being rude and arrogant or unresponsive. Indirect is when the victim is not physically present. The simplest example is gossiping or instigating someone against another person.
6. **Emotional aggression:** It is expressed in a desperate manner.
7. **Hostile aggression:** It is emotionally driven and produced by anger. It is impulsive and labelled as hot. It may result from provocation.
8. **Premeditated aggression:** It is deliberate and planned aggression.
9. **Aggression and violence towards self and towards others:** To self is drug abuse, addiction, free sex and suicide attempts. Aggression towards others includes parents, siblings, partners, friends, strangers, animals and property. It is in the form of something like homicide, rape or robbery.
10. **Accidental aggression:** It results from carelessness, and it is not intentional.
11. **Expressive aggression:** It is just an expression of aggression without any intention of harming others.
12. **Passive aggression:** It is not physically violent. It can take the form of obscured criticism of others' actions, where an individual becomes argumentative, critical of authority, complains about being underevaluated and misunderstood and resists subordination.

Some researchers have given two basic types: emotional and goal-directed. Emotional is related to hostile and reactive tendencies. Here, for example, an individual may be interested in taking revenge for their insult. The other is goal-directed aggression, like destroying public property. Sometimes, the motives are mixed. One more type is relational aggression, like covert bullying or social manipulation. Direct and indirect, intentional or unintentional, emotion based or related to mental status, social or non-social are some more types. The aggression taxonomy is given by Krahe (2013). The aggression taxonomy by Parrott and Giancola (2007) is also considered an elaborate work. In those aspects and sub-types are considered, like if response modality is considered, sub-types are physical, verbal, postural and relational.

Immediacy is indirect and direct. Visibility is also discussed as overt and covert. Response quality is of two types: action and no action. Instigation is as proactive and reactive. According to him, goal direction is either holistic or instrumental. Two types of harm—physical and psychological—and two types of duration—transient and lasting—are discussed. It considers individuals and groups as social units.

Early signs are uncontrolled anger, prejudices against particular individual, caste, religion or community. That, in turn, results in intolerance of differences in values, lifestyles and the like. Feelings of rejection and being isolated leads to social withdrawal. Sometimes, expression of violence is seen in drawing and writing. The sequence of hostile behaviour and severe rage due to minor reasons are also reported. Perceived injustice and perceived threat lead to low self-esteem and anxiety which generates anger. Frustration and humiliation are associated with feeling of insecurity resulting in aggression and violence. Even a single incidence of violence may change whole life of the victim and aggressor as well.

4.2. CORRELATES OF ANGER, AGGRESSION AND VIOLENCE

There are various causes and correlates of aggression and violence. They belong to the social, psychological, physiological, academic and economic spheres of life.

Low socio-economic strata, a traumatic environment and the company of criminals increase acceptance of aggression and violence. Cultural differences in the acceptability of aggression are well documented. High population density and low availability of resources lead to more aggression and violence. Motivation means an immediate trigger for aggression. Frustration is a common motivation for aggression. Frustration, in turn, may have some deep-rooted causes. These causes may be interpersonal, intrapersonal or environmental. Physical, mental, emotional distress, injustice, insecurity, insults, fear, rejection, neglect and disorientation are reported to be the basic reasons. Inappropriate and inconsistent discipline of parents, childhood abuse and wrong role models also result in the same. Many clinical problems regarding mental health are related to aggression and violence. Narcissistic, antisocial or borderline personality disorders combined with a breakdown in coping skills result in violence. Post-traumatic stress disorder, bipolar disorder, drug and alcohol abuse can contribute to both aggression and violence. Loneliness, mood disorder, disturbed sleep, irrational fear, anxiety, suspicion and sexual abuse were found to be the most common reasons.

Predictors of adolescents' aggression are reported to be hyperac-tivity, academic failure, delinquent peer group and the availability of drugs. It is reported in various countries that drug addiction is significantly associated to conflicts, injuries and even murders. Low anger control, poor quality of life, history of expression and experi-ence of aggression are well documented. Antisocial personality traits, depression, impulsiveness, attention problems and low intelligence are also found to be associated with aggression and violence. Sibling bullying may lead to depression and self-harm or rebellious attitudes.

Theories of violence can be broadly divided into two types. The first type is violence as instinct and violence as related to human nature, including psychobiological and temperamental vulnerabilities. The second type considers violence as the consequence of a damaged psyche.

Detailed classification gives the following five types:

1. **Cognitive neoassociation theory:** Aversive events produce nega-tive affect. This results in thoughts and responses and stimulates memories related to anger and fear. Emotional responses are trig-gered by cues and availability, like guns.
2. **Social learning theory:** Observational learning during socializa-tion leads to negative patterns of behaviour. If a father screams loudly and slaps his son, the son, in adulthood, may do the same with his son.
3. **Script theory:** Already existing, well-learned concepts which have causal links, goals and action plans guide individuals' behaviour. A specific role is selected and behaviour is linked to it accordingly.
4. **Excitation transfer theory:** Physiological arousal generated by one event is transferred to the next event occurring shortly.

5. **Social interaction theory:** Aggression is a result of social inter-action oriented towards higher-level goals. Expected rewards, costs and possible outcomes in a given culture decide the degree of aggression. It is sometimes oriented towards protecting social identity or producing compliance.

Three theories are basic: instinct theory, frustration aggression hypothesis and social learning theory. Sigmund Freud's psychoanalytic theory says aggression is a human instinct related to dread of death. The death instinct is oriented towards self-destruction. Its displacement results in aggression against others. Miller and Dollard mentioned that frustration results from events blocking a particular goal-directed behaviour. Self-esteem is threatened. Frustration of strong desires leads to aggression, according to this theory. Further, it is linked to the displacement of aggression. If an individual can't express their anger and aggression in a particular way, they will try to give it an outlet in some other way. For example, a youth who can't retaliate in front of their boss may become very aggressive and scream loudly while interacting with their mother. Bandura's theory of social learning explains aggression as acquired or learned. If aggressiveness prevails in the environment, an individual may have a readymade idea regarding how to behave in a given situation. Hence, it is the impact of parents, siblings, relatives, friends, neighbours and even teachers.

Frustration aggression theory says that all aggression is caused by frustration. When a goal is blocked, frustration results, which causes aggression. Aggression achieves catharsis. If aggression is punished, it may lead to more aggression due to a lack of catharsis. The culture of violence theory is related to the pervasiveness of violent behaviour. Structural violence is a systematic violence taught by culture and society.[5]

There are some overlapping ideas in some theories. Moral reasoning theory mentions that respect comes from fear. If there is no fear, there will be more aggression (Dalton Production, 2014; HarvardX, 2017). Different models of aggression are given by experts to explain the causes,

---

[5] violence ppt: http://www.slideshare.net

relations and contributions of various factors in aggression. Individuals with developmental disabilities and those who are lagging behind in terms of developmental tasks are aggressive. Inappropriate outlets for emotional problems may lead to frustration. Psychological problems leading to mental health issues may generate aggressive tendencies.

The genetic theory gives an example of 47 chromosomes XYY syndrome as the cause of aggressive tendencies. Genetic endowment plays a decisive role in aggressive tendencies. Now, two genes related to violent crime have been identified. The same genes are related to attention deficit hyperactive disorder and drug abuse. A meta-analysis of many studies concluded that 40 per cent of variation among individuals regarding aggression can be explained on the basis of genes. The remaining 60 per cent can be related to environmental influences.

The evolutionary biological view depicts aggression as useful for survival and reproduction. Physiological and biochemical determinants have attracted the attention of researchers for more than a century. Substantial research is available that gives detailed cause and effect relations between these factors and aggression or violence. Most studies have found that testosterone is associated with aggressive tendencies, criminality and antisocial behaviour. The pituitary gland influences testosterone levels. Not only in human beings but in other species also, males are more aggressive than females. The reports regarding crimes show that more males are involved in crimes, especially violent crimes. When the level of testosterone increases during teenage, the involvement of male members in aggression, violence and crime also increases. In 2014, Indian researchers Sharma and Marimuthu (2014) reported that male youths have high aggression scores; they experience more aggression and anger in their late teenage. Physical abuse in childhood, substance abuse, family violence, academic failure and the impact of the mass media are the risk factors. Some disorders, such as attention deficit hyperactivity disorder, mood disturbances and loneliness, may result in aggression.

As excess testosterone leads to anger and aggression in males, premenstrual hormonal disturbances in females also lead to irritation, anger, aggression and anxiety, as well as mood swings. The hormone called glucocorticoid plays an important role in aggression. Abnormalities in the serotonin system, catecholamine system and hypothalamic pituitary adrenal axis are associated with aggression. The low level of serotonin is associated with crime. As far as physiological correlates of aggression are concerned, it is reported that consumption of alcohol, amphetamine and cocaine leads to aggression.

Cognitive abilities are affected. The ability to process information and to exert cognitive control over one's behaviour deteriorates. Objectivity, empathy, prudence and thoughtfulness decrease. In this situation, stereotypes become prominent. Such neurochemical changes that are changes in neurotransmitters due to extreme anger are detrimental to an individual's health. It results in diseases like ulcers or cancer.

Anger not only hurts others but hurts the individual themselves, who is angry. The immediate effects of anger are increased heart rate, increased blood pressure, perspiration and increased testosterone. The need for oxygen increases, which leads to tightening of the chest. More release of glucose stored in the liver and muscles is reported due to it. Blood rushes to the brain and limbs. It results in headaches, acidity, abdominal pain, skin problems such as eczema, anxiety and depression. It may lead to cognitive problems such as distorted perception and thinking problems. Lesions of the orbitofrontal cortex are related to anger. In the long run, it may affect the physical and psychological health of an individual. Serotonin levels decrease, which leads to decreased happiness. An elevated level of cortisol causes damage to neurons in the prefrontal cortex. Mirror neurons produce the same effect when an individual watches anger in others. Stress may negatively affect neurons in the hippocampus. As anger starts with the amygdala, it stimulates the hypothalamus and pituitary gland due to which adrenaline and cortisone are released. Blood glucose increases. It negatively affects one's immune system. There are examples of even more severe problems, such as high blood pressure, stomach ulcers and heart diseases. Some cases of heart attacks are also recorded.[6]

The role of biology in violence is very complicated. No research on terrorism is available as it is difficult to get relevant data. The amygdala plays an important role in processing emotions and is related to violence as well. About an 18 per cent reduction in the amygdala is reported among violent individuals. Positron

[6] https://www.nicabm.com/how-anger-affects-the-brain-and-body-infographic/; http://www.psychguides.com

emission tomography studies show that frontal lobe functioning is poor in the case of these individuals. Even if it is intact, the prefrontal cortex is less active. Suppressing emotional expressions is difficult for them. Decisions are not properly made, like, for example, they are involved in gambling. One more significant finding is that low resting heart rate is found in violent individuals. Longitudinal studies show that lack of fear of punishment among children is related to violence after many years. An enriched environment may reduce violent behaviour by 35 per cent. It includes more cognitive stimulation, more physical exercise and better nutrition (University of Pennsylvania, 2014).

Studies of twins also show the contribution of heredity to violence. There are examples of adopted children reared in a conducive environment showing that their biological parents' impact is seen as they are genetically predisposed to violence (CBS News, 2013).

Do You Know the Effects of Childhood Abuse?

The prefrontal cortex controls aggression. Lesions in a part of the brain called orbitofrontal cortex of the human brain are reported to be a cause of reactive aggression. Reduced response inhibition is found in violent people. Abusive treatment in childhood affects the development of brain regions, like the amygdale, which, in turn, influences the behaviour of an individual, even in youth. Battered baby syndrome is a condition where the child's whole body is shaken with a lot of anger and aggression. Due to it, their brains are also shaken and shunting to and fro in the skull. As a consequence, the prefrontal cortex is damaged, which, in turn, results in neurocriminology, which is directly associated with aggression and violence in young adulthood.

Hence, if the prefrontal cortex is injured, it results in aggression, violence and antisocial behaviour. Antisocial personality disorder is found to be associated with an 11 per cent or more reduction in grey matter of the prefrontal lobe. Research regarding killers has proved that they have a highly activated brain but a lack of activation in the prefrontal cortex. So they become extremely aggressive.

Impulsiveness, low intelligence and low academic achievement are associated with deficiencies in the executive functions of the frontal lobe, such as self-monitoring, self-awareness and self-management, especially of impulsive behaviour. Sustaining attention and concentration, planning, abstract reasoning and concept formation are adversely affected by it.

Emotional causes are also proved in different research studies. Distress, disorientation, emotional hurt, neglect, insecurity, fear, insults and perceived injustice are predominant causes of aggression. Unpleasant childhood experiences, neglect by parents, frustration and tendencies to overcompensate for feelings of inferiority are also reported to result in aggressive tendencies. The causes are deeper in one's psyche, and one may or may not be completely aware of that. Among other causes of aggression are frustration of social goals, such as dominance, social rejection, provocation by abuse and environmental problems such as pollution, overcrowding, extreme climatic conditions and heightened physical arousal. So unpleasant experiences—physical, social and psychological—may trigger aggression.

Impulse control disorder, as mentioned in the *Diagnostic and Statistical Manual of Mental* Disorders, indicates extreme expression of anger which is uncontrollable and disproportionate to the cause. Even under conduct disorder, there are destructive behaviour, physical and verbal aggression and cruel behaviour towards human beings and animals. Alcohol intoxication, antisocial personality disorder, borderline personality disorder, intermittent explosive disorder, psychosis, attention deficit hyperactivity disorder, phencyclidine and taking mind-altering drugs are found to be associated with aggression and violence.

The mass media has proved to be one of the major correlates of aggression among adolescents and youth. Most of the research about mass media—that is, 80 per cent—is regarding aggressive tendencies among viewers. As per social learning theory and observational learning, a huge amount of aggression and violence depicted in the mass media are imitated by growing individuals. As it is shown as the easiest way to solve real-life problems, aggression and violence depicted become very effective. No unpleasant consequences of aggression and violence are ever shown in programmes on mass media. Television programmes depict a lot of violence and aggression in various ways. Programmes related to crimes, various violence-based movies and even the news contain violent actions. There is substantial aggression and violence in cartoons also. Most research indicates that there is a significant correlation between watching violence on television and violent behaviour. However, it is a controversial issue. Those who are aggressive and violent prefer to watch violent television programmes. So both depend on each other.

A very famous English movie, *The Burning Bed*, depicted a story of the abuse of a wife. It is based on a true story. After years of domestic abuse, the lady set fire to the bed of her husband. (Beautybythelady, 1984).[7] After release of the film, there were many cases of killing one's partner in the same way. There are examples of observational learning when an individual imitates the style of hurting others exactly as shown on a television programme. Playing violent video games has also proven to be related to aggression, youth violence and bullying. Violent videos and games are reported to be more detrimental as the individual is actively participating, interacting and getting awards. This leads to more involvement and aggression in the case of cognitive affective and behavioural domains.

4.2.1. Culture

The ideal image of an Indian male with reference to religion, history, politics and culture is that he is supposed to be aggressive and violent as and when necessary. If the intention behind aggression is not considered, most ideal males are very aggressive. Either they are war heroes, freedom fighters, rescuers, leaders and so on. Even in a day-to-day situation, most Indian males are substantially aggressive. They are expected to be loud, have patronizing gestures, be capable of threatening anyone who troubles young ones, girls and women in the family and so on A typical traditional family sanctions male youths for having temper tantrums, shouting and kicking and being physically and verbally aggressive. This is the way in which he is perceived to be able to protect his family and control the behaviour of family members. If aggression and violence are accepted as the best ways to solve problems in a particular culture and community, then the tendency to be violent increases. Culture of violence theory explains a particular type of violence in a specific society. It is about sanctioning violence in

[7] http://en.m.wikipedia.org

the culture of a society. Such violence is legitimized. Cultures encourage and sanction aggressive and violent acts in response to a specific situation. It is reflected in the mass media.

Sociologists have given the concept of rape culture. If in a community, rape is common, it may be due to the normalization of the general attitude of society about women. Any woman, irrespective of her age, education, socio-economic status, looks and lifestyle, can be raped. Any man can rape women, though he may not be a mental patient. Rape culture outright denies the harm done to the victim by rape. Instead of blaming the aggressor, the victim is blamed. It is interpreted as her fault. The interpretation is that she has invited rape. She deserves the same. In a country like India, many rapes are not even reported. Rape myths and victim blaming are two examples of cultural support for violence. In India, dowry deaths, honour killings, female genital mutilation, battered women and domestic terrorism are accepted by some societies and are even perceived in a dignified way and reinforced.

In brief, men are more aggressive than women for not only physiological but also psychological and social reasons. Men are more involved in physical aggression. Gender differences in verbal aggression depend on cultural expectations. Women explain their aggression in terms of excessive distress and loss of self-control. Male members think that if someone challenges their self-esteem and integrity, they become aggressive to enhance control over the opponents. Men perceive that aggression is a positive and goal-directed act. Women feel concern and guilt regarding their aggressive behaviour. Adolescent girls are more involved in indirect social aggression, such as spreading rumours, gossiping, making fun of others and ignoring them.

Narcissism, psychopathology and Machiavellianism are all related to aggression. Machiavellianism is a personality trait where an individual manipulates, deceives and exploits others for their own interest. Hostile cognitive biases accompany that. Hostile attribution bias means a tendency to perceive any ambiguous action of others as hostile. Hostile perception bias is the perception of general social interaction as being aggressive. Hostile expectation bias is a tendency to expect others to react aggressively to expected or potential conflicts.

4.3. VIOLENCE INSIDE AND OUTSIDE FAMILY: FAMILY VIOLENCE, EVE-TEASING, RAGGING AND CYBERBULLYING

In New Delhi, Suraj, an alcohol addict, age 26, killed his mother because she did not serve him dinner. She was shot dead as she disapproved of his heavy alcohol consumption (*Maharashtra Times*, 2020).

The agents of aggression and violence against women in the family are religious leaders, the media, discriminatory legislation, myths and economic dependency. In family violence in India, the basic causes are son preference, unequal resource distribution, unfair division of power and authority and unequal decision-making power. This precipitates cognitive, emotional, economic and social dependence among women due to which it is easy to harass and exploit them in every sense.

Domestic violence can take place in case of anyone, irrespective of age, education, gender and socio-economic status. Just to gain power and control, dominate and teach a lesson to their wife, mother or sister, a lot of aggression and violence is used by male members. Less education, repeated strong impulses regarding aggression or experience of violence as a victim, the prevalence of violence in the family seen in early childhood and the attitude and acceptance of discord and violence in community and culture are the predictors and correlates. Because of low self-esteem, uncontrolled anger, jealousy, feelings of inferiority and undue superiority feelings, such aggression and violence take place. If a husband has multiple partners and antisocial personality disorder or if he has doubts about infidelity of his wife, aggression and violence become a regular practice. Intimate partner abuse and marital rape are very common in developing countries. Sexual violence leads to serious ill effects. Marital rape is an extremely common way of expressing anger and taking revenge, as the wife is not supposed to even tell anyone due to social pressure. It leads to physical, sexual and psychological harm. It includes psychological abuse, physical aggression and unpleasant discourse to control partners' behaviour. In contemporary society, using WhatsApp, Facebook and similar other facilities on smartphones is becoming a matter of discord and dispute among intimate partners. It generates a lack of trust and security and increases hostility.

Since 1983, domestic violence has been legally treated as a criminal offence and laws like Section 498A protect women from domestic violence if they seek any legal help. It is widely accepted that it is the right of a male to be physically aggressive and violent, and a female has to bear it; otherwise, he will disown her. Other types of family violence are verbal and physical punishment given by parents to children and adolescents, harassment of daughter-in-laws by mother-in-laws, general deprivation such as food deprivation, excess physical effort and demands for dowry. There are cases where extreme aggression and violence are used as a weapon against a young lady so that complete subjugation is achieved. The ill effects of such repeated aggression and violence are traumatic and may spoil the whole life of the young lady.

More girls and women are sexually abused than boys and men. Boys are physically abused and emotionally neglected. Both types of abuse are seen more in poor socio-economic status. All over the world, approximately 50 per cent of the population has experienced family violence. Eve-teasing is very prevalent in India. It is harassing girls and women just for fun or enjoying the power available to male members over females. It includes sexual harassment that is openly done in public. They are touched indecently, grabbed, catcalled and abused in every sense in every crowded area. Molestation results in awkwardness, agony, shame and the feeling of being victimized among women and girls. The harasser gets sadistic pleasure and a sense of being powerful and strong. He wants to seek attention, talk to girls and prove his superiority as a male. Group eve-teasing, using too abusive language and even tearing clothes of ladies on the road are reported. Preparing videos of such harassment and making them viral is also becoming a very common trick to harass women. Calling a young lady on the phone again and again, though she is not interested and sending vulgar messages are new ways of harassing a lady. According to the National Crime Records Bureau in India, one girl is raped every six hours. Women who are forced to practice prostitution experience violence even when they are carrying.

One more very severe crime against women is acid attacks. In this case, the lady suffers very badly. Unbearable pain, long-term disabilities and costly treatment are an inherent part of it. Psychological effects are poor self-image, depression, anxiety, helplessness, hopelessness and self-hatred with self-rejection. Loneliness, awkwardness and suicide ideation follow. This leads to difficulties in getting married or continuing marital relations if they are already married.

Crime Petrol 'Acid Attack' (6 July 2013) depicts a devastating true story of a young lady who suffered due to an acid attack. As she was not interested in him, her own classmate threw acid on her face. She lost her vision completely and the hearing capacity of one ear. She had to undergo many surgeries. Laxmi Agarwal was hardly 16 years old when a known middle-aged man who wanted to exploit her sexually threw acid on her face in Khan market, New Delhi. (Trending 91, 2019). It was an extremely traumatic experience.

India Today's data intelligence unit has reported that, from 2014 to 2018, there were 1,483 cases of acid attacks in India. This does not reflect factual information as half of the attacks are never reported. The approximate incidence is 1,000 per year, according to some experts. Acid attack Wikipedia mentions that the intention is to torture, disfigure, maim or kill. The face of a young lady is targeted. It results in traumatic pain and agony. Not only the skin but even muscles, bones or eyes are permanently damaged. It may cause permanent blindness and deafness. It leads to ugliness and social stigma. Generally, sulphuric or nitric acids are used. It leads to not only physical but also social, psychological and economic difficulties. A substantial increase is seen in India every year. Although the incidence in other countries like the UK is more in cases where men are victims, in India, it has been more for women.

The seven crimes included under the Indian Penal Code are rape, kidnapping and abduction, dowry, torture, molestation, sexual harassment and importation.

Youth violence is violence by and against youth. Cyberbullying is the misuse of electronic media facilities to attack a victim. It is indirect psycho-social aggression. The most common types are sending unwanted sex-related messages, blackmailing and threatening, uploading true or fake videos.

In a study of 40 developing countries, it was found that 42 per cent of boys and 37 per cent of girls were exposed to bullying. According to a recent estimate, a million teenagers are harassed, threatened or have experienced some type of cyberbullying in one year in developed countries. Approximately 95 per cent of young users face problems like cruelty. Cyber harassers generally have some mental disorder. A victim, if they have poor self-concept and are emotionally and cognitively dependent, will not be able to tolerate it and, due to lack of proactivity, may suffer more.

It is through social media that a victim is trolled, made fun of, their privacy is violated and is harassed in different ways as character assassination. The harasser can easily hide their identity and remain anonymous. The root cause is aggression and deep-rooted jealousy. It is repeated behaviour with the intention of causing harm. Sometimes, a group of harassers join hands to do it. It is sending or posting harmful material to hurt the victim. Such harassment may include spreading rumours, posting sexual remarks, threats, defamation and posting photographs and personal information of the victim. For example, giving a photograph and phone number of a young lady and creating a fake impression that she is available for sexual pleasure. That is severely humiliating as people start calling with sexually explicit intentions. Cyberstalking is also a type of bullying where communication through electronic media is used. It is even more harmful. A troll is an intentional act of provoking or offending an individual. The intensity of all these varies. This leads to serious psychological effects on the victim. Generally, the young lady becomes emotionally upset, ashamed, frightened, guilty, anxious, frustrated and depressed. Bullying also results in loneliness, eating disorders, and more susceptibility to illness due to constant stress. It is a social stigma as all the peers and friends get that information and the victim starts seriously thinking about suicide. There is no other way to get rid of all these things, according to her. Cyberbullying is very common among teenage boys and youth. Legal procedures are also very efficient for immediately identifying the harasser, though they may be operating an account under a fake name. If a group is involved in bullying, it is called mobbing. It is worth noting that even a lady can play all these tricks against another lady. It is found even at an earlier age, like during 8/10 years in advanced countries.

It is reported in a recent survey that cyberbullying of Indian women and teenagers increased by 36 per cent in one year, while conviction rates decreased by 15 per cent.[8] Half of the victims do not report it to anyone. Everyone should know legal provisions and one's rights.

In the famous popular film *Munna Bhai MBBS* (2003), it is very effectively shown how ragging is a general practice even in medical

---

[8] www.indiaSpend.com/no jobs in villages 19/10/2020

colleges. It is humiliating, threatening and leads to stress and frustration. Most of the time, it is overwhelming physical and psychological torture. It violates the human rights and dignity of juniors. There are incidences of severe injuries and deaths as well as suicides due to ragging. The lives of such victims are shattered by it. They fall prey to mental diseases, feel helpless and hopeless. Most of the victims are depressed and sad. They experience a lot of agony and rage and can't even express it.

Around 75 per cent of the increase in ragging cases are reported in higher education in India (DH News Service, 2018). Reports like '5 cases of ragging in India that shocked the world'[9] are eye-opening. On YouTube, there are more than 25 short films showing actual shootings of ragging and regarding awareness building about ragging. The sadistic tendencies of the aggressors are gratified, and they get a sense of mastery. They think it's their turn now to harass juniors. The sense of superiority without making any effort can be achieved. About 41.5 per cent of the total homicides are youth homicides, and the criminals are also youth. There are many more injuries, hospitalizations and sufferings which are not reported.

Violence in and around bars is reported to be serious, involving weapons and resulting in injuries and legal procedures. Intoxication results in more aggressive and violent behaviour. In some research, it was pointed out that approximately 75 per cent of the aggressors were under intoxication. Even the victims are intoxicated 50 per cent of the time. Hence, fighting after drinking is very common. Excitement and thrill seeking, euphoric and unrealistic overconfidence are seen in such youth.

In developed countries, a number of youths are killed on the job due to hostility, unfair competition and a strong wish to take revenge. Targeted violence is like planned cold-blooded murder. The destruction of public property is the most common form of violence. There is hardly any awareness that it is damaging one's own nation, society and facilities available to all. Youths keep on burning public

---

[9] https://www.indiatimes.com/news/world/5-cases-of-ragging-in-india-that-shocked-the-world-278321.html

transport buses, railway trains and government offices. Sometimes, it is related to inter-religion riots and mob violence. One more additional point is that in a huge mob, punishing each individual becomes difficult for law, and hence, the violent youth can easily escape. This is seen more in urban than rural areas. In Africa, many orphans whose parents died of AIDS are violent, and the proportion of crime is extremely high. Even single-parent families have more aggressive and violent offspring.

4.4. COMMON PSYCHO-SOCIAL HEALTH PROBLEMS

4.4.1. Rebellious Attitude

A rebellious attitude is a desire to resist authority and be disobedient. The behaviour of such individuals is difficult to control. There is a state of disagreement. A rebellious attitude plays an important role in aggression and violence among adolescents and youths.

The generation gap results in communication problems between youths and their parents. Due to substantially different sets of values, goals and lifestyles, both of them fail to understand the other. As a consequence, the younger generation hides major concerns from parents. Adolescents and youths are sure that their parents may reject them and be reluctant to support them if they face any problems. It leads to insecurity, misunderstanding and poor interpersonal relations. As a consequence, their lives become free to make decisions secretly. They don't think about tomorrow due to hedonistic tendencies and immediate gratification orientation and want to enjoy life. In such a situation, antisocial elements attract their attention. They start acting without thinking about others and about themselves. Here also, there is a circular explanation. If an individual is exposed to a company with aggressive peers, they will be more aggressive. At the same time, an aggressive individual prefers aggressive groups.

Two common types of rebellious attitudes are nonconformity and non-compliance. Nonconformity is general resistance regarding social norms, traditions and ways of life. Non-compliance is about resistance to parental authority. It not only resists direction and guidance given by their parents but also the general structure of parenting. Rebellion activities may lead to serious harm. These individuals don't get identified with parents. They want to establish their identity as an independent human being. It affects close human relations negatively. Young individuals perceive it as independence. In reality, it is only doing the opposite of what the significant adult want. As a consequence of this, an individual may resist forces useful for self-support and self-development. Finally, a person may work against themselves, and it may result in harm to their self-image and self-esteem. Such individuals can't control their impulses. Their half-hearted judgments may be dangerous. High-risk excitement is very popular among rebellions. As a consequence, these individuals become substantially vulnerable without being aware. They underestimate the potential damage and only because they want to do something against their parents and spoil their future.

In India, the rebellious attitude of youth is superficial. It is restricted to some personal things. As per recent research, today's youth, though outwardly rebellious, want to appear obedient and follow all the salient traditions.

4.4.2. Delinquency and Antisocial Behaviour

In the ill-known Nirbhaya gang rape case (16 December 2012), one of the rapists was below 18 years. He was considered a minor and was sent to a rehabilitation home for three years. He was the most brutal of all the accused as he attacked Nirbhaya with an iron rod. It was because of these injuries that she could not survive (OpIndia Staff, 2020).

Delinquency is a crime committed by minor individuals. It is some offence or misconduct or illegal behaviour. The legal definition of a minor may differ in different countries. Many such misdeeds are committed as a source of excitement and may be less violent. The most common types are thefts, burglaries, road rage, assaults on women, sexual harassment, cybercrime and approximately 2 per cent are murders. Generally, these behaviour patterns are less repetitive. However, if it is repetitive, it becomes antisocial behaviour. Some parents either neglect what the adolescents are doing or indirectly encourage misbehaviour. Bad companies, models of criminal behaviour and low socio-economic status are some important correlates of delinquency.

In family, poor parenting, parental discord, large family size, maltreatment, very harsh discipline without justification, antisocial and detached parents, lack of supervision, conflict with significant adults, physical, psychological, and emotional abuse are generally seen. Such individuals have no respect for rules regulations, societal norms, and law, have personality disorders, conduct disorders, and lack of empathy. Contribution of impact of mass media as causative factor can't be underestimated. Substance abuse in young age leads to delinquency as obtaining money for purchasing drugs becomes a major concern. Immediate gratification orientation is one of the basic reasons of such antisocial behaviour. Whatever the individual wants, he wants to have it immediately and at any cost. Low or sub average intelligence, uncontrolled aggression, dropping out, unemployment are associated with delinquency. Every year incidence is increasing substantially, especially sex offences, and cyber-crimes are getting multiplied.

Different theories are put forth by researchers to explain delinquency. Freud in his theory gives psychoanalytical ideas like it is expression of id due to underdeveloped superego that is responsible for delinquency and antisocial behaviour. According to Erikson it is repeated failure to gain positive recognition from others that leads to negative self-identity and negative behaviour like delinquency. Sutherland put forth the view that impact of interaction within intimate group plays a major role in delinquency. Pavlov's theory and Skinner's theory were regarding conditioning. Bandura highlighted the role of observational learning. Some other researchers focused on moral development as a major contributing factor in delinquency.

In India, almost all delinquents are boys. Research studies have shown that approximately 2 per cent are girls. All reports by the government say that in India, both the severity and incidence of delinquency are increasing tremendously. Even inhuman rapes and murders are committed by younger individuals.

4.4.3. Self-harm

The incidence of self-harm among girls and ladies is six times more than that among males. Some researchers have also reported that, in prisons, it is 10 times higher. The prototype of other oriented aggression and violence is linked to males, and the prototype of self-harm appears to be associated with females. Women are perceived and expected to be gentle, caring, nurturing and loving. Hence, aggression and violence among them are not accepted as natural and are perceived as being the opposite of the image of the ideal woman in cultural archetype. Hence, they want to hide it. Even otherwise, self-harm is difficult to understand and justify. It is taken for granted that it indicates some psychological disease. Other oriented aggression is easily explained with reference to the expression of anger, dominance and control over others, as is cultural stereotypes of masculinity, a form of revenge and retaliation or self-protection.

Variables such as poor self-concept, isolation, hopelessness, depression, anxiety, personality disorders and attention deficit hyperactivity disorder are the contributing factors to self-harm. Low socio-economic conditions, peer pressure for self-harm, being lesbian or gay or transgender and substance and alcohol abuse are also related to self-harm. The adverse effects of negative childhood experiences such as physical or sexual abuse, parental discord and divorce and bullying are also responsible for that. Women involved in self harm have come from deprived and unprivileged environments, having fewer opportunities, more discrimination and neglect of all sorts.

4.4.3.1. Reasons of Self-harm

As suicide is the ultimate escape from problems, self-harm is a temporary relief. It is proved that:

- **It is a way to handle socially unacceptable strong emotions:** The management of emotions or regulation of affect also takes place if a lady induces physical pain; her attention will be attracted to it by the release of endorphins. That reduces emotional pain. It is a coping mechanism.

- **Expression of distress:** it is a way to communicate emotional problems. It is in anticipation that someone will help.
- **Self-punishment:** Negative attitudes towards women, in general, and towards themselves, in particular, may lead to poor self-esteem and internalization of social perspective.
- **Punishing others:** When an individual wants to punish others and they can't do so, it is always safe to harm self.
- **Empowerment and control:** Self-harm generates a sense of control on one's body and one's life. Otherwise, these individuals keep on feeling helpless and hopeless. For example, in the case of sexual abuse, the harasser uses their power over the victim's body. In such a situation, self-harm is a way of getting rid of unwanted memories of filthy touch, unpleasant feelings or disgust.

Sometimes, the victim thinks that there is something vicious in their body, and by punishing self, they can punish that evil. There is no self-respect, and they violate their human rights. Self-acceptance and self-love are also lacking. Although it is not legally a crime, it is cruel behaviour with self. It is clear that self-harm is related to the wrong treatment, neglect, abuse, discrimination, subjugation and lack of respect. It leads to anger, aggression and violence. Suppressing expression of these may lead to self-harm.

4.4.4. Impact on Victim, Aggressor and Others

The psychological and physiological effects of aggression and violence on the victim depend on severity. As there are different types, the impact also varies. However, there are some common psychological problems for victims.

The consequences of aggression and violence are physical, psychological, social and even economic. It leads to injuries, pain, medical treatment, economic loss and unemployment if work-related disabilities result from it. If it is related to the workplace, the organization may bear the cost of treatment, compensate and provide substitute arrangements. Among psychological effects, low self-esteem, loss of confidence, isolation, depression and suicidal tendencies are the most common. Victims are scared, distressed and anxious. As an outcome of stress, flight, fight and freeze responses are generated. They start abusing alcohol and drugs and get involved in self-destructive behaviour. The abused may develop a psychiatric disorder. In the case of intense aggression, victims suffer from depression, post-traumatic stress disorder, anxiety, and agony. If it is family aggression and violence, say between husband and wife, though aggressors threaten victims, if victims can't even terminate the relationship, it causes further harm.

The family members of victims face intense rage, agony, feelings of being victimized, frustration and awkwardness. On the one hand, they want to take revenge, but on the other hand, they are worried about the consequences. If the victim is to undergo some expensive medical treatment, they have to immediately make that provision. They are worried, stressed, helpless and confused. Many of them don't know anything about legal procedures. If it is related to sexual assault or rape, the family faces intense problems and is completely outcasted. There is loss of status, social stigma, isolation and a lack of social support to face the situation. Break-ups are obvious if victims are engaged or married. Nobody in the Indian community wants to marry such a lady.

There are many ill effects on the aggressor as well. There are some temporary effects of aggression. Expressions of aggressive anger are destructive, harsh, harmful, reckless and abusive. It spoils human relations. It includes mistrust, showing off, not listening to others, and not considering others' emotions. They threaten others, physically hurt people and exploit others irrespective of age and relation with them. An aggressive individual is socially rejected and stigmatized. Everyone wants to avoid them as far as possible. Even the family members want to keep away and get rid of their company. They do not freely discuss any of their problems or their problems with them. An aggressor is generally vulnerable to facing retaliation from peers, classmates or colleagues. They are abused and may miss some opportunities only because others don't want their company. An aggressor may be fired from a job again and again, experience break-ups and divorces and spend a lot of time, money and energy on legal procedures. They may feel guilt, shame, loneliness, frustration and social isolation, which lead to very poor self-image. The legal procedure includes imprisonment, trials and long-term isolation with strict disciplinary action. Detailed information regarding such cases is available in the media. This may lead to depression, hopelessness and even suicidal attempts. One of the accused in the Nirbhaya case killed himself in prison.

Some aggression results from fear. Any situation where there are no rules and regulations or is anarchic may lead to a feeling of threat, being victimized or facing injustice. Many types of social aggression may emerge from survival instinct. Confidence building and trust development may reduce such aggression.

4.5 INTERVENTION AND SELF-HELP

If aggression is chronic, the aggressor has to undergo some intervention programmes, therapies and the like. Cognitive behavioural techniques, such as social skills, anger management, stress management and problem-solving, are capable of improving the lives of adolescents and youth. Training about memory improvement and effective learning may be useful for enhancing academic achievement and getting a job. It reduces involvement in violence and aggression. Gender equality training in schools and colleges may reduce aggression and violence against women. If aggression still persists, they may have to take some psychotropic medicines.

The three types of prevention are primary, secondary and tertiary. Primary is for prevention before it occurs, secondary is immediate help, and tertiary is a long-term approach, like rehabilitation. In the case of anger, emotional catharsis may lead to emotional arousal; hence, the management of emotional outbursts is necessary. Emotional catharsis may enhance insight and reduce the burden of negative emotions such as distress, tension, anxiety and frustration. Improved relations with parents may lead to opportunities to talk freely and express innermost thoughts. Positive reinforcement and reminding them that it is for their benefit in the long run may be effective if given in a friendly manner. Training regarding various relevant social skills, such as assertiveness and positive thinking, reduces outbursts of aggression. The development of empathy may be very useful for understanding the condition of victims.

The five stage model for managing aggressive incidents gives the following stages: situation, appraisal, anger, inhibition and conflict. Situation/trigger leads to appraisal of intention. Although the situation is supposed to trigger anger, the emotional response to it plays a major role. It is the appraisal and interpretation that are responsible for anger. That, in turn, depends on the general view of the world, the impressions of others regarding the event and the mood of an individual. If the individual is already upset or angry, it will lead to more negative consequences. When extreme anger is experienced, it decreases an individual's self-control and inhibitions. Inhibitions are the results of internal and external inhibitors. External inhibitors are fear of legal action, physical retaliation, social consequences and material loss. There is anticipated embarrassment. Displacement is an ego defence mechanism which depends on inhibition. If an individual has strong inhibition about a particular target of aggression but comparatively weak inhibition about other targets, displacement occurs. If the boss is behaving in a very irritating way which triggers aggression in the mind of an employee, he will not be able to retaliate. Displacement will take place in such a way that he will show aggression towards his wife or mother. This is a chain of action and reaction. To break it, one has to cut it somewhere. If, for example, the triggering stimulus is accompanied by an apology, it will change the perception regarding appraisal. This, in turn, leads to validate anger. Internal inhibitors are moral inhibitors, guilt and self-control.

Applied behaviour analysis is a systematic study of observable and measurable behaviour. It considers the frequency, intensity, duration, latency and sequencing of aggressive behaviour. The behavioural patterns that are not acceptable to the community are studied in detail with reference to triggering factors, environmental stimuli and reinforcement or gain of the aggressor. Rescheduling of reinforcements is very effective. It can be done exactly according to the principles of conditioning. If aggressive behaviour is used to get attention, it should not be paired with aggression. On the contrary, it should be paired with soft language and sober gestures. Significant adults should try to understand adolescents and may adjust their psychological distance from them. Respecting them, giving them opportunities to shoulder various responsibilities and appreciating their efforts to behave in mature ways work. It is essential to create a conducive environment for adolescents and young adults. It includes having the optimum expression of unconditional acceptance by parents and teachers, motivating and supervising them and giving guidance to utilize their potential. Punishment is not really useful for reducing aggression, it only suppresses aggression temporarily. It leads to more problems in the long term as aggression abruptly increases. The counsellor may use the case study method to understand the causes of aggression in family, friends and educational or occupational institutes. Training and guidance regarding management of anger, conflict-solving skills, anti-bullying and anti-ragging programmes should be made available. Strict laws and their implementation regarding alcohol, drugs and weapons may prove to be effective in arresting violence.

Parents should demonstrate good emotional management and emotional intelligence while dealing with various problems in life. There should be no appreciation of aggression and violence as proper ways to solve problems in day-to-day life. Discipline should be consistent and should not be too harsh. Empathy should be generated by exercises and modelling good behaviour. If parents are not capable of resolving conflicts without being aggressive and violent, their offspring will follow the same style. Using the potential to gain appreciation, involvement in hobbies, praise and the company of non-violent friends helps. The acceptance of the individual as they are, without critically evaluating their behaviour, is essential. Aggression is also interpreted as a sign of helplessness and hopelessness. It is a cry for help. Hence, an aggressor needs to be understood. Interest groups, a healthy social environment and socially acceptable work, such as volunteering work and giving recognition, lead to less aggression.

Counselling helps an individual as well as families. Parental counselling and guidance may be useful for them to understand the effects of their child rearing practices on adolescents and youth. Hence, anger management training is essential, even for parents. Otherwise, parents may aggravate their offspring's anger and aggression by yelling and spanking them.

Around 60 per cent of aggressive and violent youths have psychiatric problems, disruptive behaviour disorder and mood disorders. Therapy needs to be selected on the basis of the exact problem, its intensity and causes. Other mental health problems, personality and life experiences of the aggressor should also be considered. In the case of domestic violence, couple therapy is generally useful. However, it may or may not work as the aggressor is generally unwilling to undergo it and is reluctant to change. Cognitive behavioural therapy helps to control one's aggression. Different coping styles, managing negative and aggressive thoughts and assessing consequences are important strategies.

Psychodynamic therapy assists individuals to become conscious of and face deep-rooted emotional causes. Expressing guilt, shame and fear may be useful for combating aggressive tendencies.

In 2010, Fernandez gave a new therapy called cognitive behavioural affective therapy to deal effectively with feelings of anger in three phases of treatment: prevention, intervention and postvention. dealing with the onset of anger, its progression and the residual features. There are some techniques to manage physiological effects also. Heart coherence training teaches specific mindfulness and biofeedback techniques to shift heart rhythm, which stabilizes the autonomic nervous system. Coherence techniques also reverse the negative effects of anger on the immune system. Hence, it is very effective.

Therapy may be useful to overcome the effects of abuse in childhood. Deep breathing and other relaxation techniques are effective in reducing aggression. Various hobbies, games, sports, music and dance help to balance an individual's emotional state. Improving self-esteem by utilizing various opportunities to gain confidence and trying to achieve various things may prove to be effective for overcoming inferiority. To improve family interaction, functional family therapy and multi-systemic therapy are used. Self-management and maturity among parents, necessary for properly guiding offspring, may be enhanced due to it.

4.6. SUMMARY

Anger, aggression and violence are all detrimental to the mental health of the victim and the individual themselves. The intensity and severity of harm to the victim vary according to different types of expressions of aggression and violence. The factors responsible for it are social, psychological, economic and environmental. Even childhood experiences and whole socialization are related to it. Interactions in family, parent–child relations, style of disciplining, peer group and their activities play an important role. There are many psychological problems and even clinical disorders linked with aggression and violence.

Effects such as physical injury, damage, lifelong disabilities, inability to work, inability to get a life partner and dependency are overtly seen. It leads to rejection, social stigma, isolation and loneliness and psychological harm such as fear, anxiety, depression, hopelessness and even suicidal tendencies.

Gender-related violence is prevalent in India, and the culture, in general, takes it for granted. Eve teasing, harassment, rape, acid attacks and marital rape are ways to exploit a lady who is a soft target. The psychological effects are very severe, from agony, frustration, depression, post-traumatic stress disorder to suicide.

Self-harm is also a self-directed aggression which needs immediate attention.

Intervention is essential to save both the victim and the aggressive individual. Guidance and counselling, therapy, social support and training regarding social skills are necessary for motivating both to lead a socially effective and individually satisfying life.

Marriage

5

5.1. INTRODUCTION

According to the very well-known psychologist, Freud, two things necessary for maintaining good mental health are work and love. From the psychological perspective, home is where one is loved, respected and cared for.[1] It is a place where we feel relaxed and comfortable. Every member is expected to enjoy independence and a feeling of cohesiveness and support from family members. Each one should work for others and get an opportunity to develop one's potential. The basic purpose should be to help each other to lead a happy life. Marriage is essentially the basic strategy for developing a family and creating a home. Marriage is the most important event in human life. It is one of the most challenging developmental tasks and a lifetime achievement if everything goes on smoothly. It is an exciting pleasure and satisfaction in youth. Social and legal sanction for sexual pleasure are added into all sorts of pleasant rituals and ceremonies. If partners get along well with each other, marriage gives ultimate support throughout lifetime. Marriage is a multidimensional interpersonal relationship. The ideal marital relationship includes emotional acceptance, psychological understanding, intellectually respecting opinion of the partner, affirming each other in a social and cultural sphere, spiritually sharing values and goals and physically caring for each other's needs.

The definition of marriage varies around the world depending on culture, religion and the general development of the region. There are many differences between the Western and Eastern worlds. It is a social sanction for sexual relations between a male and a female where

---

[1] https://meaningofhome.ca/

reproduction is considered socially and legally approved. As per traditional Indian views, no premarital and extramarital sexual relations are approved by the community and were considered as a crime till 2018. It is expected that it should be based on commitment, sharing, unconditional acceptance, love and trust, concern for each other's welfare, personal growth and respect (mynation.com, 2016). It further states that many correlates of marriage indicate positive mental health. It leads to a sense of belongingness, security, support and care, which leads to fewer accidents, fewer addictions, more holistic well-being, better success, longevity, and less mental illness.

In advanced countries, love, care, trust, passion, intellectual competence and egalitarian behaviour are expected in marital relations.

Researchers have recently proved that married individuals are happier, physically and psychologically healthy, and they live longer. They avoid risky behaviour. They combat stress in a better way and recover from illness in less time. They take care of themselves in a better way than unmarried individuals. It is proved that the possibility of developing a psychiatric illness, like depression, is 50 per cent less among married individuals than among unmarried individuals.

5.2. SELECTION OF MATE: PSYCHO-SOCIAL EXPECTATIONS, RISKS AND DECEPTION

There are many dimensions and intentions related to marriage, such as financial, religious, social, legal, physiological and emotional. The different expected roles of partners depend upon whether they are monogamy or polygamy and whether they are a joint family or nuclear family. Due to differences in geographical environment and maintenance system, the nature, types and functions of marriage are affected. For example, in hilly areas of North India, there are some tribes who depend on animal husbandry to maintain their families. To look after their pigs, sheep and goats, these men have multiple wives. In some other communities, as the resources are very limited, just to keep the family intact, many brothers have a single wife so that the offspring are from the same family, and there is no division of property, like farms. Short films like 'Polyandry still practiced in Tibet's village' (Zee News, 2013) or 'Multiple Husbands' (National Geographic, 2007) are informative and interesting.

In other areas, these practices are banned socially and legally. All over the world, women's rights are also equally proposed, but in many countries, they are not practised. Even in well-educated Indian families, there is no guarantee that the wishes and willingness of the young lady will be taken into consideration while making a decision about her marriage. Although marriage has been prevalent for generations and centuries in India, its nature, functions and expectations are changing in the contemporary world. From child marriages to late marriages, from 100 per cent arranged marriages to partial love marriages, the nature of marriage is becoming comparatively more flexible. Indian culture is resistant to change, and even today, caste, creed, community and socio-economic status are taken into consideration while making a decision about marriage. Parents and grandparents are extremely strict about this decision in traditional families and want their children to obey them without fail. While considering a marriage proposal, the difference between husband and wife is essentially maintained. The would-be wife should be younger and less educated than the husband. If she belongs to a family that is wealthier, she is welcome. The ideal bride is still expected to be good looking, submissive, soft-spoken, a serving type, interested in household jobs and pleasant. She is expected to please everyone in his family. There are hardly any exceptions in Indian culture where the bride is supposed to be confident, motivated and egalitarian.

In India, there is a very poor tolerance of negative or even positive exceptionality in life partners. Even if there is any minor disability or limitation, it becomes very difficult to find a life partner. Everyone, irrespective of their own status, wants a perfect match: healthy, wealthy and competent. It is worth noting that even a positively exceptional wife is rarely acceptable.

Meeta has recently completed a doctorate in engineering from the Indian Institute of Technology. Her parents are trying their level best to find an appropriate marriage partner. However, no one is ready to accept a well-qualified and intelligent wife, irrespective of their own education.

In contemporary society, many families and individuals give fake information to the other party, like educational qualifications, health status/any chronic illness like HIV or wealth of the family/legal cases registered. It is not socially accepted to ask for various certificates from the groom or have health-related tests performed before marriage. Hence, trust is the only way to make a decision about marriage.

Sushant has been detected as HIV positive recently. He was shocked and consulted different doctors. However, the results were confirmed. As he is well settled in his business, his family wants him to get married. He is not capable of telling the truth to his own parents. They have finalized the marriage. An equally shocking case was reported by the media in 2018 (*The Times of India*, September 18, 2018), where though the groom knew that he had HIV, he got married to a healthy woman. Now, his wife has filed a case against him.

5.3. INDIAN CONTEXT: TRADITIONS, ATTITUDES AND PRACTICES; CHANGING TRENDS: LIVE-IN RELATIONS AND SOLOGAMY

Indian social norms, traditions and perspectives about marriage depend heavily on the assumption of male superiority and justification of the subordinate status of women. For generations, the whole family system has been based on the convenience of male members and the sacrifice of women in every possible way. Even today, the impact of those unjust and inhuman ways is clearly seen.

Generally, the match criteria in India are horoscope, caste, religion, socio-economic status, profession and appearance. As per Indian traditions, a wife is supposed to surrender to the authorities of her husband and be always ready to fulfil his demands. If she fails to satisfy his sexual needs, it is not tolerated. In India, factual data is not available as ladies do not disclose these things.

The ownership of a wife is an age-old mentality in India. The sati or widow burning tradition was prevalent in India, which was banned by British governor general in 1829. The Sati Prevention Act, 1987, was the most recent form of it. The same mentality is seen even today. The traditional in-laws and husband think that they can make any decision, exploit her anyway and treat her as a slave. The Supreme Court recently mentioned that 'the wife is not a slave or property of her husband who can be asked to forcibly live with her husband' (punekarnews.in, 2021).

A 23-year-old woman committed suicide by jumping into the River Sabarmati. Just before that, she prepared a video which went viral on every news channel.[2] In Hyderabad, a 25-year-old lady engineer committed suicide over dowry harassment by her husband and in-laws.[3] A 23-year-old engineer (*The Indian Express*, 27 February 2020) hanged herself in Telangana due to constant dowry demands. *Business Standard* reported that in Delhi, a woman committed suicide due to harassment for dowry on 3 April 2019.

India, Pakistan, Iran and Bangladesh are the countries where the tradition of dowry is still prevalent. India has the highest rate of dowry deaths and dowry-related suicides, according to the Indian National Crime Record Bureau. For example, in 2012, it was reported that one bride was burned every 90 minutes. Recently, it was reported that in 2017, there were everyday 21 cases of dowry deaths reported in India. It is worth noting that the conviction rate is 35 per cent. In addition, many cases are not reported to the police, and no justice is sought. Every year, many young girls are either killed or provoked to commit suicide. Various records of crime have reported that instead of decreasing, it is increasing every year.

Dowry deaths are more frequently seen in upper- and middle-class traditional families where the age of the victim is in their early 20s. It is not related to education of the victim. In Indian marriages, wife battering, slaps, kicks, broken bones and torture are very common. Women keep quiet and their parents also do not support them. In empirical studies, it was found that if the age difference between husband and wife is more than 5 years, such injustice is more frequent. It is reported that, in the case of violence, women are helpless, depressed, powerless, timid and have a poor self-image. The tendency to under evaluate self, immaturity, lack of social skills and assertiveness are reported. The husband is possessive, dominant, depressive, suspicious,

---

[2] www.india.com>newsdesk 27 February 2021

[3] http://www.ndtv.com 30 September 2018

inferior, a sociopath or psychopath and, in most cases, an alcoholic. Alcoholism is reported in approximately 93 per cent of such cases, even at international level (Hilberman & Munson, 1978). Simple day-to-day reasons are enough to ill treat women. In a way, it is accepted by the community; hence, there is no shame or guilt.

The Dowry Prohibition Act, 1961, prohibits the payment and acceptance of dowry. The idea of ownership of a wife was so prevalent that even the law treated women as men's property. For example, previously, having sex with a married woman without permission from her husband was treated as a crime. It obviously means that if the husband gives permission, anyone can sexually exploit his wife. It is an extreme violation of the human rights of women. A wife was legally considered as the husband's property. Now, however, in September 2018, adultery is no longer a crime. It is not a criminal offence. It has stopped treating women as objects, on the one hand, and may be interpreted as an encouragement to extramarital sex, on the other.

> Preeti was just 24 years old, and this was her sixth pregnancy. Due to some gynaecological complications, five times she could not carry for more than four months. Her husband and in-laws were constantly pressurizing her to try again. Due to repeated pregnancies, her health deteriorated further. Ultimately, she delivered a baby boy who suffered from cerebral palsy.

Infertility is never tolerated in Indian society. That too, only daughters are not acceptable. It is mandatory, as per Hindu traditional Indian views, to have a son. Only the son is authorized to perform the last rituals, and only after that, parents are allowed in heaven. Many young ladies are harassed only because they can't reproduce or they have only daughters. There are examples where the lady is killed only because of gynaecological problems or divorced due to infertility. Even if it is because of her husband's physiological problems and inability to reproduce, she is the one who is blamed. In many families, infertility is perceived essentially as a shortcoming of the wife and her husband is always perceived as being perfect. He is not ready to even undergo any treatment.

Religious practices, rituals and coercive methods of marriage do not withstand legal provisions. Even today, many marriages are not legally registered and many divorces are not legally sanctioned. Even if a lady is very unhappy, she will not think of divorce due to social pressure and parental inability to support her. Sons are considered the future of the family and daughters are disowned in a way after marriage. After marriage, their original identity is lost. Recently, a few very well-educated women have retained their original names and surnames, but still there is resistance to it from the family and society.

Approximately 47 per cent of total marriages are child marriages in India, and mostly, the bride is less than 18. It was prevalent in all communities approximately two generations ago. Even today, these people think that a female child is a burden on the family, and instead of protecting her and spending money on her, it is better to dispatch her to her husband's place. The ill effects are that she can be easily harassed, prematurely sexually exploited, be forced to reproduce before physical maturity and can never think of education.

It is prevalent to practice complete ownership of one's wife. As is discussed in the section of marital rape, a wife is supposed to be used as a commodity, and her willingness, convenience and health are rarely considered. Sex is taken for granted as a privilege of the husband. A lady was set ablaze by her husband as she denied sex with him (NDTV, 2018). In another case, a wife was burned with two children because she denied sex (India News, 23 September 2018).

The law expects that every marriage should be with the consent of two individuals. Any force, coercion, fraud, misinterpretation should not be used in this consent. However, it is not always so in India. Expectations of young adults are very rarely considered while making a decision regarding their marriage. Even if they fall in love, generally, it is considered only as a hindrance to a proper, socially acceptable marriage. Honour killing is still prevalent in many Indian communities when young adults want to marry someone from other communities and go against the strict rules of their society. There are frequent incidences of parents killing both bride and groom, killing only the outsider or somehow harassing them.

Approximately 1,000 cases of honour killings are reported in India every year. Of those, 900 are from Haryana, Punjab and Uttar

Pradesh. The worldwide incidence is 5,000. Honour killing is a homicide by family members strongly under the impact of social customs and traditions about marriage. The family thinks that the individual is responsible for shame and disrespecting the family. This is against the Indian legal system and human rights (Honour killing, http://www.slideshare.net 16 Aug. 2016). The complete discussion of very ill-known cases is available in various documentation on Google and YouTube.

A father spent 1.13 crore rupees on the murder of his son-in-law, who was from a lower caste (*India Today*, 2018). A father amputated his daughter's hand as she got married to a person from another caste (India News, September 2018). In Madhya Pradesh, a young couple was beaten inhumanly and forced to consume urine as they got married against the wish of the elders in the family (Sharma, 2018). In Delhi, a young lady was killed because she wanted to marry a person from a backward caste (IndiaTV, 2014). In Telangana, a 20-year-old woman was murdered by her parents for marrying a man from a different caste (NDTV, 2018). A newly wed husband and wife were killed in Kolhapur, Maharashtra (Jai Maharashtra News, 2015). A newly married couple was shot dead in Amritsar (ABP Sanjha, 2016). Recently, on 26 December 2020, a 27-year-old man was killed as he had married a young lady from another caste.[4] It is done to purify the caste and regain the status of the family (Bhatnagar et al., 2012).

5.3.1. Changing Trends: Live-in and Sologamy

Live-in or cohabitation is a comparatively new style of establishing a relationship. In this, two individuals who are not married live together and share sexually intimate relations. Live-in relationships are not socially acceptable in most communities, religions and regions of India. Very few hi-fi societies of advanced families in metro cities may accept it, but most societies think that it is a threat to the family system. The legal system in India, however, protects women in live-in under the Domestic Violence Act and Section 498A.

---

[4] timesofindia.com>topic>honourkilling 3 January 2021

This type of sexual relationship has become common in advanced countries in the last few decades. Gradually, marriage is becoming an outdated institution. Cultures in advanced countries are becoming more open to these lifestyles. In a country like the USA, 67 per cent of married couples live together without marriage before they get married. It is convenient economically and gives an opportunity to test relationships and compatibility. If they can't get along well, they terminate the relationship. The younger generation doesn't believe in marriage. Around 10 per cent of them have children also. Along with social rejection, the effects on child development are also a matter of concern.

Researchers have reported controversial results regarding the stability of marriages after live-in relationships. However, most of them have reported that live-in leads to divorce within a few years of marriage. The percentage was reported to be double. Infidelity and abuse are also reported in live-in relationships. This type of arrangement is legally prohibited in most Muslim countries.

In November 2018, the court ordered a male partner in a live-in relationship to pay maintenance charges for the offspring as the relationship was terminated. This has happened due to deception on the part of the male as he pretended to marry the female partner but never did it legally.

The latest trend is sologamy or marrying oneself. In Europe, this new trend is emerging. According to the supporters, it affirms one's own value, which leads to a happier life. This is a self-marriage or self-uniting marriage, which is a marriage without an officiant. The ceremony of such marriages is the same as other marriages. There is a provision for guidance and support for such marriages. Self-marriages are becoming increasingly popular among well-educated and well-to-do women. There has been a lot of controversy about it since 2014, as such marriages were reported from that year. Self-marriage packages have been offered by travel agencies since 2014. British photographer Grace Gelder's and Italian Laura Mesi's self-marriages were widely publicized. In October 2018, in London, a student called Jemima got married to herself and declared that she would always live with herself. Career-oriented young individuals are, in a way, declaring that they are not interested in marriage and would like to lead an independent life.

5.4. RESPONSIBILITIES AND ROLES FOR MAINTAINING FAMILY, PARENTHOOD AND BEING SINGLE PARENT

Sangita was not well for a month after delivery. Her husband, Shekhar, had to take care of the baby also. He used to even give a bath to the baby, cook and serve and do the remaining household jobs. He had to take her to the hospital and help her do her routine activities. There are very few male members who show this type of cooperation in Indian families. However, that should be the atmosphere for optimum affection, trust and mutual support. Even in lockdown, due to coronavirus infection, in April 2020, many wives are facing problems because their husbands are not sharing any household responsibilities despite the fact that no domestic help is available. Indian males staying abroad, however, have to manage on their own, especially during child birth.

During the first few years after marriage, adjustment problems are challenging. However, various roles and responsibilities are life-long and require a lot of maturity, persistence and effort. The life of an individual changes substantially due to marriage. Economic, social, emotional and family-related responsibilities, including extended family, are the major issues. Every day, without fail, the whole cycle of family maintenance has to be taken care of. There are various expectations of a family as a unit regarding social interactions. Emotionally, it is expected that an individual should develop maturity, sensitivity, empathy and insight into the problems of family members and others too. Other family-related responsibilities are basically taking care of their own offspring, parents and other members of the extended families of both husband and wife. It is worth noting that Indian culture expects every married lady to take care of her in-laws only, and her own parents should be looked after by her daughter-in-law. A daughter is not supposed to and, most of the time, not allowed to help her own parents in terms of money, effort, time and even emotional support. This traditional attitude may contribute to the preference for sons.

Factors influencing adjustment to parenthood are: attitude towards pregnancy and parenthood, age of parents, preference for child's sex, number of children, conflict about child rearing and the child's health and temperament. There are many other indirect factors, such as socio-economic status, education, religion and general involvement in the welfare of children, that affect the whole interaction. The most important responsibility is that of expression of unconditional acceptance and love and creating a conducive environment for the growth and development of children. However, there is hardly any awareness among even educated parents about these psychologically important things.

Among Indian women, there is a tendency for clinging behaviour to marital relations. As women are taught to be dependent on men emotionally, socially, cognitively and economically, they feel safe if they stay with their husbands, even if the marital adjustment is very poor or even when the lady has to suffer a lot. There are women who stay with their husbands even though their husbands are openly involved in extramarital affairs, as there is no other way to support themselves and their children.

5.5. MUTUAL MALADJUSTMENT, OTHER PSYCHOLOGICAL PROBLEMS AND DIVORCE

Marital satisfaction is defined as a subjective feeling of happiness, satisfaction and pleasure experienced by an individual after considering all aspects of one's marriage. Some experts highlight that it is the degree of congruence between expectations a person has and the rewards they actually receive (Burr et al., 1979.) It is expected that if one spouse is satisfied, the other should be satisfied also. However, it was not found to be true in research. The correlation between the two is not perfect. If the husband insists on his needs, wishes and sexual satisfaction without considering the wife's wish, convenience and satisfaction, the husband will be satisfied and the wife will not be. Although it is seen that those who come from different backgrounds find it difficult to adjust, the basic issues are love, affection and respect for each other.

Researchers have classified marriages in different ways. Lederer and Jackson (1990) classified them into two dimensions: satisfactory and unsatisfactory and stable and unstable. Approximately 50 years ago, Cuber and Harroff (1966) gave the following five types:

1. **Conflict habituated relationship:** It is based on quarrelling, nagging and fault finding.

2. **Devitalized relationship:** For the first few years, the relationship is satisfactory, but then it becomes an empty marriage where the couple stays together because of children. There is no emotional involvement, no overt conflict, only dull and detached behaviour.

3. **Passive congenial relationship:** Right from the beginning, marital relations are maintained in an unemotional way. It is social and economic adjustment. There is no satisfaction and no overt conflict.

4. **Vital relationship:** Most satisfactory but rear relationship which depends on psychological bonds, concern for mutual satisfaction and open communication. Conflicts are resolved quickly.

5. **Total relationship:** Depends on total togetherness, no conflict and no private experience.

Due to the system of arranged marriages in India, the husband and wife know nothing about each other's personality, values, real interests, likes and dislikes and socialization. As a consequence, there are many misunderstandings, distorted perceptions and undue expectations about each other. Everyone expects the other person to help them. There is an unconscious agenda to achieve something, get a particular type of satisfaction, pleasure and achieve a particular goal. Every individual has their own emotional problems, experiences, childhood wounds and ideal picture of a sound marriage. This may not match with the partner's phenomenological world. It is essential to try to understand one's partner's psychological world and expectations. Without it, nobody would be capable of perceiving anything on common ground. On the one hand, both of them are interested in intimacy, and on the other, there is self-awareness. If an individual is not aware of one's own potential, interests and expectations, confusion increases even further.

The interaction, many a time, is consciously or unconsciously oriented towards changing one's partner. It becomes a tug of war between her needs and his needs. In Indian conditions, sexual adjustment and satisfaction are not openly discussed. If there is any discrepancy between their ideas, practices, expectations and expressing styles, both of them will be unhappy.

It is reported by researchers that women are interested in the expression of love and affection. They want to spend quality time with the partner and are very happy if the partner is sensitive and caring. On the other hand, male members are more interested in being physical and enjoying sex without much other interaction. Culture contributes a lot to it.

Due to different biochemical and physiological endowments and differential socialization, men and women develop diametrically opposite personalities. That is why they are not in a position to understand each other's phenomenological world. For good marital adjustment, they should play complimentary roles. Understanding the needs of the partner is essential. Personality traits such as openness, agreeableness and expressiveness are good predictors of marital satisfaction. Enthusiasm and genuineness in a partner's personality predict good marital satisfaction. In day-to-day situations, a lot of conflict may emerge due to the lack of understanding of a partner's perspective. It is reported by researchers that as male members are socialized in such a way that they develop less empathy, they do not accept many ideas, plans and behavioural patterns of their partners.

Age, education, religion, income and length of marriage are linked to marital satisfaction. Marital stability and satisfaction are related to active listening skills, agreement, approval, assent and the use of humour (Fisher, 1982). Trust and sharing are the two important pillars of marital satisfaction. Hiding something or partially hiding something affects marital adjustment in an adverse way. The individual feels rejected and excluded (Finkenauer et al., 2009). Money may become a crucial factor detrimental to marital adjustment.

The importance of communication can't be underestimated at any point of time in marital relations. About 80 per cent of divorces take place because of a lack of skills for proper communication. During the first year after marriage, husbands are very sensitive to the needs of wives. They are supportive; they appreciate their efforts and achievements, and they are very pleasant. However, as time passes, things are taken for granted. The wife is supposed to serve, cook and clean, take care of the young ones and old ones without a single word of appreciation. For years, she is to satisfy the husband sexually without any consideration of her own health, responsibilities, achievements and wishes. The quality and quantity of communication, time spent with each other and disclosing thoughts decide intimacy. The quality of communication is more important than quantity. Unrewarding communication patterns such as disagreement, criticism, putting down, sarcasm and rejections result in marital dissatisfaction.

> Gottman is a very well-known researcher in the field of marital relations. He has published 190 scholarly articles and 40 books on that subject. According to Gottman et al. (1995), satisfied couples maintain a 5:1 ratio, which means 5 positive to 1 negative communication. Poor communication, talking only regarding regular routine, criticizing each other and no communication of positive feelings result in marital problems. Gottman gave a theory in 1999 which puts forward the idea that positive interaction and friendship are the most decisive factors regarding marital satisfaction and stability. Gottman's book *The Seven Principles of Making Marriage Work* (2000) sheds light on many important aspects of marital relations.

Jorgensen and Gaudy (1990) define self-disclosure as 'a process by which a marriage partner expresses feelings, perceptions, fears, doubts to the partner allowing personal and private information to surface the relationship that normally is reveled in day to day interaction.' Mostly, socially unacceptable information which is intimate and negative is cancelled. According to Altman and Taylor in 1987, self-disclosure is with reference to perceptions, worldview and tastes. For example, women express their problems, personal information and distressing information. Male members neither disclose their problems nor ask for help. It is proven that a lower level of self-disclosure leads to more mental health problems. Expressing problems leads to a reduction in stress and proper emotional catharsis. It enhances psychological well-being. Those who do not share distressing information are reported to be more depressed, shy, anxious and have low self-esteem (Kelly & Johnston, 2001). In marital relationships, information, that is, mostly regarding sexual orientation, sexual exploitation, experiences of child abuse, disease and so on plays an important role.

Egalitarian views of husbands are found to be associated with marital satisfaction of their wives, but when husbands hold traditional views, wives' egalitarianism is found to be associated with poor marital happiness of their husbands.

Childhood experiences and parental marital adjustment also play an important role in deciding the offspring's marital adjustment. Those who have been experiencing parental discord since childhood think that this is the way to interact with one's spouse. Their marital adjustment is very poor. If an individual has developed compassion, high ethics, morals and values, they will compromise regarding many things to maintain good relationships. If one of the partners comes from a hostile background, the marriage becomes traumatic for the other. If both of them come from a hostile background, continuous fighting and quarrelling takes place. If both partners are happy with sexual gratification, it leads to better marital adjustment. Otherwise, negative interactions result in a lack of love and concern, and this generates apathy, incompetence, frustration and aggression. Both these things are interdependent. Sex does not take place satisfactorily without trust, acceptance and compassion. A lady respects her husband's wish to have sex only when she has concern and love for him, when he respects her and mutual relations are satisfactory. When the husband cares for his wife during sexual interaction, appreciates if she is too tired and makes her comfortable, their interpersonal relations are satisfactory. Intimacy and sexual pleasure dissolve most of the discords in marital life. There are differences in attitudes, physiological health and eagerness, degree of interest and privacy expected for enjoying sexual activities, which lead to more long-lasting and serious conflicts. If time and opportunities are rear, it creates tension and detachment.

Factors influencing sexual adjustment are attitude towards sex, sexual infidelity, past experience, desire, early marital sex, attitude towards use of contraceptives and pornography consumption. In recent years, watching pornography substantially changed one's expectations and actual behaviour regarding sex. If the partner is not interested in advanced experiments about sexual pleasure, many male members are disturbed, disappointed and frustrated. At the same time, excess sex drive and interest in sexual pleasure of husband makes his wife anxious, irritated and tired, and she wants to avoid it. As a consequence, interpersonal relations, in general, deteriorate. Hence, above average or below average sex drive, mismatching ideas of enjoying sex, energy available, privacy available and other worries and responsibilities are related to sexual satisfaction of both.

Child birth directly affects marital adjustment, especially if it is against the wish of the mother. She may become upset and indirectly hate the baby. In most families in India, a wife does not have any authority to decide anything about her pregnancy. It is decided by her husband and in-laws. This leads to unwanted pregnancies and a number of ill effects on interpersonal relations between husband and wife as well as mother and child. In many communities, a daughter's birth is most unwanted, and hence, before birth, identification of sex of the foetus and termination of the pregnancy is done even against the will of the expecting mother.

For satisfactory marital adjustment, it is necessary to have enough maturity to bear more stress, responsibilities and emotional, social and economic demands. If one of the partners is irresponsible and immature, it leads to poor marital adjustment. Indian research has also proved that there is a significant negative relationship between stress, depression and marital adjustment.

The relationship between education and marital adjustment is not simple. Previously, it was found that there was a positive relationship between the two. However, more educated and independent wife may expect more decent interaction and an egalitarian atmosphere. If not, then it may result in a divorce. The working status of the wife may lead to better marital adjustment as she is more satisfied, confident, plays multiple roles, has high self-esteem and, in a way, is independent. A housewife is more demanding emotionally, economically and socially. Housewives are more insecure, dependent, anxious and hopeless (Nathawat & Mathur, 1993). However, it depends on the expected role of the wife in a specific family and the general ideology of the husband.

International research has proved that trust is one of the most important and critical aspects of marital adjustment. Psychiatric illness, substance abuse, and anxiety are related to relationship problems. They are interdependent. Psychological problems may result from marital discord, and marital discord may result from these problems. The need for belongingness is the impetus of marriage. If the need for belongingness is satisfied, marital adjustment is good, general adjustment, health and well-being are also satisfactory. Bipolar disorder, insecurity, powerlessness, emotional instability, physical and emotional abuse, tension, anxiety, worry, suspicion and defensiveness are reported to be associated with marital dissatisfaction.

Loyalty to the partner is necessary not just for morality but for one's own safety.

Marital adjustment depends on many aspects of interaction between the husband and wife. To some extent, others, like in-laws, play an important role, especially in the case of Indian daughter-in-laws. Significant correlates of marital adjustment are the balance of power and authority, as well as respect and empathy while communicating with each other (Figure 5.1). In contemporary culture, especially in

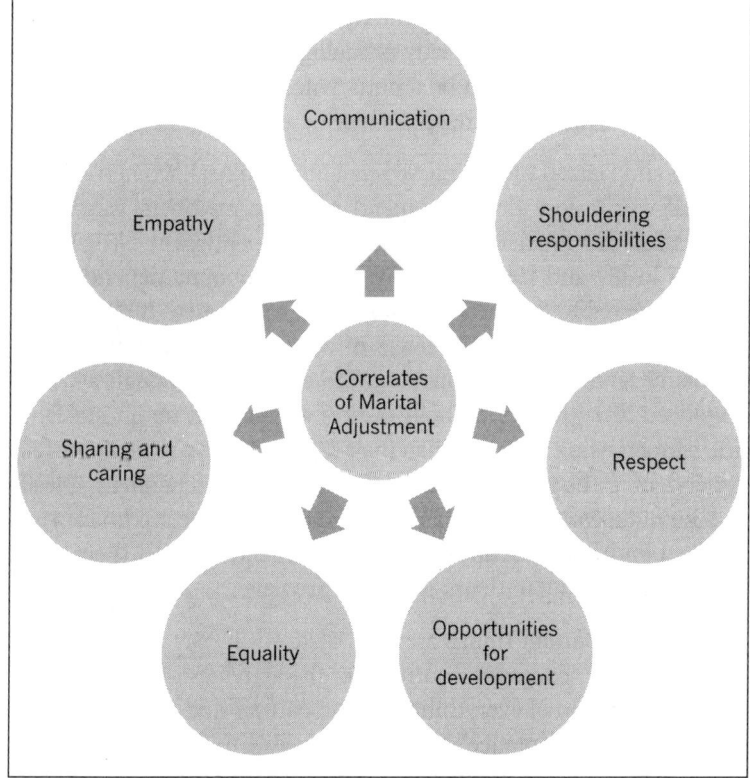

Figure 5.1 *Correlates of Marital Adjustment*

educated Indian families, an egalitarian attitude is essential to maintain good marital adjustment. Everyone needs some space to develop and some opportunities to grow. In traditional Indian culture, the housewife, even if she is well educated and motivated, does not get a single hour to pursue her hobbies, interests or to work gainfully. She is taken for granted for 24 hours and is supposed to fulfil all duties, serve every member of the family and forget about self-development. In such a case, the lady's life becomes boring and frustrating. Her marital adjustment generally deteriorates.

Research regarding housewives demonstrated that a housewife hardly gets any cognitive stimulation, and her cognitive abilities deteriorate as time passes. Everyday changes are taking place in every sphere of life, and she is not exposed to these changes, and her general confidence also decreases. Learned helplessness further diminishes her self-worth. If the young lady is intelligent, motivated and eager to work, but she is forced to be a housewife, this results in frustration and apathy, which, in turn, spoils marital relations.

Niaz and Hassan (2006) proved that in South Asia, women's mobility, self-worth and identity depend on male members' mood and permission. No financial and emotional independence restricts their choices in life and free expression of self. Economic dependence is directly related to the mental health of Indian women. It affects their self-worth, confidence and sense of competence. Economic independence is very rarely available to housewives. Although a wife is employed, sharing of household work is very rare. In traditional families, women who earn more than their husbands are also economically dependent. If the wife wants to be economically independent, it leads to a lot of discord, quarrels and even revenge. There are housewives who exploit their husbands and want to spend a lot on their lavish lifestyle. According to them, it is their privilege.

If these important things are not balanced, it may lead to marital maladjustment. Excessive control over the activities of one's partner, critical evaluation of everything that the partner does, no respect and unconditional acceptance of the partner lead to marital maladjustment. In recent years, many discords in marriage are related to doubts about the partner's activities on Facebook, WhatsApp and Instagram. Having doubts that husband or wife is involved with someone else, at least emotionally, and is engaged in constant communication with that individual, creates an unpleasant atmosphere. The lack of appreciation may be the root cause of infidelity. If the partners spend less quality time with each other, it may lead to detachment. About 45 per cent of men and 35% women have emotional affairs. Spying, keeping track and asking for details about phone calls and messages are very common problems nowadays. Married couples feel insecure. Keeping secrets, hiding things and giving partial information are the ways of interacting that create discord.

Trust is the main foundation of every relationship. Differences regarding values, philosophy of life, attitudes regarding stereotypical gender roles may lead to major conflict. Spouses in well-adjusted marriages show affection for each other, and their level of anxiety is low. If there is any problem, they discuss it with each other and solve it after considering each other's views. Agreement, affection, cohesion and satisfaction are the factors which lead to a well-adjusted marriage. In Indian society, a wife who is assertive, confident and independent may not be acceptable to the husband and in-laws. That creates stress and discord due to different expectations.

No relationship is free from problems, conflicts and disagreements. Marriage tests the way one works, respects commitments, fulfils one's duties, and communicates with family members. Some serious issues are irresponsible behaviour, neglecting one's duties and abusive relationships, both physical and emotional abuse. Boundary problems are very subtle, but their impact is substantial. If an individual is self-oriented, he will force the partner to behave as per his wish. Sometimes, the ego enlargement of one of them may result in a lot of discord. Time management plays a crucial role in marital life.

In advanced countries like the USA, 50 per cent of marriages end in divorce. The whole family system is becoming less respected and less stable. Previously, partners were expected to fulfil each other's needs, such as needs for daily requirements, safety and love and affection. In addition to that, today's marriages in modern and educated families have a requirement for the provision of personal growth and development. Now, both partners have an orientation towards self-actualization. They expect the partner to support them in achieving the same. They don't depend on each other for their livelihood but essentially expect respect, support, sharing and caring, equality, empathy and understanding.

Adjustment with in-laws depends upon undue expectations, stereotypes, family cohesiveness, social mobility, desire for independence, care necessary for the elderly and career demands of the daughter-in-law and son-in-law. The inability and unwillingness to forgive and different ideas about interaction with relatives may also interfere with marital adjustment.

In the case of disabled or chronically ill children, there are many conflicts about the sharing of responsibility. The mother is more oriented to the welfare of the child than anything else. The father, however, does not want to give up his privileges, free time and devote extra money to the differently able child. Divorce may take place only because of this issue.

In 1889, an ill-known case of a 10-year-old girl who lost her life to marital rape was a matter of debate. The National Family Health Survey found that 77 per cent of women were raped by their husbands. A total of 33 per cent of husbands accept it. About 2 crore ladies in India suffer due to its severity (YouTube, 2021). Child marriages result in added injustice as the bride is generally below maturity age, and the groom is mature. This leads to very painful sex for the young girl, premature pregnancies and no awareness of her own rights. They don't have the confidence and strength to retaliate. Even otherwise, Indian women do not have and get any opportunity to develop a proactive attitude. They are reactive and this results in a vicious circle of unhappiness and poor interpersonal relations. Many such issues which are already discussed in the chapters on abuse and gender are linked with various issues in marital adjustment.

In short, emotionally relating to each other, being honest and having self-management skills for avoiding infidelity are the basic issues.

Expressions of love and affection lead to warm relations. Deception may not be tolerated by the partner and affect marital adjustment. The criteria for successful marital adjustment are happiness of partners, good parent–child relations, good adjustment of children, ability to deal with disagreements and a feeling of togetherness. Unconditional acceptance, empathy and respecting each other help a lot.

There are many benefits to marriage for psycho-social health of an individual. The prominent ones are mental health and physical health. Psychological well-being, love, intimacy, protection from loneliness and physiological satisfaction and social interactions as a family are the major benefits. As compared to unmarried individuals, married individuals experience less distress; men show fewer stress hormones, and women experience less psychological stress. Single mothers face more conflicts, more ambivalence and lack expression of love and intimacy as compared to married mothers staying with their families. General parenting stress is more for single parents. Depression is less in the case of married mothers, especially when the relationship is stable and the partners support each other. Even children and adolescents experience less distress if they stay in an intact family.

> ### Are There Gender Differences in the Incidence of Suicide of Married and Unmarried Individuals?
>
> Less married men commit suicide. Marriage is a protection against suicidal thoughts for men. However, the same is not true in the case of women. More married women commit suicide in India due to unbearable anxiety, harassment, physical and psychological abuse and demands regarding dowry. They are treated in such a way that it leads to provoking them to commit suicide. Adolescents coming from divorced families are more vulnerable to suicide.

Happiness, positive attitude, more self-management and less possibility of developing addiction are reported among married than unmarried individuals. General trust regarding others is less in the case of single or divorced individuals. Burgess and Cottrell (1939) were the pioneering researchers who gave the first marital adjustment measure. They have included areas such as agreement, common interest and joint activities, affection and mutual confidence, complaints and feeling lonely and miserable and irritable.

5.5.1. Divorce

A divorce is the dissolution of a marriage before the death of one partner. It is the final termination which cancels all legal and social responsibilities associated with marriage. It dissolves the bonds of matrimony. In India, divorce was not allowed before the Hindu Marriage Act, 1955. Different religions are governed by different marriage acts. Hindus, Jains, Buddhists and Sikhs are governed by the Hindu Marriage Act, 1955. Christians are governed by the Divorce Act (1869); Parsees by the Parsi Marriage and Divorce Act, 1936, and inter-religion marriages are under the Special Marriage Act, 1954. The followers of the Catholic Church are not allowed to get a divorce like in France; it is completely prohibited. In some countries, such as Malta and the Philippines, there is no provision for divorce even today. The proportion of divorces in developed countries has increased substantially during the last 50 years. Single-parent families are becoming very common. Teenage marriages are more prevalent. The culture allows divorce as it is oriented towards individuals' happiness rather than social expectations.

> Recently, it was reported that the divorce rate is lowest in India compared to all other countries in the world. It is 1.4 per cent. The divorce rate is 50 per cent in the USA (Wikipedia, 2018). It is not due to happy marriages in India but may be related to social pressure and cultural taboos. Many separated couples don't get a legal divorce, and in unfavourable conditions, women commit suicide. Some couples are not interested in legal marriages, and they are in live-in relationships. Cases of divorce increased three times during lockdown due to corona.

The low rate of divorce in India is because of the distorted social image of marriage, extreme patriotic traditional ideology, the very low status of women, in general, less education and less freedom sanctioned for women to be independent. The lack of appropriate interaction, happiness and satisfaction in marital relations are very common. Women keep on tolerating injustice for the whole of their lives with substantial social pressure, expected loss of status and a lack of financial support. If a divorce takes place, the causes are infidelity, lack of proper communication, lack of equality and lack of intimacy.

Even today, most uneducated and semi-educated women respect their husbands as super beings, though they are exploitative. These women are ready to submit to their husbands' authority. Many of them are regularly harassed and abused. The whole family system is dependent on the constant devotion and sacrifice of women. For these reasons, if a woman thinks about divorce, the next moment she gets discouraged as nobody is there to support her, and she does not know how to survive independently. The rate of divorce is increasing due to the impact of other cultures and independent, competent and well-educated ladies are capable of making their own decisions.

Marriages fail because of hostility, defensiveness, criticism, nagging, contempt, abuse and exploitation. Domestic violence, stonewalling and rejection lead to psychological distancing. More ill effects of divorce are seen if the person does not want it to happen. There are various reasons behind a divorce, such as addictions, extramarital affairs, stress and strain in the family and mid-life crisis. There are examples where one of them is a workaholic. A divorce may take place due to mental and physical cruelty, sexual incompatibility and infidelity, sex addiction, dowry demands or any other exploitation like physical or emotional abuse. Researchers all over the world have found that more men are involved in extramarital affairs than women; more women are affected by abuse, and more men are workaholics. Factors such as chronic illness of the partner and terminal illnesses like cancer or infertility are a few more examples of how couples in India get divorced. Like Christian marriage, Hindu marriage does not expect the partners to support each other in illness and wellness. So just to get rid of the effort and pain associated with illness and the limitations of the partner's life due to illness, they get divorced.

The emotional stages of divorce are accepting reality, moving on, coping with extreme emotional swings, depression, sense of loss, social withdrawal resulting in loss of support from relatives, rejection, embarrassment and denial. Emotionally, the person becomes vulnerable, and anger, guilt, low self-esteem and loss of sense of identity are commonly experienced. Alienation, hostility and tense interactions make the problem worse. Bargaining, trying to find out the possibility of repair, undoing and managing the effects on self-esteem are essential strategies for overcoming the ill effects. There are pent-up feelings which disturb the individual further. The recent trend in developed countries is that less time is devoted to the maintenance of marital relations. Anger and withdrawal by a man develop anxiety and fear in a woman's mind. Men generally are critical, defensive and contemptuous and use stonewalling. All these behavioural patterns are specifically used when they feel inferior and inadequate as providers, lovers and protectors. Similar behavioural patterns are seen among women when they experience fear of harm, deprivation and isolation (Finkel et al., 2014). The effects of anger depend on to whom it is directed.

Sbarra et al. (2015) conducted some research in Arizona and proved that divorce leads to prolonged emotional distress, including clinical depression. Divorced individuals have a 23 per cent higher mortality rate.

> Even well-educated people use inhuman tricks to get a divorce in no time. In 2018, in Pune, Maharashtra, a doctor gave HIV-infected saline to his pregnant wife as her parents were not capable of fulfilling his demands for dowry, and she was not ready to give divorce.[5]

The legal procedure for divorce is frustrating and tiring in India. Legal divorce is a long process which requires a lot of effort, time and money. As a consequence, it is very difficult for a lady to bear it. If she is economically dependent, has young children, is illiterate or semi-literate or from a rural area, it becomes even more difficult. Repeatedly, she has to travel to the court and manage things for years. It is emotionally exhausting and creates more problems. Custody of children and settlement regarding money are the key issues.

Problems do not decrease after divorce. On the contrary, they increase. Due to two separate households, the cost of maintenance increases. In spite of the provision of alimony, which is mostly insufficient, women suffer as they have lower potential to earn while looking after children. As the other partner, mostly the husband, is not allowed to see the children very often, it affects his mental health and stability of personality. Recent research has demonstrated that even when an individual is unhappily married, their well-being does not increase due to divorce. It is on par with those who remain married.

The dimensions include self-esteem, personal mastery, purpose in life, depression, alcohol consumption and the like. Suicidal tendencies are also more in divorcees. Their life expectancy decreases and even their children's life expectancy reduces by four years. The possibilities of major illnesses such as stroke, cancer, infectious diseases, heart problems, arthritis and even sexually transmitted diseases have increased.

In the case of extreme conflict, a divorce is better and can have positive effects. However, if the dispute does not cause much problems for the children, divorce may lead to more harm. Children of divorcee families face behaviour problems, are more abused and consider divorce as an appropriate answer to marital problems. These children are more involved in early sex, drug abuse, alcoholism and suicide. If there is marital discord, the offspring suffer even in the long term. They face health problems and psychological problems. Anxiety, depression, addiction and premarital sex are very common among these children. Emotional divorce is withdrawal, emotional detachment and mutual hatred, antagonism and hostility. This hurts the partners depending on the injustice they have to tolerate. Children suffer most in such a situation.

Adjustment to remaining single is also a challenging task. Some common reasons for remaining single are cheating by marriage alliance, unattractive appearance, ill health, incapability, difficulty finding a partner, high career aspirations, not willing to shoulder responsibility, unhappy childhood due to parental marital discord and homosexuality. It is easy and socially less tabooed for a man to stay alone. They are free and relaxed. However, single women may not feel secure and may face many problems, such as social rejection, restrictions, pressures and character assassination. Premarital and extramarital sex can result in not only sexually transmitted diseases and AIDS, but also a lot of distrust, discord, maladjustment and many more negative effects, both physiological and psychological.

Widowhood is a traumatic situation where social stigma is still seen. After her husband's death, a lady is mostly deprived of property and is disowned by traditional Indian families. Sometimes, there is no provision to support the lady and her offspring for survival. For generations, a widow has not been allowed to participate in any religious or social function. Inhuman practices, such as shaving the head of a widow and no possibility of remarriage, were prevalent for many generations. She was treated as if it was her fault or misfortune and she was responsible for his death. A widower, however, is in better condition. Immediately after the death of his wife, his family use to start planning a remarriage. Irrespective of age, education, number of children and socio-economic conditions, it has been customary to give priority to the comfort of a widower.

In India, there is hardly any awareness about the various skills necessary for developing good interpersonal relations with one's life partner. Sharing of power and authority, labour and responsibilities, conflict management skills and mutual respect make both of them psychologically healthy and happy. Women, for physiological and social as well as psychological reasons, are more involved in emotional closeness, sharing of experiences, tenderness and security. The male may not be oriented to all these. Hence, it is a must to understand each other's perspective and develop empathy for one's partner.

The behaviour of today's modern youth is reported by researchers as a combination of partially traditional and partially modern views, attitudes and interaction patterns. They are practising the American style of life before marriage while enjoying premarital sexual relations, and being very traditional when it comes to marriage. Hence, they want their partner to be virgin and very smart at the same time. In this situation, there are chances of deception and cognitive dissonance. Most marriages are still arranged. According to researchers, the percentage is more than 90.

In a typical Indian traditional family, there is no emotional catharsis. The husband can't discuss things openly with his wife, who can't help him solve his problems. Male members generally don't disclose their problems to anyone and consider them a loss of status. For example, if the husband can't earn enough money for proper maintenance of the family, he pretends that there is no problem, though there is constant stress. Both of them are in their own worlds and can't even think of helping each other. In such a situation, marriage results in a sort of burden and may lead to a lot of unhappiness.

General interactions among the relatives of the husband and wife are based on misunderstandings, misconceptions and undue expectations related to stereotypical ideas. Her parents are supposed to spend a lot of money to please his parents even after many years of marriage. Whatever they do, many times, it is not enough, and there is some discord. This, in turn, leads to unhappiness, quarrels and poor relations between husband and wife. A lot of distress is created for the newly wed young lady. In extreme cases, she is harassed, abused, physically beaten, provoked to commit suicide or is actually killed. There is constant anxiety, frustration, depression, hopelessness and helplessness due to which the young ladies suffer from severe consequences like depression.

Of the total murders of ladies, more than 80 per cent are done by their family members. So they don't feel secure even at home. This is a major hindrance to psycho-social health. In 2018, according to the National Crime Records Bureau, 134,516 married young ladies killed themselves due to marital discord (Kajal, 2020).

Relations between mother-in-law and daughter-in-law are known to be very strained. Every now and then, the mother-in-law in some traditional families critically evaluates every activity of the daughter-in-law, restricts her activities, insults her, compels her to do various household jobs and may even compel her to terminate pregnancy if it is a female foetus, as she is the ultimate authority. The husband also can't protect his wife and generally neglects all these things. All these constant unwanted interactions lead to psychological illness. It is difficult to get the exact figures as there is hardly any research regarding these issues and individuals are not supposed to disclose their family problems to others.

Unnatural sexual practices, bizarre expectations, disorders related to sex, like sex addiction of the partner, lead to extreme mental disorders for the partner. Abusing the partner emotionally, physically, economically and socially results in psycho-social problems. Forcing the wife to wear a particular type of dress or act in a particular way may lead to frustration and hate. This type of ownership makes even lovemaking an automatic activity. Infidelity also plays an important role in the mental health of married couples. Claiming that the husband is not the biological father of the baby or paranoid suspicion affects the partner's mental health. It affects emotional balance, produces guilt and shame, awkwardness, social stigma and the like. This results in physiological and psychological problems.

Going abroad and compelling the wife to stay back and shoulder the responsibilities of the old in-laws is also a new trend. Here, the wife becomes burned out and may become frustrated and alienated. Drug addiction and alcoholism detach an individual from his partner. In India, not only low socio-economic strata youth, but well-educated and well-to-do people also give preference to such enjoyment. In such circumstances, the wife gets emotionally hurt, aloof and loses interest in marital relations. This affects her psycho-social health adversely.

Deception leads to a loss of trust and the inability to love. It also generates a sense of hopelessness in the victim. Hidden mental illnesses, like schizophrenia, may develop agony and a feeling of martyrdom as the individual discovers them. The whole life of the victim becomes worthless. These are some examples of the relationship between mental health and marriage.

5.6. CORRECTIVE MEASURES

Loyalty, integrity and unity are three basic pillars of a firm family system. The whole world appreciates the stable family system of India. Values, morals, religious faith and socially acceptable behaviour patterns are developed in the next generation because of such a permanent family bond. Although there are many problems related to marriage in the Indian community, there are many positive outcomes also. Specially, if interpersonal relations are maintained properly, marriage results in multiple advantages of varied nature, such as social, psychological, financial and the like.

There are some very significant functions of marriage. It regulates sexual behaviour by providing satisfaction of personal needs in a socially acceptable manner. The division of labour is useful for dividing work as per convenience, skills, expertise and physiological characteristics. Marriage should be an emotional union so that psychological health and stability can be achieved. To maintain a good marital relations, it is essential to understand gender differences which influence relations. Women value marital relations and give a lot of importance and weightage to them. Their happiness, satisfaction, as well as their self-worth, depend on marital relations. Women are more involved in feelings and emotions in marital relations. They communicate their ideas indirectly. They like to share and like to be listened to. This is the preference of the auditory channel. They expect the partner to honestly communicate everything. Women's needs are affection, commitment, openness and financial support. Men communicate directly, briefly and want to focus on reasons rather than emotions. Their communication is based on logical analysis and systematic predictions. They prefer visual channels. They are work-oriented, detached and they value power and authority. For them, achievements are more important than maintaining interpersonal relationships. They don't accept any help from their wives. This causes detachment and poor relations. Male members need sexual satisfaction, an attractive spouse, pleasant company for light activities, such as recreation and domestic support. They need approval and admiration.

Considering these differences, one has to make special efforts to develop good relations with one's partner. The interaction should be such that it should contribute to enhancing the self-esteem of one's partner. The most essential for that is having empathy, without which it is impossible to understand the psychological status of one's partner. The expression of respect, devoting attention, spending quality time and affirmation make the whole interaction worthy. Intimacy develops due to accepting differences, kindness, keeping promises and sharing power and responsibility. Forgiving, accepting one's own mistakes and expressing apology, appreciating and considering others' opinions while making important decisions creates a conducive environment. Respect, which is essential for healthy relations, is related to trust, cooperation, support, honesty, safety and accountability.

Marriage may provide an enhanced feeling of meaning and purpose, improved self-worth and a sense of mastery (Bierman et al., 2006). Marriage is ideally expected to generate both independence and togetherness. Both partners should have and express gratitude and appreciation. According to Chatterjee (1999), best marriages are based on intimate friendship at an intellectual and emotional level. A good support system is needed to overcome problems and their ill effects. To improve relations with marriage partner, it is recommended that one has to reduce expectations and communicate wholeheartedly. One should not try to control behaviour of one's partner. One should express that the partner plays an important role in happiness in life. Accepting each other's limitations enhances good relations.

It is worth noting that, irrespective of gender, marriage may result in happiness or unhappiness. Even a male member may be harassed, exploited and given unfair treatment. The proportion of such inhuman treatment to husbands is comparatively substantially less. However, it is equally harmful to the individual. For example, a son-in-law may face nagging, insults, excess work, financial, emotional and social subordination and the like. In some communities, they are supposed to work for their in-laws families for the whole of their lives. For example, in Meghalaya in Khasi marriage, men live with their wives and their families (Bhattacharya, 2015). If men suffer, it is also equally unfair and needs immediate attention.

Proper self-confidence, family support, the opportunity to be independent and solve problems with the help of a counsellor may result in improving the condition. Proactive and positive thinking, assertiveness, problem-solving skills are essential for that. Before marriage, it is essential to make the bride emotionally, cognitively and economically independent. She must know ways of self-defence. She should be ready to face any problem, be strong and firm. Both the genders must get an equal opportunity to develop potentials and the family members should share other responsibilities for that.

Male members should be oriented towards enhancing a sense of power only by making the other gender more comfortable, whether it be mother, sister or life partner. They should get proper guidance regarding extra strength like muscular power, more vitality and freedom and how to use it for achieving success in life rather than just getting involved in misusing it. A balance point is necessary for cultural demands and philosophy where an individual's happiness, satisfaction, and development should be given importance rather than only customs and traditions.

No achievement is greater than mutual harmony, unconditional love, acceptance and affection that we can develop with our family members and help each other to lead a happy and healthy life. In such a situation, mutual support may generate satisfaction and happiness for both husband and wife.

5.7. SUMMARY

Marriage is not only one of the most important developmental tasks but also the main source of maintaining good psycho-social health. If the partners are well adjusted to each other and the environment is equally conducive for both of them, it leads to the ultimate happiness in human life. However, in India, there are many customs and traditions which are detrimental to that.

The mutual adjustment of husband and wife depends on many things, and most of them can be modified for the better. Improving adjustment with mate depends on various factors, such as concept and image of ideal mate and discrepancy between the actual partner and ideal one. Needs fulfilment, similarity of values, interests and general background, understanding regarding the role of each one and differences in each other's concepts and demands due to marriage contribute a lot.

The stability of the family system is essentially related to the firm value system and general health of society. Hence, it is essential to rethink about inappropriate practices and various types of exploitation. No one should take undue advantage of any given situation. It is essential to practice androgyny.

Pornography Addiction and Sexual Addiction

6.1. INTRODUCTION

The galloping advancement of science and technology has changed the whole lives of the younger generation: cognitively, emotionally and even socially. The internet unfolds a whole world of knowledge and information. The number of internet users in India was around 70 crore in 2020. Since 1995, the number of consumers has been increasing every moment. India is the second largest market for the internet after China. The most vital thing in the lives of adolescents and youth is the smartphone. Emotional dependency on smartphones is highest in India. Recently, it was reported by researchers that in India, 65 per cent of smartphone users think that smartphone is their best friend. Around 47 per cent of the youth prefer smartphone to being with their loved ones. A total of 75 per cent of parents in advanced countries don't consider it safe. In Britain, a survey was conducted recently of 2,000 parents. By the age of 6, children get the facility to use the internet via smartphones; at the age of 10, it is 92 per cent, and by 12 years, it is even more than 96 per cent. Internet addiction is found to be related to loneliness and depression among youth.

The internet has generated entirely novel forms and problems of sexual and gender issues. Millions of sexually explicit conversations, apps and photographs are uploaded to the internet every day. The advanced internet facility provides multiple sex chat rooms for chatting with people having a variety of different sexual interests, like gays. Hence, the most popular use of smartphones is for pornography consumption. The proportion of adolescents and youth watching pornography regularly is increasing every day in India (Joseph, 2019).

More than 80 per cent of Indian high school students are exposed to porn (Das, 2013). Around 75 per cent of pre-university students in rural areas of India are addicted to porn (*The Indian Express*, 27 February 2013). There are many articles and videos about this cyber-sex addiction, like Cover Story: Pornography and Its Devastating Consequences on Youth and Women in India (FM Editorial, 2014). Recently, research-based books have also been published, like *Youth and Internet Pornography: The Impact and Influence on Adolescent Development* (Bel, 2019).

What do Indians do with the free Wi-Fi provided by the government at railway stations? *The Times of India* (17 February 2018) mentions that free Wi-Fi at railway stations is mostly being used for viewing and downloading pornography (also by Zee News, 18 October 2016). From 2013 to 2017, porn trafficking increased by 121 per cent in India. This estimate is more than that of any other country. After internet data became cheap, porn consumption increased by 75 per cent. The total time spent watching porn also increased by 60 per cent. About 2,800 crore times porn was searched in 2018 in India. About 800 sites of pornography are banned. Still, tricks to access porn are being used. The most preferred are violent sex videos (Zee News, 2019). Researchers in India have stated that under reporting of consumption of pornography is a serious issue even when confidentiality is ensured (Sharma, 2019).

> According to one estimate, there are more than 26 crore websites serving pornography. A new pornographic video is prepared every few minutes, and every second there are thousands of people watching internet pornography. These estimates are multiplied every month. An increase of 405 per cent was reported in downloads of porn in one year. Around 95 per cent of the spike in porn consumption is reported during lockdown in India. Around 70 per cent of students in India watch pornography by the age of 10. It is worth noting that publishing or transmitting pornography is illegal in India (Seth, 2020).

Pornography affects individuals' lives adversely in every sense. It may lead to uncontrollable sexual urges which may result in socially unacceptable expressions and crimes against women. Indian consumers are more interested in finding out and sharing porn videos depicting real-life rape. Those who upload such videos on porn sites are getting lakhs of rupees from porn sites (*Maharashtra Times*, 8 December 2019). All over the world, this business is worth billions of dollars. Such actual rape videos from India are very popular all over the world. Also, videos regarding gang rape are the most searched for and shared. Uttar Pradesh, New Delhi, Haryana, Madhya Pradesh and some states from the South are the leading states for uploading such videos. In India, some states have the highest number of viewers. They are Delhi, Punjab, Rajasthan, Jammu & Kashmir and the North-eastern states. One more trend is that such actual videos are of socially unacceptable physical relations between student–teacher, youth–sister-in-law, youth–aunty and the like. According to cyber experts, one in every 16 persons is interested in real porn.

6.2. NATURE, SIGNS, SYMPTOMS AND FACTORS FACILITATING PORNOGRAPHY ADDICTION

Pornography is printed or audio–visual material which intends to stimulate sexual excitement and, for that reason, depicts the explicit display or description of sex organs and activities. Many scientific definitions include the depiction of erotic behaviour for immediate intense emotional reactions along with sexual arousal. Cambridge Dictionary defines (2018) it contents of printed material or audio–visuals without artistic value that describe or show sexual acts or naked people in a way that is intended to be sexually exciting. Many others have mentioned videos, photographs, movies and stated that it is an open and direct way of depicting sex. Pornography shows sexually stimulating and arousing acts using real models. It shows various private parts of both men and women and depicts intercourse natural, anal and oral in various styles and positions. There are various categories, such as lesbian, gay, group sex and hardcore. Some such films may also be about child pornography, painful actions during intercourse and sexual aggression. Animals are also used for sexual experiments. Women are whipped, beaten, raped, tortured and exploited in every sense. Women are depicted as passive victims and objects of mere sexual pleasure. According to Kuhn et al. (2007), 'pornography is a communication material provided for the purpose of sexually arousing or gratifying a user in isolation from others or in company of others.' When the time devoted to porn is too much, it has a significant negative impact on not only interpersonal and intrapersonal relations, academic achievement, health and performance on job but all areas of life. It results in porn addiction. Porn addiction is an ever-growing compulsion to view pornographic material. There are no demands in terms of expression of love, involvement, responsibility or pleasant interaction. Now, the mass media, the internet, social media and the availability of smartphones make it very convenient for the viewer as it is available anytime, anywhere to anybody.

Child pornography is also very popular among viewers. Children used for child pornography range from less than 3–12 years, depicting oral sex, genital touching and penetration. Child pornography is illegal and banned in India. Approximately 3,000 sites showing child pornography are banned by the Indian government.

Various international studies have shown porn consumption to be 50–99 per cent among men and 30–86 per cent among women. The exact figures may vary depending on culture, availability of smartphones and privacy, socio-economic condition and daily routine of the individuals studied. The most important thing is the openness and honesty of participants to accept that they watch pornography. In Indian research, it was recently reported that pornography addiction starts at the age of 10, and teenagers and young adults are represented as the maximum number of porn addicts.

Although the exact symptoms depend on the severity of addiction, generally:

- There is a strong urge to view porn. It is the craving for porn which is accompanied by withdrawal features, irritability, loss of aim, preoccupation throughout the day with the same thoughts and the inability to have a normal relationship with family and friends.
- As a consequence of pornography addiction, students underachieve and employees can't concentrate on their duties. Specially, among married and unmarried couples, reduced sexual satisfaction, decreased intimacy and undue expectations from partners are experienced.

- Gradually, the time of porn viewing increases and all the remaining things become less important for an individual.
- These addicts can't accept the idea of reducing or terminating viewing of porn. They become angry, argumentative, hostile and irritated in such conditions.
- Most addicts watch porn secretly. They hide it fully or partially from family and friends. Addicts feel awkward and guilty about accepting their behaviour. So there is secrecy in relations also. Some overcompensation for hiding these things is seen in their behaviour.
- Even if the individual attempts to get rid of their porn addiction, they are unable to do so. Approximately 9 per cent of the viewers are reported to be trapped like that.
- Increasingly, more provoking porn is needed for getting same amount of satisfaction.

Researchers have also reported that 60 per cent of pornography addicts have difficulty achieving arousal with their partner, though they could achieve it with pornography. This is called porn-induced erectile dysfunction.

Researchers have reported that the perceived motives of cybersex are instant gratification, escape from tension and anxiety, a sense of approval and affirmation and disease-free sexual satisfaction. It helps to cope with the pain of childhood sexual abuse. Those who are lonely, introvert, have trouble establishing satisfactory relations with the opposite sex and lack warm maternal relations in childhood are found to be more attracted to porn. More addicts prefer violent porn.

There are some positive outcomes to watching pornography in a limited way. It is useful for managing sex impulses, reducing guilt and shame about sex and accepting it as a natural enjoyment in life. However, it is essential to give scientific information about the risks involved in exaggerated and unnatural sexual practices.

6.3. BIOLOGICAL, SOCIAL AND PSYCHOLOGICAL EFFECTS OF PORNOGRAPHY

Pornography results in various ill effects. Basically, these three effects are immensely significant.

6.3.1. Biological Effects

Substantial research has been done regarding the neurobiology of pornography addiction. Young adults are highly vulnerable to porn addiction and rewiring of the brain. Their brains are at the peak of dopamine production and neuroplasticity. Pornography overloads circuits and creates desire, dependence and desensitization. That, in turn, creates a very strong experience, forming strong memories. Porn does not activate the brain's natural aversion system. So the activity can be continued with the same liking for an unlimited time.

> The medical daily Journal of *JAMA Psychiatry* presented research in 2014 which found that porn may shrink the brain, which leads to a smaller striatum with fewer connections. This may happen when watching pornography becomes less rewarding. As similar changes in the brain are seen in the cases of depression, alcoholism and loneliness, some overlapping effects may result from these changes. For example, if a depressed person is a pornography addict, it is difficult to find the exact contribution of each condition.

Pornography addiction is associated with some specific phenomena, which are as follows:

1. Pornography activates mirror neurons system located in the frontal and parietal lobes. Mirror neurons mimic or imitate actions and help in the observational learning. The mirror neuron system stimulates and triggers arousal, which leads to sexual tension (Schmauder, 2015). As a consequence, the individual gets more involved in watching porn.
2. The neurotransmitter dopamine plays an important role in reward-related learning. Dopamine is responsible for 'arousal addiction'. The brain prefers images and is less satisfied with real-life partners. There are many couples who face serious problems because the addict partner is never satisfied with their sexual interaction and keeps on thinking of more provocative images and ideas about porn. As repeated dopamine surges result into desensitization, they try to get more exciting novel stimuli for a longer duration, more frequent porn viewing to get the same arousal. This again leads to a constantly increasing and more intense desire, which results in

addiction. Dopamine spikes during viewing of pornography last longer than normal sex.

3. Pornography addiction releases bodily endorphins, which are pain-reducing natural substances responsible for euphoria, transcendence and pleasure feelings.

4. Hormones, oxytocin and vasopressin are released during orgasm and are meant for attachment and bonding with the partner. If they are released while watching pornography, there is hardly any attachment to their life partner. Oxytocin is a natural tranquillizer and helps in dealing with stress. So if associated with porn watching, it becomes a strengthening factor for addiction.

5. While watching pornography, the neurotransmitter serotonin is released. This, in turn, causes changes in mood and results in calm, relaxed feelings and a sense of enjoyment.

6. Another important point is that norepinephrine stores memories related to sexually explicit material for years. This keeps the brain alert and aroused. The hormone, testosterone, is released and that increases sex drive. Both these things result in more vulnerability to pornography addiction.

When a person wants to escape from painful emotions, porn is used. Many porn addicts use other forms of sex, such as webcam sex, sexting, casual or anonymous sex, affairs, prostitution, exhibition and voyeurism online or offline. Sexual stimulation experienced by an individual and sexual behaviour are both regulated by hypothalamic nuclei. It is an integration centre for such information. Nuclei receive information from the mesolimbic dopamine pathway. The reward centre in the human brain, which is related to the feeling of pleasure, is activated due to pornography. It communicates with other areas such as the hippocampus, amygdala and frontal cortex related to memory and emotions and coordinates them with attention, motivation and reward. That is responsible for behaviour also. The role of the mesolimbic dopamine pathway is important in this interaction.

Childress et al. (1999) conducted a study where functional MRI scans of cocaine-addicted patients were analysed.

Visually, two different types of stimuli were presented to the addicts for just 33 milliseconds. One type was regarding drug-related images and the other was sexually related erotic images. It was observed that both the stimulations resulted in activation of the same limbic system/reward centre. Doidge (2015) has reported that internet pornography stimulates neuro-plastic changes which are responsible for the perception of positive reinforcement related to the experience.

Gray matter in the area of the brain known for sexual arousal and motivation, that is, the dorsal striatum, is negatively correlated with pornography consumption. That means more pornography consumption is correlated with lower grey matter volume in the dorsal striatum.

Many scientific articles are available regarding pornography addiction and ways to deal with it (Cherikal, 2018). Before adolescents could develop the capacity to integrate factual information into their healthy sexual identity, they are prematurely exposed to pornography. According to Benedeck and Brown (1999), this leads to modelling and imitation which interferes with normal sexual development. That, in turn, results in shame, guilt, anxiety and confusion. Such psychological status leads to harmful attitudes, aggression and sexual experiments, sexual acting out, depersonalization of women, poor social bonds and ultimately pornography addiction (Stack et al., 2004).

Pornography addiction is related to moral and ethical decisions also. In a very interesting research, it was observed that watching porn is related to morality and will power. Schmauder (2015) has reported that watching pornography and masturbating weakens cingulate cortex that is the region responsible for ethical and moral decision-making and willpower. Such researches are clearly indicating that physiological impact of pornography is directly linked with individual's moral behaviour and cognitive processes. It is also proved that biological reinforcement enhances pornography addiction.

Porn addiction is reported to be associated with various sexual problems having serious ill effects. Most common are the loss of libido, erectile dysfunction, early ejaculations, desire and practice of unnatural sex: anal and oral. Pornography addiction leads to multiple extramarital or premarital affairs and casual sex, which increases the risk of STDs, such as HIV, Hepatitis B and C, gonorrhoea, syphilis, herpes and the like.

6.3.2. Social Effects

The social effects of pornography addiction can't be underestimated. The most detrimental effect is regarding the increasing incidence of crime associated with watching pornography. It has been scientifically proven that, since 1990, violent and degrading behavioural patterns shown in pornography have negatively influenced the attitudes of addicts. It increases fantasies of rape, distorted belief that some women secretly desire to be raped and general insensitivity to rape victims increases. All these, in turn, lead to acceptance of violence against women, sex without emotional involvement and the urge to watch more violent pornography. In a way, it is a vicious circle.

Ill-known serial murderers from all over the world, including in the USA, namely Ted Bundy, Gary Bishop and Jeffrey Dahmer, confessed in their interviews that pornographic material was an influential factor in their compulsion and obsession with sexual offenses and murders.

Similar cases are also abundant in India. Thirty children were killed by a serial killer in Uttar Pradesh, Haryana and New Delhi. The killer used to watch pornography, drink and, due to uncontrollable sexual arousal, then used to find poor children. Ravinder, the killer, was a porn addict and was involved in drug and alcohol abuse too (BBC News, 23 July 2015). A very ill-known serial killer in Nithari in Utter Pradesh used to rape young girls and kill them. The murderers were involved in child pornography (*India Today*, 29 October 2014).

A whole family was killed by a school principal when he was caught red-handed while watching porn and performing some awful activity. Afterwards, he killed himself (*Mirror*, 27 February 2019). He was so deeply involved in pornography that he had accessed 97 per cent of salacious websites on his school PC and the remaining on his phone. IB Times (Nair, 2014) reported that Ram (age 19) and Manoj Kumar (age 22) raped a five-year-old girl and told that they were ... 'fired by pornography and alcohol'. In Gurgaon, a 7-year-old child was killed after a sexual assault in school. He was killed by a student in Class 11. The murderer loved watching porn and watched porn on the day of the murder. He is a porn addict and used to watch porn during school hours also. The murderer sodomized the child before murder

(Zee Media, 9 November 2017). There are hundreds of such cases reported by the media. On 4 December 2019, in the east Godavari district, a 60-year-old woman was sexually assaulted and murdered. The accused was a pornography addict. His phone was full of pornographic videos. He had watched porn before committing the crime (*The Hindu*, 8 December 2019).

Due to pornography, respect for family relations and boundaries of intimacy are both vanishing. Pornography addicts are eager to experiment and experience the thrill of various sexual acts, even with family members, including mother, mother-in-law, sister, niece and their own daughter. This deterioration of values indicates that the family system is going to lose its selfless unconditional love and emotional support, especially for women.

Recently, in December 2018, a porn addict killed his sister-in-law and niece and then raped them (*Navbharat Times*, 4 December 2018). On 12 June 2018, a 14-year-old porn addict raped his own sister in Mumbai (*Maharashtra Times*, 2018). A pornography addict raped his mother in Palanpur, Gujarat (*Maharashtra Times*, 22 April 2018). In December 2019, in Hyderabad, a man raped his mother-in-law (News 18, 16 December 2019).

By and large, love, affection, emotional support and a sense of security are expected to be achieved only as a by-product of socially sanctioned sex satisfaction, that is, marriage. In case of all premarital and extramarital sexual relations, emotional, social and legal problems arise.

Very young children are also involved in pornography and this premature exposure stimulates them sexually. Four children, ranging from 6–10 years old, used to enjoy watching pornography. They gang raped a 4-year-old girl in Kanpur (*Navbharat Times*, 3 July 2018).

Crimes related to sexual aggression against women and girls are increasing substantially all over India. The statistics regarding the same are more than enough to prove that in the last few years, it has increased 400 times. There are many incidences which are never reported, and the most obvious among them are marital rape and marital sexual aggression, which is obviously a serious abuse. Most of them are closely related to porn addiction.

Experts in the area have given alarming advice that it is essential to ban pornography to arrest human trafficking. Kidnapped women and children are reported to be exploited for sexual abuse and for working as models for pornographic films. Although it is illegal in 140 countries, human trafficking is the third major danger after weapons, arms and drugs in the whole world. For example, 3 lakh adolescents are kidnapped every year in the USA.

In short, research has found that there is a significant positive association between pornography use and attitudes supporting violence against women. An addict who is accustomed to watching substantial aggression against women gradually starts thinking that it is acceptable and natural. It is also reported all over the world that sexual aggression increases due to porn watching. According to one estimate, 88 per cent of scenes contain physical aggression, and 49 per cent contain verbal aggression. As a consequence of these attitudes, girls and women from addicts' families, from their schools or colleges, workplaces and society at large suffer.

6.3.3. Psychological Ill Effects of Watching Pornography

Pornography addiction affects every aspect of human life, from the personal level to the academic and professional level.

Due to the number of hours of secret activity, the person gets isolated, withdrawn from family and friends. There is no time to devote to other activities, which are essential for maintaining family and social contacts. As an addict gets socially isolated, impulsivity, compulsive behaviour, trouble with relationship stability and intimacy, low ability to tolerate frustration and problems with coping with emotions emerge. Risky behaviour, insecurity, frustration and anger may result. Financial losses can cause some other problems. Legal issues can also arise. Two major correlates of pornography addiction are alcoholism and depression.

It affects academic achievement, career and work as it decreases involvement in studies and productivity and performance at work. Difficulties with concentrating on lessons in spite of being physically present in the class and other concentration problems are very common. This is indirectly related to poor self-concept, self-worth and loss of self-confidence. The person becomes apathetic about future goals and has lower aspirations. Pornography results in disturbed relationships and lower sexual satisfaction as well (Sex Roles, 2012).

As the number of hours of pornography increases, emotional distancing, lack of intimacy and unrealistic expectations regarding sexual relations increase. Uncontrollable desires lead to compulsive behaviour and affect the whole personality. Pornography shapes sexual attitudes, perceptions and sex behaviour. It leads to unrealistic expectations regarding unnatural sex from the partner. That, in turn, results in the deterioration of married life, family and interpersonal relationships. The psychological ill effects of detachment, immorality and isolation, secrecy, deception, insecurity, betrayal feelings, separation and divorce are the indirect consequences which cause emotional distress. It is detrimental to not only the partner of an addict, but their children, parents, siblings and others. Other problems, such as battered women syndrome, child victims and crimes lead to extremely unpleasant consequences detrimental to mental health.

In short, disturbed intimate relations, feelings of shame and guilt, problems in every sphere of life and the loss of status in the community due to social rejection and failures result in other more serious psychological disorders, like mood disorders, and substance and alcohol abuse. In a way, the individual wants to avoid facing reality and the real challenges of life. In addition, anxiety, obsessive-compulsive disorder and learning disability are reported by researchers as risk factors for pornography addiction. Introverted and highly educated people are more inclined to develop sexual internet addictions (KLFY.com, 2018).

6.4. INTERVENTION

Skinner's seven levels of porn addiction (2017) can be utilized to assess the severity of porn addiction. If a standardized test is not available, a questionnaire may be used for assessing the necessity of helping and treating.

In India, watching pornography is, by and large, socially unapproved and tabooed. An addict may feel awkward and may not be comfortable accepting that they are a porn addict. So the first stage is to accept that one is suffering and then to approach a knowledgeable and experienced professional for help. An individual should communicate honestly and share everything with the therapist, which may help to treat them properly.

Some useful strategies for psychological intervention are as follows:

1. **Self-monitoring:** The addict may be asked to write down their experiences during and after each session of porn viewing. They should also write about and examine the consequences of each pornography engagement episode. Introspection and objectively understanding as well as accepting the experiences and their effects on mental status and physical conditions may help. An individual should objectively evaluate the impact of involvement in work and studies as a consequence of that. This will lead to insight into the problem. Setting limits and goals by self may be more useful for self-discipline than any other external control. The use of cognitive restructuring, delay of gratification, long-term planning, enhancing self-efficacy and self-confidence and giving reward and reinforcement to self for reducing time spent watching pornography are essential for regulating behaviour.

2. **Acceptance and commitment therapy:** Instead of being defensive, addicts must be encouraged to accept the facts and be objective about their problems. Here, the addict should not avoid and hide the problem. An addict should be given appropriate support to have the courage to face it. This leads to a commitment to behaviour that facilitates thriving. Accepting what is out of their control, practising mindfulness and then commitment to act to improve their life may effectively reduce addiction.

3. **Self-discipline:** Opportunities to enhance self-esteem and self-image, addressing emotional problems, limiting computer and mobile use and blocking pornographic sites are basic steps for enhancing self-discipline. Open discussion with parents and guidance given by teachers may help in developing a balanced view regarding age-appropriate surfing. As children grow older, parents should share some ideas and actually surf with them. Keeping an eye on what the adolescents are surfing without physically controlling them is a must.

4. **Cognitive behaviour therapy:** Counsellors may use it to change thoughts and behaviour. However, as there are strong associations with physiological and biochemical factors, it should be supplemented with drug therapy.

5. **Proper psycho education:** It should include scientific information not only about sex and physiology but also about pornography, its ill effects, risks and losses in detail. The relationship between pornography and sex addiction also be made clear. The WHO has reported that difficulty in managing sex impulses is one of the major causes of mental health problems among Indian students.

6. **Psychodynamic psychotherapy:** This therapy, for porn addiction, explores the core conflicts that drive dysfunctional sexual expressions. Themes of shame, avoidance, anger and impaired self-esteem and efficacy are common.

7. **Family therapy:** Family members may be encouraged to understand and help adolescents and youth. Couple therapy may restore trust, minimize shame/guilt and establish a healthy sexual relationship between life partners. It may assist the life partner to understand the emotional problems of the addict. Pharmacotherapy may be used to decrease the urges or cravings and preoccupation associated with sex and pornographic addiction. Mood stabilizers are also used for the treatment of patients with bipolar disorder and compulsive sexual behaviour. Regulating sexual hormone function, lower serum testosterone levels diminishes sexual drive and desire.

Inspector Pratibha Sharma, investigating officer of the Nirbhaya case, mentioned that 'easy access to pornography is damaging the entire generation' (Trivedi, 2019).

6.5. SEXUAL ADDICTION: CAUSE, SYMPTOMS AND RISKS

As sexual satisfaction is a natural physiological need, some experts put forth the view that the dividing line between normal and abnormal sex drive and behaviour related to it is difficult to decide. However, uncontrollable and exaggerated sexual activity is seen in the case of sex addicts. Hypersexuality or sex addiction is a serious problem among contemporary youth. Its evidence was found as early as the year 1700. It is known by various names, such as erotomania, nymphomania in females, excessive sexual drive, satyriasis, Don Juanism and paraphilia. It includes loss of control or limited control of excessive sex urges, fantasies and behaviour, which, in turn, results in many more problems. It was included in the Diagnostic and Statistical Manual of Mental Disorders-IV-TR for the first time. It is also included in the International Statistical Classification of Diseases and Related Health Problems 10th version 2010 (Section F 52.8). As mentioned in it, sex addiction is 'a situation where experience of distress is highlighted due to a pattern of repeated sexual relationships involving a succession of partners used only as things'. It is out of control sexual behaviour which leads to distress. The term sexual addict indicates compulsive behaviour regarding sexual acts despite their negative consequences. These consequences may affect someone else or the person or both. It may be limited to compulsive masturbation or viewing pornography or may extend to getting involved in socially unacceptable sexual acts such as exhibitionism, voyeurism, failure to resist sexual impulses or even rape. It results in difficulty in normal functioning in social situations.

Even in the International Statistical Classification of Diseases and Related Health Problems 11 (2018, 6 c 72), it is described as a compulsive sexual behaviour disorder. It is characterized by a persistent pattern of failure to control intense, repetitive sexual impulses or urges, resulting in repetitive sexual behaviour. It leads to substantial distress and impairment in personal, familial, social, educational, occupational and all important areas of life.

As sexual addiction is a blanket term, it includes different types of problematic behaviour. All over the world, it is estimated that it affects 3–6 per cent of people. For example, in the USA, approximately 30 million people are sex addicts. It affects both men and women. Sexually deviant behaviour is classified into two types: nonparaphilic and paraphilic addiction. In nonparaphilic addiction, fantasies and sexual behaviours that are supposed to be normal are included. In paraphilic addiction, fantasies and behaviours related to sex which are unacceptable to society are incorporated. Hence, consumption of pornography is grouped under the paraphilic group.

6.5.1. Causes of Sexual Addiction

According to experts, it may be a symptom of other psychodynamic diseases such as depression, compulsive personality disorder and loneliness. Biochemical imbalances and social as well as family-related problems also trigger such types of behaviour. Family dysfunctions, broken families, families with criminal records, lack of proper love and affection, extremely low socio-economic status and valueless peer groups are some correlates of sex addiction. Some researchers have proved that there is a lack of self-confidence and intense guilt among these addicts. They get involved in sex just to feel good.

Carnes, a very well-known researcher in this field who has published many articles and books on this issue, has given the addiction cycle (2001). There are the following four phases:

1. **Preoccupation:** It is a mental state characterized by obsessive search for sex.
2. **Ritualization:** It is patterned ritualistic behaviour oriented to sex.
3. **Compulsive sexual behaviour:** Uncontrollable sexual behaviour.
4. **Despair:** Powerlessness of the individual regarding their sexual behaviour. It is considered the end point of the cycle and the beginning of the next cycle. It leads to unmanageable stress in every area of life.

Unpleasant childhood experiences like sexual or emotional and physical abuse, unhealthy relations with parents and inappropriate behaviour of parents have long-lasting ill effects. Carnes put forth the idea that childhood experiences and the family environment are responsible for sex addiction. It is worth noting that 81 per cent of sex addicts experienced sex abuse in childhood, and 97 per cent experienced emotional abuse. It is also reported that 72 per cent of sex addicts suffer from physical abuse. Hence, it is generated by some intense unresolved trauma, high stress, self-hatred and shame.

Almost 87 per cent of the families of sex addicts have some other addiction. Some members of their family have an addiction related to drugs or alcohol. About 77 per cent of families are rigid and conservative or give inadequate emotional support. It means only 13 per cent of sex addicts come from families without addiction. Some current psychiatry researchers have concluded that seeking pleasure and reducing anxiety are two major motives for sex addiction. It is triggered by sadness or depression, and the output is extreme shame. Some drugs to increase dopamine are given for Parkinson's disease and may increase hypersexuality. Hypersexuality is similar to both impulse control disorder and substance abuse disorder. According to one estimate, approximately 5–6 per cent of people are affected by sexual addiction as per Diagnostic and Statistical Manual (DSM) IV criteria. Some theories about sex addiction have given factors which may be responsible for it. They are as follows:

1. Genetic factors.
2. Sexual abuse or substance abuse in childhood.
3. Traumatic head injury.
4. Endocrine dysfunction, low level of serotonin.
5. Any other psychiatric disorder such as depression, anxiety, bipolar or conduct disorder or impulse control disorder.
6. **Brain pathology:** Some research has also proved that fibres connecting the sex area of brain are different among those who have sex addiction. Multiple sclerosis and stroke patients have over involvement in sexual behaviour due to conditions in their brain. Disorders of the brain's frontal lobe such as tumours, lesions, seizers or dementia result in reduced inhibition. This enhances their vulnerability to sexual addiction. Sometimes, the rush of dopamine due to sexual activity resulting in a feeling of pleasure is mistaken as central to survival. The frontal cortex, which is associated with logic and morality, is impaired by the influence of the midbrain. All these, in turn, enhance sex addiction.

Male members are more vulnerable to sex addiction. Social sanction and freedom are related to it.

Generally, sexual addiction results in multiple sex partners. The Coolidge effect indicates that there is renewed sexual interest if a new, more receptive sexual partner is available. Hence, different sexual partners increase interest in sexual pleasure. It was experimentally proved after conducting a number of experiments on rats.

The same effect is seen in human beings. As a consequence, an addict is strongly involved in sex with multiple partners. It is accepted and proved that males in late adolescence to mid-20s are more vulnerable to becoming sex addicts. Sex addicts have a fear of being abandoned, so they cling to unhealthy relationships also. They feel lonely and isolated when they are alone. They think they are incomplete and their lives are empty without such interaction. Very frequently, they are afraid, feel guilty and get involved in sex to maintain the temporary balance of their minds. Although comparatively fewer females are affected, they also face various problems due to sex addiction. They are sexually exploited by a number of male members, subjugated to character assassination and social rejection and have health risks. There are many risks, such as sexually transmitted infections, other injuries, loss of social status and emotional ill effects. Sometimes, serious legal complications may also emerge. About 75 per cent of ladies face problems with unwanted pregnancies.

In India, many so-called religious leaders, god-men and fake gurus are actually found to be sex addicts, and recently, some of them have also been arrested for multiple rapes and exploiting ladies in various ways. According to recent research, it is seen that 38 per cent of men and 45 per cent of women sex addicts are suffering from venereal disease as a result of their uncontrolled sexual interaction.

6.5.2. Symptoms of Hypersexuality

- These are intense and recurrent sexual fantasies, sexual behaviour and sexual urges, compulsive masturbation and cybersex. Cases reported by researchers have mentioned that some of them had more than 900 sex partners, more than 6,000 partners for sex chat. Even when the addict tries to control these thoughts and acts, it is of no use.
- These fantasies, urges, drives and actual sex behaviour result in distress and impairment as they are substantially intense and frequent.
- Such things are given as a reaction to some negative emotions such as boredom, stress, anxiety and depression, impulse control problems, lack of emotional regulation and obsessive–compulsive disorder.

- Although the individual is aware of potential risks and problems of physical, emotional and social harm to both self and the others involved, they neglect that and get involved in multiple affairs, casual sex, such as one night stand and multiple partners. They recklessly practise unsafe sex.
- Deterioration in academic and job performance due to excess time spent in such sexual thoughts and actions.
- Inability to respect the boundaries of sexual partner is a significant sign of sexual addiction. One more equally important finding is inability to feel fulfilment in sexual urge accompany sexual addiction.
- The addicts are always involved in attracting others, starting new romantic relations and being in love with someone new.
- Dissociation of sex with emotional satisfaction is essentially a very important symptom of sex addiction.
- In advanced stages, sexual rage disorder also results, where the addict becomes anxious, distressed, restless and violent if sex is not available.

Although it is difficult to have a clear bifurcation of symptoms of interest in enjoying sex and sex addiction, researchers have given some directions. According to the Semel Institute for Neuroscience and Human Behaviour (2012), sexual addiction can be considered as a mental health issue only when:

> The individual experiences repeated sexual fantasies, behaviours and urges that last up to six months and are not resulting from other conditions like substance abuse, manic episodes, and side effects of any medicine. As per some research these addicts also have intimacy disorder. It means that they have fear of bonding, they don't want to shoulder any responsibility of maintaining good interpersonal relation. Hence they don't want to get married.

6.5.3. Risks of STDs

Even in advanced countries, new patients with STDs are approximately 20 million per year and half of these are young individuals ranging from 15 to 24 years old. In a country like India, due to lack of awareness, the incidence must be even higher. Many cases are not diagnosed and remain untreated. Homosexuals and some minority groups are reported to suffer more. As it spreads rapidly, it is very risky for others as well. All over the world, girls and women are reported to have greater risk of more complications because of two reasons: The first is that exposure to semen is substantial and for a longer duration if no protection is used, and second, vaginal tissues are fragile. More infected women are unaware that they are infected as they are more likely to be asymptomatic. Some of these infections, such as herpes and HIV, also have properties of latency or window period. During this period, the infected person does not experience any symptoms and even some tests fail to show them. Hence, knowing the history of the sexual partner regarding various sexually transmitted infections is very important and difficult at the same time.

6.5.4. Categories of STDs or Infections

STDs can be classified into three broad categories (Figure 6.1).

1. **Ectoparasitic infections:** Scabies spread during skin-to-skin contact, sexual and non-sexual.
2. **Bacterial infections:** Some STDs are caused by bacteria. Some of them are as follows:
   a. **Gonorrhoea:** It is caused by the bacterium Neisseria gonorrhoea, which survives only in mucous membranes having substantial warmth and moisture, like those of the cervix, urethra, mouth, throat, rectum and even the eyes. It spreads only sexually and from mother to baby during delivery. All sorts of unprotected natural and unnatural sexual interactions may cause it.
   b. **Syphilis:** A bacterium called the treponema pallidum, which survives in the mucous membranes, spreads. Syphilis is transmitted during sexual contact and spreads to the cervix, penis, anus and lips. Congenital syphilis may be transmitted through the placenta during pregnancy.
   c. **Chlamydia:** It is the common name for infections caused by a bacterium called chlamydia trachomatis. As the symptoms are mild, it is not identified easily.

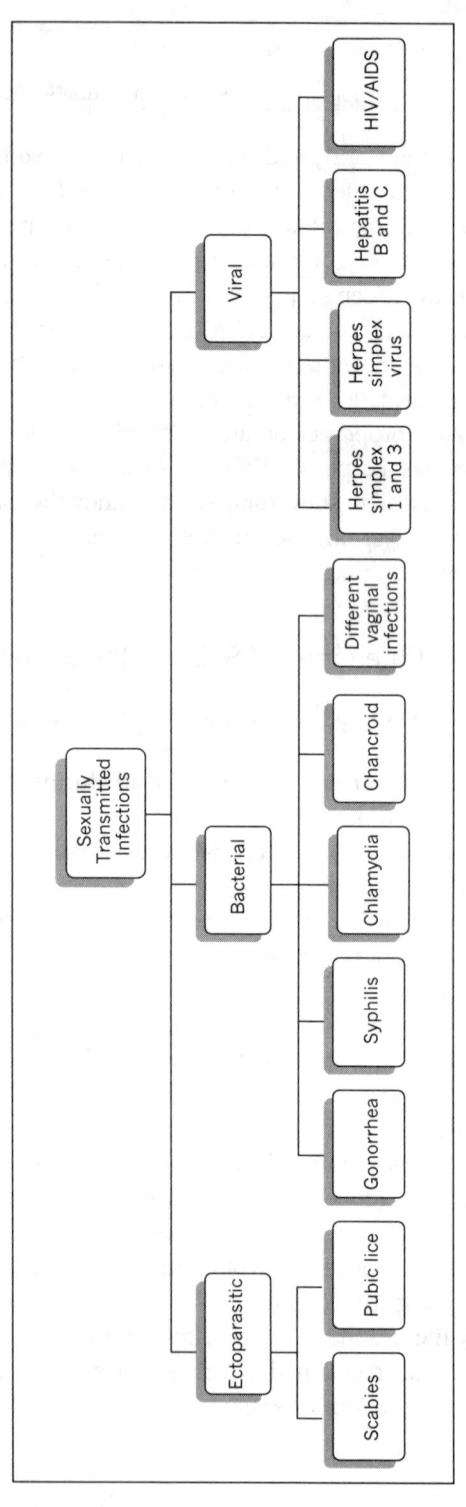

Figure 6.1 *Sexually Transmitted Infections*

3. **Viral or sexually transmitted infections:** Some of these are as follows:

   a. Herpes simplex Type 1 is contagious and is not curable. It is transmitted through kissing or sharing eating or drinking utensils and causes cold sores or blisters to the mouth or lips. It may affect the genitals. Herpes simplex Type 2 spreads due to sexual interaction and can infect the mouth and lips.

   b. Human papilloma virus has more than 100 varieties. Some of them (40) can infect genitals, anus, mouth and throat during unprotected sexual behaviour of all sorts.

      Some high-risk infections are responsible for cancers related to the cervix, vagina, vulva, anal and pennies. In developed countries, this problem is so common that they have developed a vaccine for the same.

   c. Hepatitis B and C are spread due to high-risk sexual behaviour. Hepatitis C are also spread by intravenous drug administration and transfusion of infected blood.

'The most dangerous infection is AIDS.... Everyone should know about it.'

HIV and AIDS are serious concerns all over the world. AIDS is caused by a viral infection with HIV. This virus is primarily transmitted through body fluids, including semen and vaginal fluid, breast milk and blood. The infection takes place during vaginal and anal intercourse. Homosexual and bisexual practices as well as drug use with sharing of needles result in this dangerous infection. This infection is permanent and fatal. There is a dormant stage during which there are no symptoms, but the individual may spread the disease.

HIV attacks the T-lymphocytes, which leads to gradual deterioration of the immune system through destruction of T helper lymphocytes, leaving fewer of them to fight off infections. Various opportunistic infections make the patient too weak to survive after a few years. Detection is possible between two weeks and six months after infection, depending on which test is used. Those who have other STDs have a higher risk of getting infected. The exact incidence in India is difficult to calculate due to social stigma and lack of awareness. According to one estimate, 20 per cent of patients are completely unaware that they are infected for a substantial period of time. When it comes to the last stage where the individual suffers very seriously, there is complete social isolation, and social stigma is severe. High-risk sexual behaviours in adolescents and youth, such as multiple sexual partners, irregular use of condom and consumption of alcohol during sexual activity, increase the risks of HIV infection. Such a decline in T helper lymphocytes takes 3–5 years.

AIDS develops within 8–10 years among HIV patients if not treated properly. Common symptoms are fatigue, fever, headaches, sore throats and chronic swollen lymph nodes in the neck or armpits. Afterwards, substantial weight loss, cognitive confusion, dizziness, blurring of vision, hearing problems, severe diarrhoea for a month, night sweats, oral candidiasis, gingivitis and oral ulcers are experienced. Pneumonia, a rare type of blood vessel cancer, lesions and cervical cancer among female patients are very common. Other STDs may develop and become resistant to treatment, like genital warts or syphilis. New ways of prevention of STDs are being developed by researchers.

6.6. EFFECTS ON THE INDIVIDUAL, FAMILY AND SOCIETY

Sex addiction affects the individual's physiological, psychological, social and moral health. As this is out of control behaviour, one faces many problems regarding intra and interpersonal relations. Serious psychological distress results in impairment of salient roles in family, educational and occupational institutes, and social and religious interactions. An individual's functioning in every aspect of life deteriorates. On the one hand, the person gets involved in sex addiction to reduce anxiety, depression and sadness, and on the other hand, it leads to overwhelming guilt and shame. As they have to utilize a lot of time for sex and related activities, there is no time for hobbies, friends or any social interaction. They are perceived as being bizarre, aggressive and hostile by others. Hence, they never get respect and acceptance in their family and society. Due to temporary and ever-changing relations with numerous sexual partners, there is no stability, sense of security or peace of mind. Sexual partners are perceived only as sex objects, a commodity. The addict becomes restless, anxious and more involved in sexual satisfaction. The loss of trust between life partners because of infidelity, deception and a complete lack of empathy leads to no emotional involvement and love. No trust, unconditional love and compassion can develop in such a relationships. Due to less involvement in jobs, an economic crisis may emerge. The addict may get involved in violating others' rights and that leads to legal issues.

Sexual addiction not only results in harmful effects on the addict themselves but also substantially increases various problems for their family and society. The wife of a sex addict is raped several times during the day and night, becomes helpless and either leaves the husband or faces major health problems. She may feel humiliated, angry, alienated, isolated and depressed. The whole family suffers due to the eccentric behaviour of the addict that is socially unacceptable. The addict is involved with multiple sex partners and does not consider any risk to self and life partner due to it. They never think of the inconvenience to their family while exploiting all the resources available for addiction, such as money, time and space. This, in turn, may lead to loss of status and disturbed interpersonal relations with relatives. It also affects the image of the family in a negative way. A sex addict is an opportunist, and hence, they may prove to be dangerous for the whole society. He may try to take undue advantage and sexually exploit neighbouring girls and women, relatives and acquaintances. In the workplace, the addict will show indecent behaviour and sexually harass girls and ladies. As a consequence, sex-related crime increases, and the general atmosphere becomes insecure.

6.6.1. Crime Related to Sexual Addiction

In Hyderabad, a lady doctor called Priyanka Reddy was gang raped and set ablaze in the month of November 2019. Those criminals were repeatedly involved in such types of extreme crimes and had already gang raped and burnt nine ladies before that (*Maharashtra Times*, 18 December 2019). A few years ago, it was reported that among 242 sex offenders in Tihar jail, 75 per cent were repeat offenders. They admitted that they had already raped before they committed the crime for which they were punished. They are not registered as sex offenders. Most of them thought that repeating offenses was normal sex. Those who were released from prison raped the victim again and killed her.

A similar case is that of a criminal from Shirdi, Maharashtra (*India Today*, 14 January 2013). He was released from jail on 28 May 2012 after two jail terms, one for seven years and the other for 10 years for rape and murder of minor girls. When he was set free, he again did the same, raped and killed a girl on 28 December 2012. Such sex addicts do not respect the law, and it is difficult to rehabilitate them.

On 22 August 2013, a 22-year-old lady photo journalist was gang raped in the premises of Shakti Mills, Mumbai. The rapists were sex addicts.[1]

Some foreign countries, like the USA, have banned sexual addicts as they are not allowed to go to gardens, schools and libraries, can't drive bus and taxi while on probation. In some other countries, every year evaluation of their attitudes, behaviour and intentions is done. There are different legal provisions for punishments. In South Korea, chemical castration of rapists is done if the victim is minor.

There is a department of sexual medicine in King Edward Memorial Hospital and Seth Gordhandas Sunderdas Medical College, Mumbai. Every month, only 25–30 cases are coming for treatment from all over India. This is not even 0.1 per cent of actual cases of sexual addiction. If not treated, it leads to more sex crime.

6.7. AWARENESS, SEX EDUCATION, INTERVENTION AND MANAGEMENT IN INDIA

The lack of awareness, illogical explanations, unscientific methods of treatment and extreme social stigma, which lead to a lack of trust and sharing with others, are serious problems in the Indian situation. Uneducated and poor youth don't consider the risk at all. Partially, educated and even some well-educated and rich Indian male members think that having multiple partners and not using any protection, like condoms, is prestigious for males. Even going to various sex workers is considered as a matter of pride. These distorted perceptions and harmful attitudes generate more risk. Not only advanced countries but

[1] https://en.wikipedia.org/wiki/Shakti_Mills_gang_rape

also in India, many well-known players, actors and supermodels have accepted that they are suffering from sex addiction.

Scientific information regarding sexual matters, various diseases related to unsafe sex, unnatural sexual practices and the harmful psychological and physiological effects of pornography addiction and sex addiction should be given in detail to teenagers. As pornography is available on the web, all scientific information about the risks of sex addictions is also available on the web. However, boys and youth do not extract appropriate information from it.

NCERT has developed new syllabi which include sex education for 1–12th standards. All relevant scientific facts are included in it and are made easy to understand with the help of film, role play and other aids. For example, for the first standard, the concept of sexual abuse in childhood is to be discussed. Although CBSE and ICSE have included sex education in their syllabi, state boards in 12 states have completely ignored it.

Undue curiosity regarding sex and lack of proper knowledge regarding personal safety lead to impulse control problems and enlarged risks. In April 2018, the current government declared that sex education is going to be a part and parcel of the school curriculum for every child. It will include details of sexual and reproductive health, good touch, bad touch, sexual abuse and STDs. In addition, nutrition and mental health are also going to be discussed with the students. It may enhance understanding among students.

The incidence of sex addiction is increasing substantially in India and it is difficult to arrest it because there are no rules and regulations and no factual information is available to health-related authorities of the government. There are various misconceptions about how STDs spread. In India, there is no awareness about the ill effects and risks of oral and anal sex practices. No one knows how many Indians practice protective behavioural patterns. There are increasing cases of throat cancer among young men and women and the origin may be oral sex. As far as cunnilingus, that is, oral sex on female, is concerned, it is considered only as a foreplay, which is also equally responsible for the spread of infections. Lack of awareness regarding dental dams, which protect the individual during oral and anal sex, leads to more risk. One-night stands are common nowadays among youth and sexual activities are performed under the influence of alcohol or drugs. In such a situation, the individuals involved are not bothered about safety. This is a hook-up culture. Before the age of 18, the risk of infections is greater, and it also increases when one or both partners inject drugs.

Case studies reported by researchers are useful for understanding the life of a sex addict. They mentioned that these addicts had sex with hundreds of partners. The calculation of the risk of infection is difficult even in the case of only one addict. Hundreds of sex partners may again infect thousands of others and this multiplication is never ending. They are mostly bisexual and are equally interested in having sex with both genders. Hence, it has to be unnatural also.

6.8. INTERVENTION AND MANAGEMENT

A person suffering from sexual addiction will deny that there is any problem and something needs to be done. They will try to rationalize and justify their behaviour and thinking. Two things that are necessary to reduce sex drive are involvement and to nurture appropriate interpersonal relations. There are self-help organizations, such as Sex Addicts Anonymous, Sex and Love Addicts Anonymous and Sexaholics Anonymous. They run their programmes, like Alcoholic Anonymous, and offer self-management and enhancement. In India, considering the severity of problem, more self-help groups, like Anonymous, and helplines, as well as free services are necessary.

'Sex Addict Anonymous' was established 8 years ago in Delhi and a medical professional who has recovered from sex addiction is playing a major role in it. There are only 78 members. According to experts, it is a denial of reality, as in the dense population of India, 5 per cent of cases means millions of patients in every city. Residential and in-patient programmes are also available for specialized services. Establishing sex de-addiction centres is necessary in all parts of the country. As sex addiction is a socially tabooed issue, an addict feels extreme shame and guilt. Increasing awareness of the larger public and developing special centres for ladies are essential to help them.

Psychological counselling has become a must for better coping strategies, knowledge about viruses and to reduce the spread of disease. These patients generally suffer from depression and suicidal tendencies. Management of anxiety, stress and negative thinking become the topmost priority. Identifying the causes and triggering factors of the sudden increase in sexual impulses and compulsive sexual acts may be useful to reconsider conditioning to decrease the sexual outbursts. Cognitive behaviour therapy is given to change the thoughts, feelings and behaviour that lead to dysfunctional interactions of an addict. Psychodynamic therapy may be used as it creates insight into conscious and unconscious thoughts and ideas. Comorbid and hidden mental health problems also need to be treated.

It is estimated that 40 per cent of sex addicts have some other psychological problems. Treating both simultaneously with psychotherapy and pharmacotherapy gives the best results. Managing harmful behaviour and relapses becomes essential. Medicines to reduce sexual urges are available, but side effects should be considered before administration. Family's support should be developed and relations rebuilt. It is difficult to accept such individual with all their problematic behaviour and to develop empathy for them. Still, counsellors may try to develop good family relation with the help of family therapy. Rational Emotive Behaviour therapy is also recommended.

In Uttar Pradesh, in a village called Prem Ganj, some AIDS patients were found. People became aware and, in 2018, decided that they would check the HIV infection of all the brides and grooms and make sure that none of them are infected. Accordingly, producing the normal health report is a must before marriage. This is the best policy, and if it is practised all over India, it will reduce infections through marriage and child birth.

Developing and strengthening relationships with family and friends may also help a lot. If there is enough love and affection, emotional support and unconditional acceptance, the person may achieve better self-worth and social image. They may not need to struggle hard to feel good. The company of family members and their understanding may prove to be the most effective intervention. Once the frequency of sex decreases, withdrawal symptoms, such as intense discomfort, anger and irritability, emerge. Proper treatment is essential to recover from these symptoms also. Engagement in better activities which are constructive may enhance positive thinking and motivation to lead a socially acceptable life. Hobbies, interesting work, socially relevant activities, helping the needy and using different potential and aptitudes for self-acceptance as a worthy person are the most basic and effective strategies.

6.9. SUMMARY

The advancement of science and technology has resulted in some new psychological problems, like internet addiction. Pornography addiction, in particular, leads to an uncontrollable urge to watch pornography, neglecting all the important aspects of human life. There are many harmful effects of pornography consumption which disturb the addict's whole life, including academics, performance at work, emotional balance, social life, duties and responsibilities regarding family and friends. Their sex life gets upset as they want to imitate various ways of enjoying sex.

Sex addiction is an uncontrolled sex urge. Exaggerated sexual activities, without paying any heed to social approval, norms and etiquette, make the addict feel guilty and ashamed. There is a substantial risk of STDs along with HIV and AIDS due to multiple partners. Sex addiction affects the present and future of individuals and families. These individuals are involved in sex-related crimes. They don't respect any relationship or authority but want to have sex with anyone who is available. As this is a comparatively recent consideration, in India very few experts are working in this field, and due to extreme social stigma, very few patients accept it and are interested in getting help. Both pornography addiction and sex addiction are serious problems in the Indian community and need immediate attention.

Sexual Abuse, Sexual Harassment and Rape

7.1. INTRODUCTION

Daisy Irani, a very well-known talented child artist, was raped at the age of six. The rapist was supposed to be her guardian and accompanied her on an outdoor film shoot. He threatened her and beat her. (YouTube, 2018).

In Kanpur, Uttar Pradesh, a husband threw acid on the private parts of his wife as she denied sex. It happened in the village of Bahrain in November 2017 (NDTV, 1 November 2017). On the same day, a 100-year-old lady was raped when she was sleeping in the courtyard of her house. The old lady was so shocked that she died within a few minutes.[1]

According to a recent survey conducted by Thomson Reuters Foundation based on opinions of 548 international experts, India is the most dangerous country in the whole world for women. Indian women are sexually exploited and are subjected to oppressive treatment. They are forced to work excessively (Goldsmith et al., 2018).

Sex is a crucial natural pleasure in human life. Power plays an important role in any sexual relations. As far as physical strength is concerned, men are more powerful. In the case of misuse of power, various crimes, injustice and inhuman treatment given to women and children become very common. Hence, things are taken for granted, and even when the girl or woman is denying it, sexual activity continues.

---

[1] https://www.indiatoday.in 24 October 2018

7.2. SEXUAL ABUSE AND ITS EFFECTS: PSYCHOLOGICAL TRAUMA

Sexual contact by an adult with an individual below 17 years of age is sexual abuse. The intensity of such abuse may differ, and in some cases, it is equivalent to rape. It is undesired sexual behaviour or molestation by an individual upon another. It is taking undue advantage and forcefully misusing power so that the other person is exploited. If such an act is for short duration, the force is applied on the spot or it occurs rarely, it is sexual assault. It is very common to abuse children all over the world.[2]

It was reported in February 2018 that every 15 minutes a child is sexually abused in India. It is worth noting that many sexual abuse cases are never reported; hence, these statistics are only an under-estimation. In 2012, the Indian government passed a law to protect children from sexual abuse, called 'Protection of Children from Sexual Offences or POCSO'. However, in day-to-day life situations, its application becomes difficult (*Hindustan Times*, 2018). It is essential to consider sexual abuse in detail because, though it takes place mostly in childhood or adolescence, the ill effects on the personality and emotional well-being of the victim are seen throughout their life.

Sexual abuse occurs in the case of both boys and girls, and extreme emotional ill effects are equally harmful for both. Even some male celebrities, such as Akshay Kumar and Anurag Kashyap, have shared their experiences regarding childhood sexual abuse. On YouTube, one may find many short films and videos about sexual abuse and its impact on the victim, such as 'Child Sexual Abuse: Trauma and Recovery after Child Abuse' (youtube 30 January 2015) and 'Depression and Child Sexual Abuse: Dr Rosaleen McElvaney' (Aware, 2017). 'Komal: A Film on Child Sexual Abuse' (PIB India, 2016) by the Ministry of Women and Child Development depicts child abuse and its impact. In Satyamev Jayate (2012), 'Child Sexual Abuse', a pro-gramme presented by Amir Khan, a case is shown where a male child is abused and raped from 7 to 18 years of age, that is, 11 long years. It is

---

[2] https://en.wikipedia.org/wiki/Sexual_abuse

reported that many Bollywood celebrities were sexually assaulted in their childhood, such as Kalki and Anoushka Shankar.

Approximately 33 per cent of child abuse incidents are identified, and very few of them are reported to the police. Before the age of 8, 20 per cent of total abuses take place. It is reported that 15 per cent of the total abuses are done by juveniles. Those who are abused before the age of 12 may develop eating disorders. In 90 per cent of cases, sexual abuse of children is done by known individuals. They are family members, relatives, neighbours, friends and acquaintances. More than 10 per cent of the total children in any society are abused sexually.

7.2.1. Types of Sexual Abuse

There are four types of sexual abuse, which are as follows:

1. Complete sexual act, that is, intercourse.
2. Incomplete sexual acts or attempted but unsuccessful intercourse. However, it may include touching, kissing, fondling, etc.
3. Abusive sexual contact touches or hurts sexual or private parts.
4. Sexual abuse without contact or non-touching abuse is verbal sexual abuse and intentional unwanted exposure of obnoxious sights. This can include cyber abuse, such as abuse on WhatsApp and Facebook, showing pornography, taking photographs of victims in indecent positions, voyeurism, talking about sexually stimulating things on the phone, sending vulgar messages and pictures.

Any unwanted or forced sexual activity, inappropriate sexual behaviour in front of children and sexual acts with somebody who is drunk, drugged or unconscious are included in sexual abuse. Not allowing the partner to protect themselves from STDs or unwanted pregnancy are also sexual abuses resulting in physical, social and psychological problems in the long term.

Children are more vulnerable to abuse and molestation. As they are weak, submissive and obedient, it is easy to get them, threaten them, abuse them or even kill them. Infants can't report what has happened and can't identify the abuser.

It is difficult to define sexual abuse and include all forms of it. That is why the exact incidence is difficult to find out. In developed countries, like the USA, a child is raped every 26 seconds. Approximately 33 per cent of women and 18 per cent of men have a history of childhood sexual abuse (Hall & Hall, 2011).

There is a general misconception that only girls are abused sexually. Actually, both boys and girls are sexually abused. However, due to the stereotype of male superiority and patriarchy, boys never share their problems with anyone and don't seek any help. In 2007, the Ministry of Women and Child Welfare found that 53.22 per cent of children in India suffered due to sexual abuse. The percentage of boys was 52.94 and that of girls was 47.06 (Ministry of Women and Child Development, 2007). It is extremely awkward for a boy, a male adolescent or adult to accept that he has been sexually abused or raped. There is social stigma; hence, they prefer to hide it from the world. Emotional problems remain hidden for the whole of their lives.

7.2.2. Signs and Symptoms of Sexual Abuse

Due to ongoing physiological development, there are many curiosities and emerging interests. Sex is a taboo, and children hide their concerns. It makes children and adolescents more vulnerable. It is easy to persuade adolescents due to their growing interest in sex. The victims of sexual abuse want to forget about it and do not remember or discuss it with anyone else. In sexual abuse, the abuser keeps the victim under constant threat so that he can repeatedly keep on exploiting the same individual. The victim is even otherwise reluctant to tell parents and significant adults. Researchers and counsellors have reported that, especially when the abuser is a known and so-called respectable individual, the victim's family members, even parents, do not trust the victim. They blame victims for inviting them. The victims experience a lot of shame and guilt due to taboos and misconceptions. They also feel that their family will treat them as filthy and dirty and will withdraw love and affection. They are afraid of separation from their loved ones. Hence, they prefer to keep it as a secret. The abuser may take undue advantage of the victim's fear, awkwardness, guilt and shame to compel the victim to keep mum. An impression that the victim is also responsible for whatever has happened, and they will have to face a lot of rejection if others get the factual information, may be used for keeping things secret.

'My Parents Never Told Cops about My Rape' (The Quint, 2019) depicts the experience of childhood sexual abuse from the age of 6–13, and its impact on the individual even as an adult.

'I Am Not Just a Girl' (YouTube, 19 July 2016) reports a real experience of a 15-year-old girl who was abused by her own maternal uncle which included all sorts of physical abuse also.

Generally, the abusers have an attractive personality, are friendly, confident and charming. They can win the trust of the victim within no time. By and large, the general impression of them is that they are leading a socially acceptable life. However, it is proven that they are aggressive and impulsive. They have poor social skills, low intelligence and an unhappy family history. Their self-esteem is low. They themselves were abused in childhood. They are generally pornography addicts. They sexually exploit children one after the other. Sexual abuse is equally practised in all socio-economic strata. Sexual abuse can take place even among two individuals of the same age.

To start with, an abuser pretends that they care, admire and have fatherly feelings and affection for a victim. Then they gradually start telling sex-related jokes, stories, showing pornography, playing sex-related games and touching the victim, pretending that there is no inappropriate intention behind it. They don't have any guilt and assume that the victim enjoys it. The victim is so young that she sometimes can't even understand the purpose behind it. Young victims don't know the proper words to express what has taken place. Most of the time, the abuser is from the victim's own family or extended family. This is called incest.

7.2.3. Psychological Effects of Sexual Abuse

The general consequences of sexual abuse are feeling humiliated, dehumanized, angry and helpless. It diminishes self-respect and self-confidence. These victims feel defensive, avoid intimacy and are constantly engaged in thoughts of revenge. They face problems such as hyperactivity and agitation, sleep disorders, nightmares, self-deprecation and unexplained stomach aches and headaches. There is obsession or aversion regarding sex and perfectionism and work holism. Other problems are feeling hyperactive and unclean. The victim becomes over defensive, experiences panic and fright.

Childhood sexual abuse is found to be related to anxiety, depression, self-blame, eating disorders, somatic concerns, repression and denial. These victims experience problems related to intimate relations and sexual relations in adulthood. Most of the victims have body image problems and dissatisfaction with their appearance. Ratican (1992) reported that feeling dirty, ugly and obesity are common symptoms. More females experiencing sexual abuse have somatic complaints. Gastrointestinal problems, pelvic pain, difficulty swallowing and head-aches are reported by researchers. The emotional ill effects are similar to war-related trauma. In some cases, dissociative problems are seen as protecting the victim. That coping mechanism is used even in adult-hood. It includes confusion, disorientation, flashbacks, nightmares and emotional insensitivity. Repression and denial are associated with amnesia, neglecting the impact of abuse and the feeling that one should forget it. The most common effect is depression in the long run. More self-harm, self-destructive thoughts and actions are seen. The more intense emotional signs of sexual abuse are post-traumatic stress disorder, suicidal thoughts, and abusing medicines, drugs and substances.

Emotional and cognitive problems are also among the first signs and immediate consequences of child abuse. Irrespective of the age of the victim, the emotional and physical ill effects of sexual abuse are long-lasting. They can't trust any relationships, have sexual difficulties and never feel secure and relaxed while interacting with others. They face problems like depression in the long run. Their self-esteem is low. Their self-image is damaged. They are more conscious of their appearance. They are oriented to abusing substances and overeating, which affects their whole future. Child abuse increases the chances of dropping out of school.

Immediately after abuse, unbearable physical effects are seen depending on the actual cruelty. It includes extreme pain, sleeplessness, bleeding, urinary tract infection, STDs, including HIV, and sometimes pregnancy at an early age. Some of the victims can't even walk properly without pain.

Organizations Working for Protecting Children
Childline India is a non-government service available for 24 hours to save children from any type of exploitation and protect their rights. They get 25 lakh phones from children needing help in one year. These services are available in 200 cities. It is worth remembering that within 1 hour, essential help is made available. The needy and distressed child should call a toll free number 1098.

Sexual abuse in the case of preschool children results in regression, bed wetting, thumb sucking and they are afraid of sleeping alone. In school-age children, phobias, sleep difficulties and acting out sexually are reported. Headaches, stomach aches and avoiding problems are very common among these children. Approximately one in every six women is sexually abused. The behavioural effects of sexual abuse are that people distrust others and themselves. They feel self-hatred and aloofness, alienation from their own body, isolation and social withdrawal. The victim becomes passive.

Women who experienced childhood familial sexual abuse have more depression and anxiety. The intensity of abuse, the young age of the victim and repeated abuse increase the distress. Victims' general support, perspective and resources play an important role. The traumatic experience of sexual abuse results in premature and forced sexual activity, which causes many psycho-social problems. Even as adults, they have problems with interpersonal relations, such as lack of trust, fear of intimacy, fear of being different and being passive. They get involved in abusive relationships (Ratican, 1992).

Satish, a good-looking and frail adolescent, was raped many times during his school days when he used to stay in a hostel. After marriage, he could not initiate any sexual activity. There was hardly any arousal that he could achieve. He has been only passive during sexual intimacy. His wife was frustrated and, for years, could not get any sexual satisfaction. In addition to that, he was very defensive and aggressive as that was the only compensatory mechanism. Finally, she filed for a divorce.

The sexual difficulties of these victims are well reported by researchers. They are avoidance, fear, lack of interest, anger and disgust. They perceive sex only as an obligation; they are not aroused by it. They are aloof and think about something disturbing about sex. Their sexual behaviour is never appropriate. Women experience pain. In general, arousal disorders and low sexual desire are common. These significant ill effects of sexual abuse are seen even after a number of years.

As the severity of sexual abuse increases, an individual's ability to adjust to intimate relationships decreases (Feinauer et al., 1996). In childhood, if someone the child loves abuses the child sexually, the victim thinks that the people they love will hurt them. This link between adult victimization and childhood sexual abuse is shown by Kessler and Bieschke (1999).

7.2.4. Intervention

The best way to protect children and adolescents from sexual abuse is to make them aware and give them proper information about it. It is essential to train them about the various skills necessary to protect self. Parents should trust the child, encourage them to tell the details and be strong enough to take some corrective steps. Communication between parents and their offspring should be so open that they will be able to share their experiences and worries with parents. Abuse is generally neglected, especially when the abuser is a family member, like the grandfather or uncle. However, it is essential to arrest it and give justice to the child. Victims should be helped to develop enough self-confidence and assertiveness. Individuals who are aware of their own rights, know the nature of sexual abuse, respect themselves and know the way to get help themselves are less vulnerable, according to Hall and Hall (2011).

While treating post-traumatic stress disorder of sexually abused victims, cognitive behavioural therapy is effective. The victim is helped to recognize negative thoughts and their impact. With therapy, they are helped to get rid of them. Family therapy and play therapy work very well. Parents and teachers should develop empathy for the victims and give assurance and enhance a sense of security in their minds. The victim should be encouraged to learn how to face the public, which can be achieved only when they accept reality. During this stage, the victim has to learn to overcome the trauma. In the integration stage, there are some stimuli that trigger memories of abuse. The victim gets disturbed but knows how to overcome that. Emotional support, unconditional love and affection and helping to get rid of the harasser and negative thoughts are the most essential strategies.

7.3. SEXUAL HARASSMENT AND CONSEQUENCES

Do You Know?

A very well-known scientist, Marie Curie, was the first woman to win the Nobel prize. She received the Nobel prize twice. After the death of her husband, her colleagues harassed her and were involved in her character assassination.

Women's sexual harassment in the workplace has been a burning problem all over the world. Although it has been existing for generations, scientific evidence is available from 1832 onwards. The term 'sexual harassment' was coined in the mid-1970s by North American feminists. Since 1970s, there has been a substantial research in the UK, Australia, the USA, Canada, Sweden, Holland, Denmark, Japan, etc. As compared to that in India, there is still a paucity of research and a lack of awareness among the general population. Sexual harassment of women in the workplace is the obvious violation of the human rights of women.

At present, 154 countries have laws to prevent sexual harassment of women in the workplace. According to the Ministry of Women and Child Development, there is an 80 per cent increase in complaints of sexual harassment in the workplace (News B, 20 October 2019).

A 33-year-old lady officer at BHEL killed herself due to workplace harassment by a senior and six colleagues (PTI, 2019) in October 2019. In a video, a 'lady constable harassed by Uttar Pradesh police officers' depicts disturbing experiences regarding the sexual harassment of a young lady constable where she is not getting any justice (Crime Tak, 2020). BBC News on 15 January 2020 reports that an Indian businessman has been sentenced for molesting a former

Bollywood actress on a flight. He will be imprisoned for three years. A major general was fired from the Indian Army in August 2019 under the provisions of IPC Section 354A and the legal provisions of Armed Forces Section 45 under the charge of sexual harassment.[3] It was a case of court martial. In 1988, a lady IAS officer, Rupan Bajaj, was molested in a gathering of elite people by the Director General of Police, K. P. S. Gill, and there was hardly any action taken against him in spite of filing a legal case which continued till July 2005. Rupan Bajaj could not get any support from anyone, and the whole incidence was underevaluated (Wikipedia). It took 31 long years to change the scenario substantially.

It is essential to note that even men can be harassed sexually and otherwise, but the proportion of reported harassment is comparatively less. #MeToo has resulted in the declaring sexual harassment experiences of many celebrities.[4] It started in late 2018 in India. Many prominent personalities are victims and harassers too.

Sexual harassment is so common that the majority of girls and women experience it sometimes in their lives. Indian researchers have reported that approximately 90 per cent of working women experience it repeatedly. Approximately half of them were harassed by their own colleagues and bosses. If it is an educational institution or workplace where an individual is being harassed, the ill effects are more serious: educationally, psychologically, socially and physiologically. Many times, sexual harassment is an inherent part of the work environment which remains hidden and is considered as natural and unquestioned.

7.3.1. Nature of Sexual Harassment

Sexual harassment is a form of sex discrimination as it would not have occurred but for the person's gender. It is not mutual; on the contrary, it is unwelcome, and is a result of the abuse of power and rude and demanding behaviour of the harasser. It is an unwanted repeated sexual advancement which cause a lot of discomfort and

[3] timesofindia.com, 17 August 2019

[4] timesofindia.com 6 November 2017

psycho-social problems for the victim. It is a form of male dominance which is especially detrimental to working women. There is a lot of ambiguity regarding the definition of sexual harassment. However, generally it is accepted as a very unpleasant experience for the victim. The Equal Opportunity Commission has given a definition of sexual harassment which says,

> Sexual harassment is caused by repeated and unwanted visual, verbal, behavioural sexual advances, sexually explicit derogatory statements or sexually discriminating remarks because of which the worker feels threat, humiliation, offence, and distress, which in turn interferes with job performance, emphasizes person's sexuality over her role as a worker and creates unpleasant working environment.[5]

Sexual harassment is any unwanted attention of a sexual nature that creates discomfort and interferes with performance.

The scientific definition of sexual harassment includes leering and sexually suggestive facial expressions in visual harassment. In verbal harassment, ridicule, embarrassing remarks or jokes, unwelcome comments about dress or appearance, sexually discriminating remarks and deliberate abuse regarding work are included. In behavioural harassment, sexually suggestive non-verbal expressions, unwanted physical contact, demands for sexual favours and sexual advances are seen. Indecent touch, brushing the body, teasing, body shaming, looking at various body parts of women, patting, pinching, using awful expressions to suggest sexual interaction with the help of objects, fruits or even tongue are frequently reported by ladies. Different types of sexual aggression and flirting are used. Some harassers sexually touch their own private parts in front of women and manipulate things in such a way that it is extremely awkward for the women.

The two main types of harassment are work-related harassment and sexual harassment. Both of them overlap and the distinction becomes difficult. Most of the time, sexual harassment has a hidden and covert intention, while work-related harassment is an overt expression. Such victims are given excessive work which is insignificant and are

---

[5] https://www.humanrights.vic.gov.au/for-individual/human-rights

supposed to complete it with perfection within a minimum time. They are insulted, shifted to other departments, fired or demoted. In spite of all their hard work, they are never considered as an appropriate candidate for promotion. Extreme non-cooperation is seen in such interaction, where the harasser boss spoils the confidential report of the victim.

Different subtypes of sexual harassment are equally unpleasant. Third-party harassment is one of them. In this case, the harasser makes sure that the victim is around and starts discussing and cracking jokes related to sex life of someone else. The lady feels extremely awkward and ashamed. In a way, the harasser is neither talking about her nor talking to her, but the intention is clearly the same.

Quid pro quo harassment is another type of harassment where the supervisor demands sexual favours in return for extra facilities, better treatment, less work and more promotions. If a victim is not ready to submit, he threatens her with extra work, firing, demotion and unwanted transfer. This is an obvious misuse of power. Giving excess, insignificant, and tedious work to the lady, insulting her in front of others, telling her to do something just to indicate that he is her boss, extreme expectations, and seeking her company though not required to do the work are similar behavioural patterns. Hostile environment harassment is the basic but hidden harassment. Such behaviour by a male member becomes offensive to a lady and the work environment becomes unpleasant and hostile. This includes suggestive facial expressions and gestures, sex-related jokes, sexual touching, embarrassing questions, unfair comments, vulgar and sexually suggestive language and pornography. Sexual propositions are also reported in such a environment. Touching the victim's body, hair, dress, leaning over the victim, standing too close, brushing against her body parts, kissing when she is unaware and unwilling and suggesting interest in her personal life disturbs the lady substantially.

There are many misconceptions about sexual harassment. Especially male members think that such interaction is natural, and women like it. Women are pleased to see that someone is interested in them. They like flirting. The lady is responsible for it. As a consequence, women who are harassed feel ashamed, guilty, awkward and are reluctant to express it. As they are confused and don't know what to do to stop it, they neglect sexual harassment. It is proven that sexual harassment increases after neglecting it. No resistance is taken to mean no objection and agreement. It results in more serious sexual harassment. This is a vicious circle.

There is a substantial gender difference between reported perceptions regarding sexual harassment. Most male members discard the idea of sexual harassment and label it as 'office banter' even when it is a serious abuse. Almost always, men banter and women are bantered at. Men and women have different standards of decency, good manners and appropriate behaviour. In some research, a video tape was used to depict interaction between men and women. Men label a few types of behaviour as sexual harassment and gave a broader definition of socially acceptable behaviour. For men, it is harmless fun to keep the atmosphere light and pleasant.

Sometimes, the harassers are not aware of their unpleasant and indecent behaviour. It is their general style of interacting with ladies and they don't consider that their colleagues are well educated and equally competent as they are. Generally, men in power harass women subordinates. General masculine power over women is role appropriate and power role multiplies the stereotypical gender role. It is because of the relation between sex and power that makes it even more difficult for the woman to face it.

7.3.2. Factors Contributing to Sexual Harassment

Irrespective of marital status, education, appearance, age, experience and designation, any woman can be easily harassed in any organization. In addition to physiological limitations, there are some issues related to nurture. Specific biased gender socialization and the typical personality patterns emerging out of it are responsible for sexual harassment. Due to internalization of social values, women develop self-imposed, self-attributed fearfulness and impose restrictions on their own activities and aspirations. By and large, the work environment is male-dominated and skewed in favour of men. Women have to put in extra effort to prove their competence. Women are oriented towards interpersonal relations. They put others' needs first. They have empathy, are sensitive, kind and emotionally responsive. The work-related stereotypical personality of a woman is such that she has low self-efficacy, negative thinking and an external locus of control. Low aims and aspirations, low motivation and self-defeating attribution styles are proven all over the world. She works for others. She is cognitively dependent on others and wants to follow rather than lead. She has an emotionally oriented-adjustment style, low self-confidence and low self-worth. Due to her wish to be pleasant, she avoids confrontation. She is helpless and is easily discouraged if the environment is not conducive. Women can exercise less power, get fewer opportunities and are given less respect. They are less capable of making decisions independently. They have a fear of success, which is accompanied by a fear of character assassination, loss of femininity, isolation and neglect. In organizations, women are expected to be both, masculine and feminine. Their looks and femininity count for getting employment, and they have to work in a masculine fashion and compete with their male colleagues.

There are many theories which try to explain various aspects of sexual harassment. The harasser may have low self-concept, unfair intentions, may be unhappy with his married life, may be attracted to the lady and knows that she will never accept it. As a consequence, he tries to get some sadistic pleasure by harassing the lady. Even otherwise, men find it difficult to desexualize women.

7.3.3. Effects of Sexual Harassment

The consequences of sexual harassment are physiological, psychological, especially emotional, cognitive, social and interpersonal. They are classified as short-term and long-term problems, psychological and physiological problems and personal and work-related issues.

1. Psychosomatic problems: Short-term psychosomatic problems are emotional issues, such as fear, anger, anxiety, guilt, shame, tension, stress and depression. Nervousness, powerlessness, isolation, denial, frustration, insecurity, confusion, embarrassment, betrayal and self-blame are experienced due to unpleasant experiences. It

also results in poor self-concept, maladjustment, and decreased creativity.

Physiological effects such as lethargy, headaches, nausea, insomnia, gastrointestinal distress, dermatological reactions, weight fluctuations and nightmares are reported by victims. The long-term effects are detrimental to mental health, such as restlessness, fatigue, drug dependence, sleeplessness, illness and issues of interpersonal relations with family and friends. In addition, phobias, sex-related problems and panic reactions have a serious impact.

Long-term physiological effects range from weight loss to coronary heart disease.

2. **Work-related effects:** Short-term problems are avoidance and apathy, lack of concentration, absenteeism, reduced job satisfaction and decreased job performance. The long-term problems are the loss of opportunities for promotions, low efficacy, being labelled as being less capable, unreliable and unwilling to work hard. This results in unfavourable evaluation of performance and withdrawal from work. It is reported in research that it is a major contributor to stress at work.

7.3.4. Personal Action and Legal Provision

Confrontation is essential. The victim should be assertive. Her body language should be self-respecting and strong. She should clearly mention in front of other colleagues that she does not like the behaviour of the harasser. Getting support from other colleagues, some non-government organizations, legal advisers and a counsellor becomes essential. Considering the ambiguity of the nature and definition of sexual harassment, it is difficult to prove that sexual harassment has taken place. Social rejection, character assassination and isolation are the consequences of confrontation. More than 50 per cent victims leave their jobs.

In 1997, the Supreme Court gave a judgment which is known as the Vishaka judgment. Sexual harassment is accepted as a violation of constitutionally guaranteed fundamental rights. Three years of imprisonment with a fine is recommended for the harasser. The Indian Government Gazette Act, 2013, is the current legal provision for sexual harassment of women at the workplace. According to it, it is essential to submit a written complaint regarding sexual harassment to the local complaints committee chairman. Every organization should have an internal committee working to prevent sexual harassment. There is one local complaint committee appointed by the government. Indian Penal Code Section 509, which has many subsections, is applicable to it. The loss of career opportunities, psychological trauma, distress, suffering, pain and medical expenses for treatment are considered. No information is disclosed to the media.

The legal provisions to punish harassers are very strict and punishment is substantial. Some harassers are fired from a permanent and high-status jobs also. For example, a senior judicial officer was fired by the high court in Karnataka for sexually harassing four women in his office. In January 2016, a second additional district and session judge was fired due to sexual harassment. A leader was arrested in July 2016 for the character assassination of a lady leader from another political party. In developed countries, the provisions are so perfect that the harasser is punished without delay.

A 35-year-old US-based Indian man has been sentenced to 9 years in jail for sexually assaulting a passenger next to him on a US flight. (BBC News, 2018). A 58-year-old Indian was travelling on a US flight on 30 July 2016. A young white lady next to him was fast asleep when V. Rao started touching her in an indecent manner. He was arrested immediately when the flight landed. For parole, he had to pay $50,000 dollars. He was imprisoned for some months and sent to an alcohol treatment centre for some more. The maximum punishment for such cases is two years imprisonment and $250,000 dollars as a fine for compensation.[6]

Women should develop self-respect and accept their potential. They must make decisions independently. They should have enough confidence to deal with new challenges. Women should be assertive and proactive while interacting with others. They should put in extra efforts to solve their own problems. At the same time, women should not discuss their personal and family problems with male colleagues. They should have an attitude and behavioural pattern declaring androgyny.

[6] www.justice.gov>news 2 August 2016

Male members should be more careful and formal while interacting with the opposite gender.

In developed countries, approximately 20 per cent of the total complaints are related to harassment of men.[7] Some of them are harassed by men and others by women. Men feel more awkward and think that it is a loss of masculine image to accept that they are sexually harassed.

7.4. RAPE: NATURE, THEORIES AND CONSEQUENCES

Different disciplines are involved in research regarding rape, such as psychology, physiology, sociology, anthropology, law and science regarding animals. Rape is the fourth most common crime against women in India. Around 98 per cent of rapes are committed by a known person, according to the National Crime Records Bureau. Most of the rapes are not reported. Extremely serious cases are only reported.

Rape was defined scientifically in 1927. However, it included only vaginal intercourse. It did not include unnatural intercourse styles, which are quite common in the contemporary world due to pornography and similar other models. It did not include oral or anal penetration, penetration with objects, rape of females by females, non-forcible rape and the rape of men. In 2013, a new Federal Bureau of Investigation definition of rape went into effect (Federal Bureau of Investigation, 2013)

Rape is now defined as 'the penetration, no matter how slight, of the vagina or anus with any body part or object, or oral penetration by a sex organ of another person, without the consent of the victim' (The United States Department of Justice, 2012). Amendment of criminal law in 2013 says that rape is 'penetration of penis into vagina, mouth or anus of a woman, or make her to do so'. The age of consent is different in different countries, from 14 years to 18 years.

Sexual assault is defined as unwanted penetration, forced oral or anal sex, masturbation, touching, fondling or kissing. It would also

[7] thewashingtonpost.com 8 April 2018

include forcing someone to view sexually explicit materials, like pornography.

Rape is defined with reference to the following conditions in the case of females:

- Against the wish of the victim.
- Without her consent or obtaining consent by threatening her or deceiving her that he is her husband or will marry her or by inducing intoxication.
- With or without consent when the victim is below 16. If the wife is less than 15 years old, even intercourse within marriage is rape. Otherwise, marital intercourse is not considered rape in India.

It is estimated by researchers that a rape takes place in India every 14 minutes (Zee News, 2019). The total reported cases in 2019 were 405,861 in India. According to a national report on the security of women (2019), Uttar Pradesh is the most insecure state for women as the crime against women is the highest, that is, 15.6 per cent. The second is Maharashtra.[8]

In developed countries, like the USA, sexual violence affects millions of individuals. Every 73 seconds, an American is sexually assaulted. About 433,648 rape cases are reported per year. Young children are at the highest risk. One out of every six women has been raped or attempted to rape. About 94 per cent of women experience post-traumatic stress disorder and drug dependence is also more.[9]

Although there are strict legal provisions against rape, over 2.4 lakh cases related to rape and sexual abuse are pending in the courts of India. Out of these, 66,994 are from Uttar Pradesh, which is the highest number (Asian News International, 5 March 2020). It is difficult to arrive at any exact conclusion as most of the rapes in India are not reported due to fear of retaliation and social stigma. According to the National Crime Record Bureau (2006), 71 per cent of crimes are never reported. There are thousands of cases of rapes where extreme inhuman brutality is seen.

[8] Maharashtra Times.com 22 October 2019

[9] https://www.rainn.org/statistics/victims-sexual-violence

Aruna Shanbaug was just a 26-year-old nurse working at KEM Hospital Mumbai. She scolded a ward boy for misappropriating the money given for feeding live stock. He raped her, sodomized and strangled her with a dog chain due to which oxygen supply to her brain was hampered. She was in a coma for the whole of her life, that is, 40 long years from 1973 to 2015 in a vegetative state and died in the same hospital (Wikipedia).

Now, young boys are more involved in sexual exploitation of girls due to premature exposure, like pornography. On the other hand, the incidence of young girls being raped is also increasing. An 8-month-old infant was raped by her 27-year-old cousin (*India Today*, 2018) in Delhi. She had to undergo major surgery (you tube, 30 Jan 2018). *The Indian Express* (2019) reports that a 13-year-old boy is being held for rape and murder of his 5-year-old cousin. A 6-year-old girl was raped in Mumbai.[10] In Gurugram, nine young girls below the age of 10 were raped and murdered in November 2018 (Times News Network, 22 November 2018). A three year old was raped by her relative in Mumbai (*Maharashtra Times*, 4 January 2020). In Pimpri, Pune, within one month, five young girls were raped (*Maharashtra Times,* 17 August 2019).

Irrespective of the relationship between victim and rapist, many rapes are taking place. This is responsible for intense insecurity for girls and women, even in their own homes. In Mumbai, in January 2020, a father raped his own daughter by blackmailing her (*Maharashtra Times*, 5 January 2020). It was reported by News 18 on 3 December 2019 that a father raped his own 16-year-old daughter for two months in Buldhana. He used to give her sleeping pills. A similar case in Raipur was reported on 30 December 2019 in the *Maharashtra Times*. In this case, the criminal raped two daughters. In Kaithal, Haryana, a rapist father was sexually exploiting his 13-year-old daughter for five years (News18 Lokmat, 25 January 2020). News18 Lokmat (18 August 2019) describes in detail how a daughter was raped for two years by her own father, and when she started resisting, he killed her.

---

[10] Maharashtra Times.com 4 December 2019

There are examples where even a grandfather raped his own grand-daughter for a number of years. In Bhopal, maternal grandfather and uncle raped a 6-year-old girl in front of her 3-year-old brother.[11] In Patna, a grandfather raped his granddaughter (*Maharashtra Times*, 25 December 2019). In June 2018, in Mumbai, a 14-year-old boy raped his own sister as he was addicted to porn. The sister became pregnant.[12] A brother raped his own sister in Pune (Times Now News, March 2017); a 15-year-old sister was raped for 4 years by her own two brothers in Meerut (NDTV, October 2018), and a 14-year-old daughter was raped by her own father in Thane (NDTV, 20 September 2018). *The Times of India* reported on 15 September 2018 that a daughter-in-law was raped by her father-in-law, and her sister-in-law made a video of the same. It was to take revenge because her father could not give expected dowry. News18 Lokmat reports on 16 December 2019, a mother-in-law was raped by her son-in-law in Hyderabad. On 25 January 2020, News18 Lokmat reported that a man had been raping his own 13-year-old daughter for five long years.

ABP News (28 December 2019) highlighted the news that 16 girls were raped in Muzaffarpur in a girls' shelter home; in addition, one girl died after rape. On 1 August 2018, in Maharashtra, a pregnant lady carrying for 8 months was gang raped in front of her husband. In Hisar, Haryana, 24 girls were sexually exploited in school by a physical training instructor (*Maharashtra Times*, 18 December 2019).

Gang rapes are also committed very often. On 20 March 2020, four rapists in the Nirbhaya gang rape case were hanged to death. Nirbhaya, a physiotherapist, was gang raped brutally by six rapists in Delhi in December 2012. She was tortured in such an inhuman way that, after a few days of extreme suffering and struggle, she died.[13] There are many other cases where criminals are involved in extreme violence. It was in November 2019 that a young lady veterinary doctor was gang raped and then burned alive in Hyderabad.[14] Afterwards, all four of

---

[11] freepressjournal.in 9 April 2021

[12] http://www.pressreader.com>in 11 June 2018

[13] http://www.bbc.com

[14] abplive.com, 30 Nov 2019.

the victims were shot dead in an encounter by police. 'News 24 Uttar Pradesh' depicts the Unnao case where after rape the victim was set ablaze, she ran 1 km and cried for help (YouTube 26 December 2019). On the 25 January, a 70-year-old lady was gang raped (as is reported by News18 Lokmat, 26 January 2020). In July 2018, in Kanpur, a 4-year-old female child was raped by four male children ranging from 6 to 10 years of age. These children told police that they had learned these sex-related acts from porn videos on mobiles.[15]

In Haryana, a lady police sub inspector was gang raped inside the all-women police station in Palwal, Haryana, in September 2018. There are many other incidents where either male police officers were the rapist or female police personnel were raped. A girlfriend was raped by her boyfriend and his four friends in Patna (Odd Naari, 5 January 2020).

Resistance is never tolerated by rapists while the act of rape. In Muzaffarpur, a 23-year-old lady was burnt alive as she was resisting the rape attempt (*Maharashtra Times*, 10 December 2019). In the same city, another lady was subjected to acid attack as she did not withdraw a case filed against the four rapists (*Maharashtra Times*, 8 December 2019).

Inhuman Cruelty during Rape

A brutal gang rape and murder on 3 Jan 2021 by a priest and two others in Uttar Pradesh was really devastating. In Badaun, a 50-year-old woman was gang raped and tortured to such an extent that an iron rod was inserted into her vagina, her lungs, legs and ribs were broken. Her flash was literally bitten. She died due to excess bleeding (News18 Lokmat, 6 January 2021, The Quint, 2021). BBC News on 18 July 2018 reported that an 11-year-old girl was gang raped by 17 adult males in Chennai. They are security guards, electricians and plumbers of a huge building in a posh residential area. A 16-year-old girl who was admitted to ICU was gang raped by five in Uttar Pradesh (Sharma, 2018). A girl who became pregnant due to rape was sentenced to death by burning alive. Caste justice Panchayat of the Adivasi community in Jharkhand declared this 'justice' (Aaj Tak, 25 October 2018).

---

[15] http://www.ndtv.com> 4 July 2018

A lady police officer and her 16-year-old daughter were raped (*Navbharat Times*, 5 October 2018). It was reported in the news in *The Hindu* on 6 December 2018 that a lady was raped and chilli powder was inserted in her private parts.

In Uttar Pradesh, a girl was raped and set ablaze on 15 December 2019 (*The Hindu*, 2019). The 23-year-old woman resisted the attempt to rape; hence, she was burnt alive in Muzaffarpur (*Maharashtra Times*, 10 December 2019). A married woman was raped by an acquaintance; video shooting was done, and she was threatened that it would be made viral (*Maharashtra Times*, 13 December 2018). *India Today* (May 28 2012) reported that a rapist released from jail again raped and killed a girl in Shirdi.

Many girls are raped in schools and hostels of government-aided institutions. In Solapur, Maharashtra, a college girl was gang raped by five (*Maharashtra Times*, 2 February 2020). A married lady who was accompanying her paralyzed husband was gang raped by a ward boy in a hospital in Jalgaon (*Maharashtra Times*, 21 February 2020). In Pune, a rapist on parole again tried to rape the victim and kill her (ABPLive, 8 February 2020). A ninth grade student was raped by a teacher in Beed (News18 Lokmat, 8 December 2019). In Hisar, Haryana, 24 girls from a government school were sexually exploited (*Maharashtra Times*, 18 Dec. 2019). A mother and daughter were gang raped in Amarawati on 17 December 2019 (Live Blog, 2019). A mother killed her own son, who used to rape his own sister. There are multiple factual stories on Google and YouTube where brothers rape their sisters (like Dailyhunt, 26 February 2020).

A very serious case of a serial killer is worth noting. He has raped 65 individuals, which includes young girls, boys, adult male members and even third gender. In the Pollachi sexual harassment case, 50 women were exploited (Oddnaari, 2021).

In research in India, 42 rape victims were studied. It was seen that 90 per cent of the rapes were situational. Half of the rapists were known individuals or acquaintances. In some other research, this percentage is as high as 94 per cent. A total of 58 per cent of rapes were done by single individuals, 21 per cent by two and the remaining 21 per cent were gang rapes. In most of these cases, there was no violence. About 70 per cent of these rapes took place in the residence of the victim or that of the criminal. The age range of the majority of victims was from 15 to 20, and that of the criminals was 23 to 30 years (Ahuja, 1992).

Rapists are punished only in 11 per cent of cases, according to records. That too, it takes years to complete the legal procedures, trials and declare punishment. There is a substantial increase in juvenile criminals. About 32,500 cases of rape were registered in 2017, approximately 90 per day. Of those, only 18,300 were disposed of. A total of 127,800 cases were pending at the end of 2017 (Reuters Staff, 2019).

In India, approximately 7,500 minors are raped each year. This figure is increasing substantially every year. It was reported by a researcher that in 38 per cent of rapes, the victim was less than 6 years old. Other rapes of minors are not reported, which may be overwhelmingly more than expected. If the case is reported, the young child gets all sorts of unfair treatment everywhere, in the family, school, society at large, and even in legal procedure. Some of them are so unwanted and neglected that they become victims of human trafficking and are forced into prostitution by their own parents. The victim is not strong enough but is passive and helpless. Sometimes, even unwanted sex is also consensual. Male members compel their girlfriends or fiancés or women to be ready for sexual relations as they are afraid of losing the man.

Social aspects to be considered about rape are during war or riots. It is very common for women from other nations, religions or territories to be raped. Even otherwise, male members of high status can manage to rescue themselves from legal punishment as well as social stigma after they rape. Women from very low status or those who do not have family are vulnerable as there is no one to support them in getting justice.

McKibbin et al. (2008) have given different types of rapists. These types and some more types are as follows:

1. **The disadvantaged rapist:** Such a male hardly gets sex. There is no worry about loss of status as there is nil.

2. **Opportunistic rapist:** He tries to convince the woman. If not, then he rapes.

3. **Power rapists:** They are motivated by the idea of domination and control.

4. **Anger rapists:** They are motivated by anger and use it in overt ways. They may use excess force or even weapons.

5. **Sadistic rapists:** Such rapists are motivated by sexual and aggressive fantasies.

6. **The rape aroused rapist:** The rapist who is sexually aroused only by rape rather than by any other sex-related activities.

7. **Psychopathic rapists:** These rapists have psychopathic problems.

8. Rapist who thinks that the victim has already had sex with another man. He does it to take revenge and wants to win the sperm competition.

Researchers have reported that 60 per cent of men accepted that they would rape under specific conditions if there was no legal punishment. In research, 356 college male students were asked if no one knew and no legal action was taken, would they commit a rape? Approximately the same percentage of students said yes, they will (Briere & Malomuth, 1983). In contemporary society, this percentage must have substantially increased. It is also proven that a substantial number of men have common fantasies related to rape. Some think that any man can rape in a given situation. Research like 'Why Do Men Rape'[16] and the one by Pandey (2017) shed some more light on the mentality of men in general and rapists in particular. Pandey interviewed 100 convicted rapists in India and found that most of them were dropouts and had not even completed primary schooling. Hardly 3/4 of these hundred were repenting about their behaviour. Others were trying to deny that rape had taken place or were trying to justify it (Update News, 2017). They did it because of general attitudes towards women and socialization practices based on the idea of male superiority. They were just ordinary men.[17] She also concluded that

---

[16] https://www.researchgate.net/publication/325271704_Why_do_men_rape_Understanding_the_determinants_of_rapes_in_India

[17] https://www.ted.com/talks/madhumita_pandey_why_i_study_rapists_and_their_motivations

rape is about power to overcome threatened masculinity due to, for example, financial incompetence. Their sense of honour is hurt by something and they want to overcome that feeling of being inferior. This 'toxic masculinity' in India needs to be changed, which depends on the change in mind set from the beginning.

Many experts think that rape is about dominating the victim, taking revenge or abusing power rather than about sex. The personality of a rapist is one of the most important research areas. Rapists are generally single males. The age range is between the ages of 15 and 30 years. Researchers also reported that rapists have high levels of impulsivity and aggression, sexist views about women, and high levels of rape myth acceptance. Individuals involved in sexual assault and rape often have histories of personal violence. It may be child physical abuse, child sexual abuse, dating violence, or intimate partner violence. They watch pornography for a substantial period of time every day (Bouffard, 2010). Most rapists repeat the crime many times. Recent research has found that the majority of rapes are done by serial offenders. It may be on an average of six rapes (Lisak & Miller, 2002).

7.4.1. Theories of Rape

It may enhance understanding of how researchers view rape and the root cause behind it. Some important theories are as follows:

1. **Psychopathology:** According to this theory, mental illness, uncontrollable sexual urges or intoxication are basic reasons for rape. Actually, the potential for rape may exist in many more so-called normal individuals also. There is a lot of research evidence about the theory. For example, in Britain, a paedophile, Huckle, raped many babies, and experts think that he raped 200 (YouTube, 2016).
2. **The victim precipitation theory:** It is based on the idea of an invitation for sex. It says that rape takes place because of specific type of behaviour of the victim. According to it, others may be safe.
3. **Feminist theory:** These theorists perceive rape as the domination of men over women. It is the threat that compels women to behave according to their traditional subordinate role. It helps to keep her 'in her place'.

4. **Sex role stereotyping theory:** Men are supposed to be strong and aggressive, and women are expected to be submissive and passive. This encourages rape as it becomes easier to oppress women. Women are perceived as 'possessions'.

5. **Sociological theory:** It says that rape is an expression of power differentials in society (Martin, 2005). The easiest way is to overpower women by rape. If a man can't prove his superiority otherwise, he proves it this way. At that moment, the rapist perceives that he has control over the whole world.

6. **Evolutionary theory:** It says that male members want more sex to spread their seed, and on the other hand, women are more selective. This difference is responsible for rape.

Some rapes are done under the influence of drugs or alcohol. Instead of using force and facing resistance, nowadays, rapists are using different ways to achieve their criminal intention. Some drugs are mixed with soft or hard drink and given to the lady when she is completely unaware of that. These drugs produce drowsiness, dizziness, memory loss, low blood pressure, sleepiness, talking difficulties and impaired motor functions. If higher doses are consumed, convulsions, vomiting, loss of consciousness and coma or death can occur. These tablets quickly dissolve and are not traceable as there is no taste, odour or colour. There are many drugs of this sort which are used for rape. Some of them are also capable of producing loss of memory of that specific event. In that case, the victim is completely unaware and, in no way, can identify the rapist. It is essential to ban these drugs strictly. Nowadays, sadism and masochism are increasing. Ties to tie hands, handcuffs and ropes are used to tie the lady while rape. Even a female robot is available to have sex in some advanced countries. However, more popular is a very expensive robot which resists and denies sex. It gives the pleasure of rape to the man.

It is also worth noting that there is more social stigma for the victim than the accused. Some communities think that it is a sign of masculinity and those who are from upper cast and higher socio-economic status should use their power in this way. It is a matter of pride for them.

7.4.2. Culture

In rape culture, rape is accepted as an everyday occurrence and even a privilege of males. Victim blaming, reluctance of authorities to go against cultural norms of male superiority, delay in legal procedures and outcasting of the victim and her family are accompanied by rape myths. There are rape myths that ladies who are characterless invite rape. Only such ladies are raped, hence they deserve the same. As a consequence, the victim feels that she is responsible. She feels guilty and does not go to police for justice. Society justifies men's behaviour as they are aggressive and impulsive, and hence, it is not perceived as their responsibility. The world hypothesis says whatever happens to any individual is linked to her or his own actions.

In some cultures, there are widespread myths that raping a young girl child will cure HIV and other STDs.

For generations, in some cultures, rape has been accepted as a punishment. For example, in Cheyenne Indians, if there is any doubt about infidelity of the wife, the punishment is gang rape by invited relatives.

In many cultures, like the Marshall Islands, a woman is considered as property of a man, and he can use her anyway he likes and sexually exploit her any way. Gusii society in Kenya evaluates the power of man on the basis of pain that he can produce during intercourse. If the female has difficulty walking the next morning, the man is recognized as powerful. In some cultures, the boy has to rape a girl to prove that he is grown-up.

South Africa is among the countries having highest reported rape rates in the world. About 50 per cent of women are raped there. It is due to acceptance of violence against women in that culture. Even their leaders are involved in rape. This includes gang rapes. In that case, the woman has to face a lot of social rejection for accusing a leader.

In some parts of India, gang rape is a punishment given to a woman if her male family member wants to marry an upper caste or tribe girl. Such punishment is given in public.

There are many more types of populations who are suffering excessively due to issues like molestation and rape. These include disable, mentally retarded, lesbian, homosexual, bar dancers and similar others, transgenders, prostitutes, street children, very poor and so on.

7.4.3. Marital Rape

A young woman was divorced because she was not ready for unnatural sexual relations (*Maharashtra Times*, 10 December 2019). http://mlokmat.com gives a self-explanatory story of divorce given to a mother of 10 children after 25 years of marriage only because she denied sex to her husband. This family is from Agra. He wanted to rape her and could not tolerate her denial. As the wife denied sex, her husband killed her and cut his own sex organ (*Maharashtra Times*, 7 July 2019). In advanced countries, like the USA, where people openly accept rape in intimate relations, it is reported that 45 per cent of females and 30 per cent males are forced to get into sex.

India is one of the 36 countries where marital rape is not a crime. Approximately, 2.6 billion women live in countries where marital rape is legal. Under the clause of exception, it is clearly mentioned that 'sexual intercourse or sexual acts by a man with his own wife, the wife not being under fifteen years of age is not rape' (Section 375 of Indian Penal Code). Although majority of sexual violence reports are within marriage, it is justified as private affair of husband and wife based on traditions and social structure. Here, the rights of a woman are overpowered by undue privilege of her husband. If husband and wife are separated, then rape becomes punishable but not in marriage. Even the Domestic Violence Act, 498A, does not include rape. It is worth noting that in National Family Health Survey, it was seen that 54 per cent of women said that violence by husband is justified (The Better India, 2017).

A total of 150 countries have laws against marital rape. Of those, some do not differentiate between rape by husband and rape by someone else. In India, it is difficult for any authority to talk openly about such injustice and be strict regarding equality. It is a very critical issue related male ego. Indian marriage is taken as legal permission to have sex any number of times irrespective of consent, willingness, health and mood of wife. Wife as young as 8 or 10 years old or even 59 years old are compelled to bear the unpleasant experience or even the torture. Once married, men think that any sort of sex they indulge in is allowed. There is no sensitivity to her pain, weakness, over exhaustion and even monthly problems due to menstruation. Although it is a crime in developed countries, India is not in a position to treat it as criminal offence. At the most she can charge the husband with offence, like cruelty, or get protection under the Domestic Violence Act. The society does not want to give power to women to say 'no'. Even very well-educated men are completely unaware of the fact that sexual intercourse without the consent of wife is unfair, unjustified and it spoils interpersonal relations.

Subordination, subjugation and submission of wife are approved by most of the religions, social norms and standards of interpersonal relations all over the world. Traditionally a husband was supposed to have every control over wife's sexuality and basic purpose of marriage was perceived only as male member's convenience to have sex as per his demands. This chronic abusive relation is based on unfair cultural practices and societal ideologies, with apathetic legal system. In India traditional views about marriage, distorted interpretation of religious doctrine, male dominated culture, subjugation oriented socialization of women enhance self-oriented and insane attitude of male members. They consider wife as a commodity and something that should be exploited to any extent. It is essential to consider that even when it comes to pregnancy, she can't decide when to have it. She can't protect herself and ask the partner to use condom though she wants to avoid pregnancy. There are cases where the husband has STDs, the wife is aware of it and still she can't escape from it. Even AIDS patients exploit their wives and as a consequence the wives also get infected.

All religions expect that a woman should be submissive and should submit herself to the authority of her husband. Around 1970, feminists in Western countries put forth that women must have a right to decide about sexual interaction and her consent is essential. Even today, 51 per cent of women are raped by intimate partners. Although marital relations are changing gradually, change in positive direction is very slow, and its proportion is very meagre. Majority of homes are still operating as per the traditional way most convenient for male members. Even authorities have submitted an affidavit to Delhi High Court that if marital rape is criminalized in India, it will destabilize marriage system. It was stated that there is a possibility that such law will be misused. It may be used as a tool to harass husbands. The Justice Verma Committee was supporting it, but there was lot of resistance.

The basic question is whether law against marital rape will destroy 'sanctity of marriage'? A well-known Supreme Court lawyer tweeted that 'there is nothing like marital rape. There will be more husbands in jail than in house, our homes should not become police stations'. It obviously means that our social leaders are also taking things so casually as if it does not exist (*The Indian Express*, 19 August 2017). Union leader and minister for women and child development, Maneka Gandhi, remarked that laws against rape are the issue which is internationally accepted. However, it can't be applied to Indian society due to illiteracy, poverty, customs and mind set of the society. A very thought-provoking video on YouTube is 'Why Is Marital Rape Still Not a Crime in India?'[18]

> The Delhi High Court recently, in July 2018, mentioned that marriage does not mean that wife should always be ready for sex. While defining rape, according to the court, it is not essential to use physical force for rape, especially in marriage. Today, the whole concept of rape needs to be changed. Male and female partners both have equal right to say no to sex.

7.4.4. Men as Victims of Rape

Although in most of the cases victims are females, sometimes, harassment, molestation and rape take place with boys and men. There are very few research studies and awareness is also less regarding ill effects of such type of oppression on personality and whole life of a victim. One study found that a lifetime prevalence rate of sexual assault in men is 13 per cent. Male rapes account for approximately 8 per cent of all non-institutional rapes in the USA.

---

[18] https://www.youtube.com/watch?v=9Ld9K5J9ptc

Are Men Really Invulnerable?

In India, there is no legal definition of male rape victims. At the most, it is accepted that they can be sodomized due to unnatural sex as 'act against god' (Section 377 of Indian Penal Code). The Protection of Children from Sexual Offences protects male children but not male adults. In a survey, it was found that 71 per cent of male members were abused in childhood or adolescence. The government data reveals that 50 per cent of child sexual abuse victims are boys of 5 to 15 years. About 60 per cent of them are raped repeatedly. One in every five males are raped or molested at least once in life. They don't talk about it due to embarrassment and as it questions masculinity of the victim.[19] In the USA, millions of men, that is, 1 in every 33 men have experienced rape or attempted rape. Transgender students are at high risk.

On 27 September 2019, a young man was gang raped in Thane. A 34-year-old man went for a walk where five men gang raped him and tortured him by inserting certain things in his anus. He was seriously injured and was operated immediately. On 12 December 2019, *Maharashtra Times* has reported that a 22-year-old young man was gang raped by four men in Mumbai. In 22 years, there is 4 times increase in sexual crimes on male children.

A woman is reported to rape many girls by using sex toy (*Maharashtra Times*, 9 November 2019). Female rapists are also reported to get involved in sexually aggressive behaviours, including forced sex with verbal coercion (Anderson & Savage, 2005). Women use psychological pressure such as verbal persuasion or emotional abuse rather than physical power for rape of a man.

The majority of men are assaulted for the first time before the age of 18. Sexual dysfunction is common in male rape victims, and it leads to unhappy marriages. Such ill effects are seen for a number of years after the rape (Walker et al, 2005). Some studies have found that male rape victims increase their post-rape sexual activity to reaffirm their manhood. Gay men are reported to be more frequently victimized than other men. Mostly, man-to-man rape is anal sex, then oral sex. This is more of a power game than sex. It results in anger, hostility,

[19] https://hindi.gonewsindia.com/latest-news/health/sexual-abuse-of-males-shrouded-in-the-shadows-553

shame, low self-esteem, self-blame, anxiety, depression and increased vulnerability. The scenario regarding male rapes is even more difficult to study scientifically. Male members essentially keep it as a secret. In Indian male-dominated society, doubts about a man who is raped are more humiliating. They are perceived as being homosexual, unmusculine and third gender. Hence, the physical injuries are also difficult to disclose. A step mother used to rape her son for two years.[20] In developed countries, it was reported that approximately half of the male victims were victimized by women.

According to the Indian Penal Code, 2013, all sexual acts between the same sex are a crime as per Section 377. Punishment for that was the same as rape. However, in 2018, same-sex marriages will be exempted from it. Scientific research on male rape was done in 1980. In sexual violence, the concept of 'made to penetrate' is used in a common form. The Centers for Disease Control and Prevention reported that in 2012, there were 1.7 million cases. Psychologist Crome concluded that only 10 per cent of the male-to-male cases are reported. Society, legal system and the family are ill equipped to support these victims. Similarly, female-to-female rapes are never reported. Male victims face problems related to mental health, such as depression, post-traumatic stress disorder, addictions and suicidal thoughts and attempts. As their sexual identity is questioned by them, their self-image depicts an inadequate man.[21]

7.4.5. Consequences of Rape

Rape is an extremely humiliating, insulting and disgusting experience which leads to intense embarrassment. Here, someone else exploits one's body in a highly offensive manner, and uses it as a commodity to be consumed. It is a physical act but simultaneously equally intolerable at a psychological level. The consequences are so intense that it is very difficult to overcome them. All the ill effects of sexual abuse and sexual harassment are seen in the cases of these victims; however,

---

[20] m.lokmat.com 13 March 2020

[21] https://en.wikipedia.org/wiki/Rape_of_males

the intensity is much greater. It is physically and psychologically painful and traumatic. If oral sex is forced, then there are problems regarding difficulty swallowing, swollen throats and infections in the mouth and throat. In the case of women, common physical effects are vaginal and anal bleeding and irritation, internal bleeding, bruising, fractures, pains and aches, difficulty in locomotion, internal complications, gynaecological problems, sexually transmitted infections and unwanted pregnancy. This makes the victim even more helpless and hopeless. It is worth noting that most of them can't return to their original functional and adjustment level. There is overwhelming self-pity, sadness, guilt and shame for the whole life.

Among the psychological impacts of rape on victims, the first is extreme shock. There is rape trauma syndrome, post-traumatic stress disorder, including severe anxiety, uncontrollable thoughts, nightmares and severe anxiety. Depression with prolonged sadness, hopelessness, unexplained crying and lack of interest in social activities are reported. All these things result in suicidal thoughts and attempts. Inability to concentrate on work, cognitive problems, such as memory problems, disorientation and inability to make decisions are reported. They can't develop good, cordial and trusting relations with others. There is emotional numbness, helplessness, fear and a sense of being worthless.

Due to social norms, social stigma and the subordinate status of women, many victims do not report it to anyone. They blame themselves for trusting the rapist, being with them or for consuming alcohol and drugs. They are afraid of the possibility that their report will not be taken seriously, but it will only lead to breaking confidentiality. There is always a terror that the rapist will retaliate and take revenge as well as repeat it. The victims become insecure and dependent on someone. This enhances the vulnerability of the victim. Due to the shattering experience of rape, some victims are completely frozen emotionally. They can't resist even at the time of rape. The law and society think that the victim never retaliated and think that they were willing to have sex. Silent rape reaction is when the victim stops sharing anything, suffers a lot but keeps mum about the rape. Those are the ones who have experienced sexual molestation in the past.

7.5. PROTECTIVE ENVIRONMENT, SOCIAL AND FAMILY SUPPORT AND INTERVENTION

Any civilized society should develop an awareness regarding human rights. Practising androgyny, enhancing empathy, unconditional positive regard for children and clear communication with each other may help to reduce many emotional factors contributing to such injustice. Acceptance of self and others should be practised from childhood. This may result in a more conducive environment for everyone, irrespective of age and gender.

A 19-year-old adolescent male killed himself in September 2018 in Raipur. The police were confused about the reason behind it. A minor girl solved the puzzle and told police that she was gang raped in front of the boy by some antisocial youth. He was beaten and was forced to watch the gang rape as he tried to protect her. Out of agony, frustration and hopelessness, he killed himself.[22]

This true story is enough to understand how others are also affected with the victim of rape. It is common that rape victims commit suicide, but the others are also affected equally.

The effects of rape on victims are extremely serious; however, family members and dear ones are also shocked by it. Parents, siblings, close friends and life partners all suffer emotionally and socially. There is an overwhelming social stigma due to which they feel ashamed, hopeless and withdrawn. They are treated unfairly and are humiliated by others. It is difficult to get justice immediately, and the family is further demoralized.

Counselling rape cases is a very skilful job. Due to the agony experienced by such victims, even the counsellor may be emotionally moved. However, the counsellor must be emotionally stable and mature enough to express critical empathy. The most significant thing is the emotional catharsis of the victim. The counsellor should have all the necessary skills to understand a victim's mental status, listen effectively and generate confidence in their mind. Equally important is to create support from family and society. Society

[22] Chattisgarh://timesofindia 13 September 2018

penalizes the victim and she has to face social stigma. It is essential to make people aware of the fact that it is not the victim's fault and she should not be blamed.

Intense family therapy should help the victims and their families to accept reality. The role of the family in helping the victim to regain routine activities and everyday interactions is very important. Continuously reminding the victim about her problems should be avoided. Medical aid should be made available immediately as there is a lot of pain, discomfort, agony and suicidal thoughts. Precautions must be taken and testing for pregnancy, AIDS and other STDs should be carried out. Legal support is equally important. There are anti-rape female condoms which are available in advanced countries. It hurts the rapist, and they have to rush to the hospital immediately. There are rape prevention programmes for both genders in colleges and universities. Economic help through various provisions by government and non-government organizations should be arranged.

Rational emotive behaviour therapy, cognitive behaviour therapy and techniques, such as thought stopping and relaxation, are effective for dealing with psychological problems. In exposure therapy, which is a behavioural therapy, the victim has to combat painful memories of abuse. The prevention of anxiety, depression, post-traumatic stress disorder and panic attacks need both medicines and counselling. Complete rehabilitation requires provision for some meaningful activities to maintain self-worth, such as work, study and hobbies. Even pets are effective in improving the conditions of the victim. Unconditional acceptance and whole-hearted compassion are the most effective ways to help the victim. In the Indian community, no one is ready to accept the victim as a marriage partner, and those who are married are also disowned immediately. More awareness and sensitivity needs to be enhanced in the Indian community.

7.6. SUMMARY

Sexual abuse, sexual harassment and rape are the most unpleasant experiences which are shocking for the victim. If the victim is comparatively young and is not in a position to explain what has happened, it is the responsibility of parents, teachers and significant adults to make behavioural signs and symptoms meaningful. They should help the individual to come out of the trauma and be more confident and fearless. Sexual harassment is so common that 90 per cent of girls and women experience it at some point in their lives. If it is an educational institution or workplace where the individual is being harassed, the ill effects are more serious psychologically, socially and physiologically.

Rape shatters victims' minds completely, and they suffer from various serious physiological and psychological disturbances. Sometimes, it is a lifelong stigma and psychological disorder. Marital rape is not taken seriously in Indian society. As a consequence, numerous women suffer for the whole of their lives. If male member is raped, it is difficult for him to lead a normal life and have a satisfactory married life.

The examples given here are just representative, and there are thousands of cases worth mentioning to understand the agony and suffering behind them. It is essential to have empathy and understanding to be with the victim and support them.

Alcohol and Substance Abuse

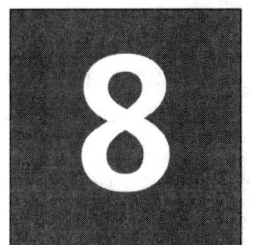

8.1. INTRODUCTION

This is the fourth time that Karan has been admitted to the intensive care unit (ICU) in a well-known multi-speciality hospital. His liver function is deteriorating, and there is an accumulation of fluid in his stomach. Liver cirrhosis is now pretty serious. Doctors repeatedly warn him not to consume alcohol. However, he is not ready to follow. He is still consuming alcohol every day, and the family members cannot control him.

Addiction has been prevalent all over the world for generations. The history of addiction is reported to be substantially lengthy, that is, for 8,000 years. It may not be possibly proved that it existed before that, though it must be. There are many communities, primitive and advanced, educated or uneducated, coming from low or high socioeconomic strata, perceiving drugs and alcohol as an inherent part of human life and celebration. It is widely accepted that it works as a medicine for many health problems as well as anxiety and tension.

What is the cost of abusing alcohol in terms of the toll of injuries, disorders, violence and human life?

A total of 28 per cent of all deaths due to alcohol result from injuries resulting from accidents, self-harm and violence, according to WHO. It is reported that 21 per cent result from digestive disorders, 19 per cent due to cardiovascular diseases and the remaining because of cancer, infections and mental disorders. Alcohol consumption has doubled in India within few years (WHO, 2018). Every 96 minutes, one Indian dies as a result of alcohol addiction.

8.1.1. Nature of Addiction

Along with alcohol, various drugs are also abused by individuals of all ages. According to WHO, a drug is any substance which modifies one or more functions of a living being if it is consumed. A psychoactive drug is one that alters mental functioning. According to Mitchell (2014), drug abuse is improper or illegal use of a drug, taking it in excessive doses when no medical reason exists. Many of them were developed and are being used as remedy for some illnesses or for reducing pain, for example—opium.

WHO defines drug abuse as a state of periodic or chronic intoxication, detrimental to the individual and the society, produced by repeated consumption of drugs. Three things are essentially seen in it: compulsion, increase in dose for the same experience, and psychological and physiological dependence.

> Average age of young addicts is less than 18, while legal drinking age is 25. Approximately 88 per cent are below that age. Dhawan et al. (2017) have reported an all-sided scenario of India in 2017. It describes results of a study of 4,000 children using substance from 100 cities all over India. Age group 10–19 constitutes 22.8 per cent and age range 5–9 years constitutes 12.5 per cent of the population involved in substance abuse. Male–female ratio is 1,000:882. The youngest child in the sample was 5-year old (NDTV, 2017).

It is reported that there has been a 30 per cent increase in drug addictions in India in the last decade (*India Today*, 2019).

There are different types of psychoactive substances. They are:

1. Alcohol
2. Opium
3. Cannabis
4. Cocaine
5. Hallucinogens like lysergic acid diethylamide (LSD)
6. Inhalants such as white ink and petrol
7. Amphetamine
8. Sedatives
9. Nicotine
10. Other stimulants like caffeine

If classification of drugs is done according to their effects, there are four types: narcotic analgesics, stimulants, depressants and hallucinogens. The first type, like opium, relieves pain. The second stimulates and speeds up the functions of the central nervous system. The third, depressants, slows down the functions of the central nervous system. Hallucinogens affect perception, emotions and mental processes.

Another classification is according to the origin of the substance. Some are natural, some are semi-synthetic, others are synthetic and some designer drugs. The designer drugs are also synthetic and have a very high addictive potential.

In spite of its ill effects, why is one attracted to addiction?

There are various reasons and correlates of alcohol and substance abuse. As far as youth are concerned, the starting point is curiosity regarding the thrill of consuming substance or alcohol. This is the stage of life where especially male members in Indian culture are attracted to exciting experiences. They are also interested in expressing that they can act independently according to their wishes and go beyond parental control. In a way, it is a rebellious attitude. In a group of friends, they want to prove that they have the daring to experience these things. At this stage, their impulse control is low. Stress management and tolerance of failure are poor. They want to get rid of unwanted realities such as childhood trauma, loss, family discord and emotional upsets. Most of them think that this is the best way to overcome fatigue and grief. Specifically, if youth are confused regarding life goals and disappointed about education, career and love affairs, it is the most common activity to indulge in. Some personality disorders are responsible for addiction. Substantial research has been done regarding it; for example, Mitchell and Potenza (2014) have shown relationship between addictions and personality traits such as impulsivity and sensation seeking.

'Drug Abuse in India' (Study IQ Education, 2018) gives substantial information about Indian situation. Many other YouTube videos, like 'Straight Talk with a Drug Addict' (Real News of India, 2015), give first-hand information regarding perception, causes and consequences of drug addiction in lower socio-economic strata addicts.

Easy availability, peer pressure, permissive atmosphere and modelling are the social factors resulting in abuse. Family history of such abuse may be related to both genetic factors and imitation orientation, leading to addiction. Some biological and biochemical factors are also responsible for such addictions. For example, role of dopamine and norepinephrine is vital in the case of some types of addictions. Sometimes, continuous use of a specific drug as medicine may lead to addiction.

> Salil was depressed, lonely and was leading a worthless life. After his love marriage, a legal case was filed against him and his influential father-in-law managed to win the case. Salil was imprisoned for a few months. His wife was forced to remarry and he was shattered, helpless, hopeless and experiencing agony. After casual exposure to Corex, which is a cough syrup, he started consuming it without any medical reason. Then, it resulted in addiction, and consumption of many bottles in a day became a routine. It was beyond treatment, and the addiction finally took a toll on his life.

Similar addictions to various medicines and painkillers are also very common. Addiction to sleeping pills is equally dangerous.

According to the International Classification of Diseases 10, the first-stage acute intoxication is a transient condition when an individual consumes alcohol or substance, which results in disturbances in the level of consciousness, cognition and perception. As a consequence, it affects behaviour. These effects decrease with time. Recovery is complete if there are no further complications or permanent damage. In extreme cases, even coma, convulsion or delirium may result.

> Soma was the only child of an affluent family. She had been involved in cocaine addiction for the last six months. Her father, who was an army officer, discovered it and immediately restricted her activities. She could not get her dose and started suffering badly. She was severely affected, had constant vomiting, was completely exhausted and could not breathe properly. She was so upset that she started screaming loudly and begging for her dose of smoke. The parents were firm. Somehow, she ran away from home and went to her addict friend. As both of them did not have money, she had to surrender herself for just two doses.

After substantial period of high dose consumption repeatedly, if the individual stops consumption, withdrawal takes place. Depending on the severity, it lasts for few hours to few days. It leads to compulsion for further use of substance.

Third stage is dependence syndrome. During this stage, consumption of substance becomes a compulsion. The desire to consume it becomes so strong that it becomes the topmost priority of the individual. It is very difficult to control the desire. Increased consumption is necessary for achieving the same pleasure. This, in turn, results in damage to other organs like liver in case of alcohol.

Fourth stage is harmful use. In this stage, irrespective of damage done to internal organ and in spite of individual's awareness, one continues consumption of the substance.

Substance abuse and mental health disorders go hand in hand. In a developed country like the USA, 20 per cent of people are affected by both. It is also responsible for substantial percentage of morbidity and mortality. Only 32 per cent of patients get proper care. In a country like India, it is difficult to estimate the exact percentage of addiction, as it is traditionally accepted as a part of life. There are many families who give opium to young children so that they sleep calmly, and their mothers can complete household jobs. There are both men and women who use tobacco in various forms, such as bidi, cigar and *hukka*.

There are alarming changes in behaviour, which are useful for identifying whether adolescents are getting addicted to some substance. If there are some remarkable changes in an adolescent's behaviour, parents and teachers must take it seriously: Suddenly, adolescents become lazy, neglect academic or job performance, personal neatness and hygiene; their absenteeism on job or college increases; the person sits alone inside a closed room for hours and is reluctant to share any feelings; aggression increases; psychological distance increases from parents and family, only few friends become favourite or close; some money and other valuables disappear from home intermittently; the individual asks for huge amount of money without giving proper explanation regarding it; the adolescent or youth avoids family functions and get togethers; they are reluctant to face the authority figures at home and in organizations, disagreements, conflicts and arguments increase; general health of the individual deteriorates; the sleep patterns become odd; they sleep for many hours even in daytime without food and do not accept that it is bizarre; on checking their college bags, matchsticks, injection syringes and needles, and silver papers are found. As far as physical changes are concerned, addiction changes the whole personality. Physical appearance also changes: lack of cleanliness, stained fingertips, cigarette burns, skin rash and needle marks on forearms are obvious; drowsiness, slurred speech, fatigue, loss of appetite, restlessness, drooping eyelids, blank face, unsteady gait and weight loss are generally seen. Withdrawal symptoms are also obviously seen.

8.2. THEORIES OF ADDICTION

There are three basic theoretical perspectives regarding why people get involved in addictions. First is neurobiological, biological and biochemical perspective. The second is psychological and third is socio-cultural approach.

Neurobiological theories explain the effects of drugs on the brain. The most common systems involved in primary action on the brain are the dopamine and opioid system. Researchers have reported that alcohol, nicotine and cannabis are directly related to the dopamine level. Increased level of dopamine is very pleasant and has the reinforcing effect. Opioids such as heroin, morphine and codeine cause tolerance and dependence. Opioid system is associated with satiation and consummatory aspects of reward, such as rest, sedation and blissfulness.

Biological theories: These theories are regarding changes in brain due to addiction and genetic characteristics. Vulnerability of an individual depends on genetic endowment. Dependence on alcohol among siblings of alcohol dependents is 50 per cent. It is worth noting that 36 per cent of relatives of alcoholics are diagnosed as having alcohol use disorder, as compared to 15 per cent of the normal. Similar results are reported by researchers for other addictions.

Genetic characteristics are related to multiple genes or incomplete expression of major genes.

Biochemistry-related theories: Neuroadaptation are changes in brain that take place to oppose drug's acute action after drug administration. These changes include brain chemistry. Actually, tolerance of the effects of drugs and withdrawal are both the result of neuroadaptation. In withdrawal symptoms, there are physical as well as psychological and motivational symptoms such as dysphoria, depression, irritability and anxiety. They contribute to vulnerability to relapse and also have significance related to mental health.

Endocrine theory: According to some experts, dysfunction of endocrine system is responsible for addictions like alcoholism.

Psychological theories: Psychological theories see the compulsion of addiction similar to other syndromes such as obsessive-compulsive disorder and gambling. There is impaired control regarding abuse and tendency to continue it despite problems. There are different perspectives:

- Psychoanalytical theory says that repressed urges, childhood trauma or unmet needs may result in addiction. Sometimes, self-punishment may be the hidden intention behind it. Addiction may result from conflicts in the unconscious mind.
- The behavioural model, depending on conditioning principles, says that the individual's action of drug dependence is instrumental in the effects of drug that are perceived as reinforcement. There are other benefits of psychological and social nature of drug consumption which are equally reinforcing. Cue exposure theory is based on the same principle. Some cues associated with drug consumption may elicit the same response when only the cues are present. This may include external as well as internal cues.

Personality theories: Eysenck, in 1997, gave a concept similar to addictive personality. In the psychological resource model, it is explained as—addiction develops because it fulfils some purpose. That purpose is related to the individual's personality. There are some individuals who cannot tolerate and cope with unpleasant experiences such as failure and rejection. Their expectations are very high, but they want an easy way to achieve that. Research has indicated that psychoticism and neuroticism are seen among those who abuse alcohol, heroin, benzodiazepines, nicotine and similar substances. It is reported that persons who are anxious, moody, irritable, impulsive and aggressive are more likely to get involved in addiction. Among adolescents, those who are rebellious and less conventional are more likely to develop addictions.

In some popular movies, like *Kabir Singh*, extreme alcoholism is depicted as a result of failure in love affair. In real life, also, many superstars from film industry are reported to be addicted to alcohol and substances.

Some videos on YouTube, like 'Top Ten Alcohol Addicted Bollywood Celebrities', give us more details. Similar information is available for Bollywood and Hollywood, such as '10 Celebrities with Alcoholism'[1] and 'Top Ten Alcoholic Celebrities in India'.[2]

Similar sites for drug addiction are also ample, like '12 Celebrities Talk about Drug Addiction'[3] or '10 Bollywood Names Linked with Drugs'.[4]

Cognitive theories: Self-regulation theory says that planning, taking into account social and physical factors, goals and acting accordingly play an important role in addiction. The individual uses drugs and alcohol as external stimuli for maintaining physical and psychological balance. These individuals crave satisfaction right now and may neglect the long-term problem it may result in.
Sociological theories: Sociological theories say that it is a social activity. Hence, social stimuli, including friends, family members and neighbours, are responsible for such abuse. It creates an opportunity for an individual to try new things and get involved in drugs. Social as well as religious attitudes are responsible for drug abuse.
Cultural theory: The attitude of society towards drinking, other means of releasing tension and general expectations of the individual resulting in tension, are the three aspects of social influence causing addiction. If social pressure is intolerable, the possibility of addiction increases.

Some researchers have observed that both strong genetic component and environmental aspects are responsible for addiction.

[1] https://www.healthline.com/health/celeraty-alcoholics 26 May 2017
[2] https://www.mensxp.com/entertainment/gossip/9242 8 October 2015
[3] www.cosmopolitan.com., 23 oct. 2017
[4] http://www.freepressjurnal.in, 24 Jun 2016

Deviant behaviour theory: According to this theory, addiction is a rebellious act against norms. If addiction is socially unacceptable behaviour, the individual gets satisfaction that they are behaving against the authorities. Conduct disorder, antisocial personality, company of peers involved in inappropriate behavioural patterns, addictions in family members, inappropriate parental attitude, family discord and low socio-economic background show significant correlation with addiction.

Rational choice theories: Why individuals engage in self-destructive behaviour on their own, or voluntarily, is the basic issue. According to some experts, due to weakness of will, they behave against their own judgments. Even if they understand that they should not, they continue consumption of addictive substance. That means they are knowingly trapped in addiction. It may be related to immediate-gratification orientation. The individual wants excitement.

8.3. TYPES OF ADDICTION AND THEIR EFFECTS ON PHYSICAL HEALTH

The National Drug Dependence Treatment Centre of the All India Institute of Medical Sciences (AIIMS), New Delhi, conducted a countrywide investigation regarding incidence of various addictions in India (National Drug Use Survey, 2019). It was observed that 14.6 per cent of people in India, that is, 16 crore people, consume alcohol. The male–female ratio is 17:1. Approximately 5.2 per cent of people are suffering due to alcohol dependence. Bhang, ganja and *charas*, that is, some forms of cannabis, are used by 3.1 crore of Indians, that is, 2.8 per cent of Indians. 72 lakh individuals are seriously affected. Opioids are being consumed in different forms by a total of 2.06 per cent of people. Heroin is used by 1.14 per cent, pharmaceutical opioids are used by 0.96 per cent and opium is used by 0.52 per cent of people. Sedatives and inhalants are used by 1.18 crore people. It is worth considering that there are more addicted children and adolescents abusing inhalants than adults. It is exactly double, that is, 1.17 per cent of the individuals in the younger group and 0.58 per cent among adults. If we consider the total percentage of people using different types of addicts, it is approximately 25 per cent in India.

About 8.5 lakh people inject drugs; Of those, 46 per cent are opioid-injecting groups, and most of them use risky practices. Comparatively, less prevalence of cocaine, amphetamine and hallucinogen consumption is seen in India.

Some states, such as Delhi, Chhattisgarh, Tripura, Manipur, Sikkim, Andhra Pradesh, Maharashtra, Uttar Pradesh and Punjab, have more addicts. It is estimated that 1 in 38 addicts get some treatment; 1 in 180 get inpatient treatment. Even in the case of other addictions, 1 in 20 get any treatment.

According to a national survey, 40 lakh youngsters below 17 years of age are drug addicts and 30 lakh are involved in alcohol abuse in India (*Maharashtra Times*, 2019). This information was given in Parliament by the Ministry of Social Justice and Empowerment. Inhaler is being used for abuse by 30 lakh youngsters and 20 lakh more are involved in opium and painkillers' abuse. Approximately 4 lakh young addicts are using amphetamine-type stimulant, 2 lakh use cocaine and similar other stuff producing half-conscious state.

AIIMS declared that 5.7 crore people in the country are addicted to alcohol and 0.72 crore to cannabis.

Approximately 30 per cent consume desi or local liquor. Highest rate of alcohol abuse is in Uttar Pradesh.

8.3.1. Alcoholism

Dinesh never wanted to be an engineer. It was only because of the compulsion by his father that he completed the course and is now working as an engineer. He does not like his job at all. In addition, he could not get along well with his wife, as he expected compensation for his dissatisfaction from his family. He started drinking with friends occasionally; gradually, the frequency increased, and finally, it was every evening that he used to drink—a lot. After that, his behaviour became reckless and aggressive; his interpersonal relations were completely spoiled, and his health started deteriorating.

The term alcohol originates from the Arabic word *al-kuhul*—meaning finally divided spirit. It is a depressant. Various brands have 40 to 60 per cent alcohol. Alcohol dependence is one of the most common addictions. As defined by Keller (1979), it is a chronic illness, psychic, somatic or psychosomatic. It is repeated drinking that interferes with health, social or economic functioning. Different stages, such as early stage, middle stage and chronic stage, are given by experts. In the early stage, increased tolerance, temporary loss of memory, preoccupation and avoiding talking about alcohol are seen. Tolerance means the effect of alcohol is reduced gradually. Hence, taking more alcohol becomes essential to get the same experience. In the middle stage, loss of control, justifying drinking, grandiose behaviour or showing off and chain drinking are seen. In the chronic stage, continuous and binge drinking results in paranoia.

> Alcohol consumption starts with a pleasant experience and continues to avoid unpleasant experiences.

According to a researcher named Jellinek (1952), who is known for his research on alcoholism, there are the following five types of alcoholism.

1. **Alpha alcoholism:** This type of excess drinking is related to the reduction of physical and emotional pain. For some time, at least, the individual can forget about their problems, but there is no loss of control.
2. **Beta alcoholism:** Drinking addiction leads to complications such as cirrhosis, gastritis and neuritis.
3. **Gamma alcoholism:** It is characterized by the inability to control drinking. It is progressive in nature. The individual is physically and psychologically dependent on alcohol.
4. **Delta alcoholism:** This causes increase in tolerance, withdrawal symptoms, and inability to abstain, but not loss of control of the amount of intake.
5. **Epsilon alcoholism:** It is compulsive drinking or spree drinking.

Some ego defence mechanisms are used by addicts of all sorts to be comfortable with their addiction. Though the addict knows that it is detrimental to their health and performance, they try to defend their addiction. It helps them to maintain their coping, though distorted. First of all is the denial of reality. The addict will deny that they have any problems, or their addiction is spoiling their life. They will deny that they are neglecting their duties and spending a lot of time and money on that.

Regression or childish behaviour such as refusing certain things, avoiding some people and showing no interest in activities to improve their condition is common. Rationalization regarding addiction and justifying it while arguing with others are seen. They may blame it on the hard work they have to do for the whole day, tension due to economic problems and the like. Blaming others, acting out, procrastination and such other inappropriate and unhealthy defence mechanisms are used by addicts.

> Vilas is a student who comes from a very well-to-do family. After 12th, he was admitted to the best college in a nearby city. He was staying at the hostel. He was enjoying life without any restrictions from his parents and became very popular among friends. Just for enjoyment and curiosity, he started taking drugs. Gradually, it resulted in a habit, and the habit became an addiction. It spoiled his future. He used all his resources and, one day, had to sell even his books, bed and other belongings for his addiction. His family disowned him, and he had nowhere to go.

There are different types of complications associated with alcoholism. The whole nervous system of the addict gets affected. Some examples of such ill effects are cerebellar degeneration, dementia, hallucinosis, delirium, neuropathy and Wernicke–Korsakoff psychosis. There is an increased tendency towards suicide and suicidal ideation. The gastrointestinal system is also affected substantially. Consumption of alcohol leads to feeling full. It contains lots of calories, but there is no nutritional value. Hence, malnutrition and deficiency of vitamin B are seen. Memory deficits, polyneuritis or nerve problems result due to it. Numbness in peripheral muscles, fatigue, high blood pressure and heart problems are also seen in some cases. Gastritis, esophagitis, peptic ulcers and cancer of the stomach are some serious ill effects. Pancreatitis, malabsorption syndrome and protein-losing syndrome are also very common. Liver problems such as fatty liver, liver cirrhosis, hepatitis, liver-cell carcinoma or cancer and liver failure may result in danger to the life of the addict.

Alcoholic myopathy, coronary artery disease, sexual dysfunction and many more ill effects are reported. If a pregnant lady is an addict, foetal alcohol syndrome is seen among newborns. Low birth weight, delayed growth, heart defects, bones and joint deformities, and subaverage cognitive functions are the major common problems among these babies. Hence, their entire future gets affected. The whole life of an addict gets affected. Addiction leads to disturbed interpersonal relations, divorce, loss of job and a tendency towards criminal acts.

Cognitive functions also deteriorate. Intoxication leads to increased reaction time, more distractibility, slow thinking and poor motor control. The thinking process, decision-making, accuracy and awareness of sensory experiences decrease. The balance of the body cannot be maintained, and muscle control diminishes. This results in various accidents, especially if the addict is driving a vehicle. General self-control diminishes, and the individual behaves in a socially unacceptable way.

During withdrawal, there are symptoms, such as a hangover, tremors, vomiting, nausea, weakness, irritability and anxiety. In extreme conditions, delirium trimex takes place. Intense depression, extreme fear, bizarre hallucinations, uncontrollable behaviour and medical complications may lead to a risk of life.

8.3.1.1. Treatment of Alcohol Addiction

1. **Behaviour therapy:** As there is no therapy to alter the pleasant experience and changes in neurotransmitters taking place after consuming alcohol, aversion therapy is used very commonly. A mild electric shock or nausea-producing drug is given to the addict at the sight of alcohol. There are many ill effects of it. Alcohol consumption leads to vomiting, giddiness, rash and, sometimes, even vomiting blood or hematemesis. It may lead to life-threatening complications. Hence, such medicines should be given under proper medical supervision. This may reduce the desire for consumption of alcohol. Self-control skills, relaxation techniques, assertiveness training and giving positive reinforcement as per conditioning principles are also useful.

2. **Psychotherapy:** Group and individual psychotherapy are effective. Awareness of the addict regarding ill effects and risks, and regarding their responsibility for their own life and others' may be

increased. A very well-known group working for alcohol addicts is Alcoholics Anonymous. In such groups, the addicts openly share their problems and learn from each other's experiences.

3. **Psycho-social rehabilitation:** It is worth considering that no one has sympathy for addicts. Hence, social rejection is obviously seen. It is necessary that the addict should be able to regain reliability and trust by consistently proving that they are wholeheartedly trying to improve their behaviour.

Instead of suddenly terminating consumption of alcohol, controlled drinking can be practised for some time. The addict should keep a record of what stimulates them to drink and when they mostly drink; this helps to change the circumstances. If it is in the company of friends, they should be taught assertiveness to deny the drink. They should be encouraged to face reality and problems as well as stress. Every morning, they should take an oath that they will not drink today. The goal is specific and sounds achievable. It trains addicts to enhance their emotional, cognitive and social skills, so that they can work and lead their lives independently.

8.3.2. Opioid Use Disorders

Two Indians die every day in India due to drug overdoses, especially sleeping pills and painkillers (*Times of India,* 2018).

The plant of opium is called the plant of joy. Opium has been used for generations for addiction and painkilling purposes. There are several derivatives such as morphine, codeine, heroin, hydromorphone and many others. Morpheus is the name of the Greek goddess of sleep. Morphine is stronger than opium and heroin is even stronger than morphine. Some of them are injected and some others are consumed by smoking. Heroin is one of the most addictive drugs. Intoxication may lead to hypotension, bradycardia, respiratory depression and low body temperature. In the case of severe conditions, even coma may result. The withdrawal symptoms are tachycardia, sweating, hypertension, body aches, cramps, vomiting, nausea, anxiety and anorexia. It is more serious in the case of heroin.

Complications are Parkinson's disease, neuropathy, degenerative changes in the brain and the like. Sharing needles for injections is known to cause AIDS, skin infections, viral hepatitis, tetanus and many other ill effects.

Behaviour therapy, interpersonal therapy, cognitive behavioural therapy, motivation enhancement therapy, family therapy and group therapy are used to help the individual. Psycho-social rehabilitation is also essential to prevent relapse.

8.3.3. Cannabis Use Disorder

Cannabis is derived from the hemp plant. It is called hashish or marijuana. Comparatively, mild physical dependence and mild withdrawal symptoms are seen in this case. Insomnia, irritability, restlessness, nervousness, decreased appetite and cravings are the withdrawal symptoms. The psychological dependence experienced is mild to severe.

Mild intoxication produces very pleasant experience. The individual feels like they were floating in the air and experiences euphoria. Light headedness, tachycardia, photophobia and red eyes are the major ill effects. Cognitive problems are depersonalization or de-realization and synaesthesia. Synaesthesia is a sensation caused by a sense modality and is experienced by another sense modality. It is something like smelling the sound and hearing the sight. Increased sensitivity to sound is also reported. Severe intoxication may result in hallucinations.

Depersonalization is complete detachment from oneself in all spheres: cognitive, emotional and behavioural. Depersonalization/de-realization is a dream-like experience. The person feels emotionally numb. They think that they are not in a position to control their own actions and even communication. In this case, an individual experiences their own thoughts, behaviour and emotional ups and downs from a distance, as if it is taking place in a dream. DSM 5 includes it.

Addicts are detached from their senses and, hence, cannot interpret environmental stimulation. Hence, they cannot make it meaningful, for example, what others are saying, whether there is any danger around and they are unaware of their own hunger, thirst and libido. It is completely a distorted perception of the world, for example, the size and colour of objects, time perception and the magnitude of sound are experienced in an unrealistic and bizarre way. All the events around are perceived as if they are reeled rather than real life. Such patients are, sometimes, confused regarding whether they are existing and alive or not. They may think that these experiences result from some serious irreversible brain damage (*Psychology Today*, 2019).

Psychological complications are severe. They are as follows.

1. **Amotivational syndrome:** Apathy, loss of interest, inertia, lethargy and a complete lack of motivation and ambition
2. **Mental health issues:** Acute anxiety, fugue-like state, paranoid psychosis, suicidal ideation, hypomania, schizophrenia, hallucinations and delusions

   A fugue is a state of reversible amnesia. Here, the individuals may forget even their personal identity, memories and personality. This may last for an unpredictable time. They start their lives with a new identity.
3. **Cannabis psychosis:** Disorientation and confusion
4. **Other effects:** Mood disorder, memory impairment, pulmonary malignancies, decreased testosterone and other hormonal problems

8.3.4. Cocaine Use Disorder

Immediately after consumption, cocaine produces a pleasurable sensation.

It is derived from the coca bush. It has been used as an analgesic since the 1860s. There are different ways in which it is consumed. It is taken orally, by smoking or parenterally.

Acute intoxication results in hypertension, tachycardia and papillary dilation, nausea, vomiting and sweating. The addict experiences elevated mood, hypervigilance and increased speed of speech. The physical effects are mild as compared to the psychological effects of cocaine. Psychological dependence is more severe. During the first few hours of withdrawal, agitation, anorexia, depression, sleepiness, craving, exhaustion and even anxiety are the symptoms experienced by such addicts. In case of complications, delusions and hallucinations, seizures, respiratory depression, arrhythmia, myocardial infarction, anoxia and lung damage are observed.

Crack is the most harmful type of cocaine. If a pregnant lady consumes it, there are severe ill effects on the foetus.

With medicine, psycho-social management, supportive psychotherapy and cognitive behavioural therapy are necessary to prevent relapse.

8.3.5. Amphetamine Use Disorder

Amphetamine has been used as a medicine since 1932 for treating asthma, rhinitis and coryza. It is also used to treat obesity, depression and Parkinsonism. Sometimes, students take it to reduce fatigue and the need for sleep.

Intoxication may lead to tachycardia, hypertension, cardiac failure, haemorrhage, tremors and even coma. The psychological effects are anxiety, insomnia, restlessness, irritability, panic disorder and hostility. Hallucinations and delusions may accompany them, while withdrawal, apathy, depression, fatigue, asthenia and sleep disorders are experienced with some other symptoms.

Use of antidepressants and supportive psychotherapy are recommended.

8.3.6. LSD Use Disorder

It has been known since 1938 that LSD is capable of producing hallucinations. Although psychological dependence and tolerance may take place, physical dependence or withdrawal symptoms are not seen.

Intoxication may lead to depersonalization or de-realization, intensification of perception, synaesthesia or confusion between senses, illusions and hallucinations, incoordination, tremors, giddiness, tachycardia, increased temperature and euphoria. Intense sensory perceptions, which are pleasant as well as fearful, are reported. The individual perceives as if their body parts are detached from each other. Paranoia may also result. Sometimes, anxiety and depression are seen in excess doses. Panic attacks are seen in acute intoxication. Withdrawal symptoms are stress and severe physical illness. Visual hallucinations are reported as a complication.

Medication and supportive psychotherapy are essential.

8.3.7. Barbiturate Use Disorder

Since 1903, it has been used as a tranquilizer and anaesthetic. It is useful as a sedative and an anticonvulsant. It is used for hypnosis also. Physical and psychological dependence develop soon. Tolerance is also quick. Intoxication results in uninhibited behaviour, slurring of speech, irritability, labile mood and memory and attention impairment. Even ataxia and suicidal ideation are seen. Withdrawal symptoms are severe. The individual suffers a lot. They experience hypertension, restlessness, tremors, seizures and delirium. After 72 hours, coma or death may occur. Medication, supportive psychotherapy and social rehabilitation are essential.

There are some more addictions, such as benzodiazepines, phencyclidine and inhalants or volatile solvent, and the ill effects are more or less similar.

In India, toddy and arrack, fenny and similar other addictions are prevalent.

8.3.8. Nicotine Addiction

One of the pioneering researchers, Sigmund Freud, used to smoke 20 cigarettes every day for years. Then he suffered from cancer of mouth. A major portion of his jaw was removed. He could not even swallow without pain. Still, he used to smoke excessively; ultimately, he died in 1939 due to cancer. A great neurologist, who has given very basic concepts in psychology, could not control his addiction.

The most common addictions in India are caffeine and nicotine. They are legally available. People are not aware of the fact that they cause all the ill effects like any other addiction.

Do you think smoking enhances positive mood and style? What happens to one's health? Smoking reduces the life span by approximately 13–14 years.

Smoking increases the risk of cancer and respiratory diseases as well as cardiovascular disease. Tobacco contains a very powerful poison, nicotine. If consumed in pure form, it has the capacity to kill human beings within a minute. The smoke from cigarette is absorbed into the blood stream and affects the brain. It is more harmful than other drugs like heroin. It is reported that more than 40 per cent of heart patients are smokers. Even passive smokers are at risk. It means the individual themselves are not smoking, but someone is smoking near them, and the smoke is inhaled anyway. Different illnesses are linked with smoking, such as cataracts, pneumonia and, along with cancer of the lungs, it causes cancer of the stomach, pancreas, cervix and kidney. If nicotine is found in a mother's milk or if babies are exposed to passive smoking, the possibility of sudden infant death syndrome increases. If women smoke, the possibility of conceiving decreases by up to 40 per cent. If at all they conceive, it results in low birth weight of babies. In India, smoking is a casual pass time activity. People are not aware of its ill effects, though the government is trying to increase awareness. Among the low socio-economic strata, even ladies are involved in smoking a crude form of cigarette called beedis, using tobacco in *hukka*, chewing tobacco directly and using it as a tooth powder. Rapid smoking technique is used for producing aversion.

It is worth noting that animals avoid eating tobacco leaves.

As the drug trade is illegal in India, lots of deception takes place. Mixing it with some other substances or harmful chemicals and other malpractices are very common. In India, the percentage of drug addicts, especially among high-school and college students and youth, is increasing substantially. Parents can not recognize it easily. There are very popular ways and forms to consume drugs, such as Kutta Goli and candy drugs. Especially, the north-eastern states have an overwhelming percentage. To fulfil requirement for money for drugs, addicts get involved in theft, crime and other illegal activities and prostitution.

Street children, truck drivers and daily-wage earners are involved in addictions for enjoyment and overcoming fatigue. Some others do it for glamour, to increase creativity, courage and to combat monotony and inhibition.

> In December 2019, as Delhi's cold wave made it difficult for the street children to survive, NDTV reported that approximately 100 homeless children stayed at the Delhi railway station and used white ink for inhalation. According to them, it gives them a lot of warmth from within (NDTV, 2009).

On the basis of this example, it is clear that the exact incidence depends on region, socio-economic status, education, religion, family and peers. For example, in tribal communities in Nagaland, Mizoram and Manipur, addiction is the highest. The opium-producing region in Madhya Pradesh also has a similar scenario. Alcohol is a regular food item in some communities.

Drug abuse basically leads to an increased possibility of HIV infection in two ways: the first is through using the same needles for injecting drugs by many individuals and the other is through sex. When an individual is under the impact of drugs, they may not have awareness that they should protect themselves while having a sexual interaction. They do it without thinking about who is the partner also. This may directly lead to infection.

8.4. CORRELATES OF DRUG ABUSE ALONG WITH CONSEQUENCES

Although it is a well-accepted fact that drug abuse is harmful, people, especially adolescents and youth, easily get involved in abuse of different sorts. Various reasons for abuse originate from the simple idea that it makes individuals happy, and they forget about their problems and tensions. There are social correlates such as peer pressure, social isolation and alienation, changing lifestyles and migration. So, on the one hand, lack of social interaction and, on the other, the wrong company may be associated with addiction. Alcohol consumption is considered as a symbol of social prestige in contemporary society. The number of ladies from the affluent class involved in alcohol consumption is increasing constantly. Again, here also, those who are from very low socio-economic strata get involved due to tensions, worries and fatigue, and the higher classes are interested in enjoyment and show-off. Personal problems such as failure in academics, unemployment, boredom, isolation and unsuccessful love affairs are common among Indian youth. In the case of younger addicts, curiosity, lack of awareness and ignorance have a strong relationship with addiction.

Addictions are related to the health of the addict, their family and even their next generation.

The long-term physical effects of addiction are degeneration of nerves in the arms and legs, destruction of brain cells and damage to the liver. Glue sniffing is reported to damage the kidneys and develop leukaemia. Heart-related problems, malnutrition, hepatitis are related to drug injections. If the expecting mother is an addict, then growth retardation and failure of brain maturation of the foetus may result, which may lead to spontaneous abortion.

More serious issues are of national and international significance. Almost all criminals are under the influence of some addiction at the time of committing a crime. In a country like India, it is very common to see family violence after the husband consumes alcohol. It is taken for granted and is not even mentioned in related news. In very few cases, it is specifically mentioned, like 'An Alcoholic MP Man Held for Repeatedly Raping Eight-year-old Daughter'.[5]

Substance abuse is affecting youth all over the world. Terrorism, the arms trade and drug trafficking enhance each other. New ways, new drugs and more dangerous and risky patterns are emerging every now and then.

India Today (2016) reported that juvenile crimes are directly linked to drug abuse. Sharma et al. have published a research paper in the

Indian Journal of Psychiatry, 2016, regarding 'Substance Use and Criminality among Juveniles-under-enquiry in New Delhi'.

It indicates that the drug–violence relation is complicated because of intoxicating doses and neurotoxic effects as well as withdrawal effects of alcohol, heroin or even inhalants.

Addiction results in accidents, domestic violence, crimes and similar social problems. National and international terrorism, excess stress on police force, increased health problems like HIV and AIDS are glaring correlates of addiction.

There are many discussions by experts on YouTube explaining the relationship between crime and addiction, like 'The Relationship between Drugs and Crime' (Kaitlyn, 2017; National Institute of Justice, 2012).

Economic insecurity, neglect and rejection by family and friends are also directly related to addiction. Cheating, lying, manipulating, unreliability and resentment are known correlates. Guilt, inferiority, anger and apathy are generated because of addiction. Contact with reality diminishes. Disturbances in interpersonal and intrapersonal relations may lead to divorce. Families of addicts and the community at large suffer due to family violence, other crimes and injuries.

Nearly 12,000 people die every year due to intoxicated drivers, and an average of nine lakh people are arrested for driving while intoxicated.[6]

There are a number of incidences where the relationship between alcohol consumption and crime becomes obvious. On 4 December 2019, in Thane, Maharashtra, an alcohol addict set his wife ablaze because of a minor reason: She did not serve him enough quantity of non-vegetarian dishes. She could not survive and, during treatment, passed away on 11 December 2019 (*Maharashtra Times*, 2019). In a way, every crime is related to some addiction; whether it is related to property, sexual offence or murder, the culprits are mostly addicts. Many thefts result from extreme and unlimited money required for purchasing drugs (National Institute of Justice, 2012; OnlyIas, 2019).

[6] timesofindia.com

The family members feel awkward about the drug addiction of their own offspring or siblings and want to hide the fact from others. This, in turn, results in guilt and shame. Social isolation of the addict, rejection and social stigma are resultant of that. Social stigma is so severe that there is a need to change social attitudes, as help from others becomes essential.

8.5. INTERVENTION AND OTHER ISSUES REGARDING MANAGEMENT

The goals of the intervention programme are as follows:

- Identifying and recognition of addiction
- Understanding
- Acceptance
- Accepting responsibility for overcoming the problem
- Modification of behaviour
- Adapting to new, healthy ways of life

There are three treatment stages: intervention, rehabilitation and maintenance.

Stage 1 is intervention, A social support team should be ready to assist an addict by giving them all sorts of support and encouragement. On the one hand, the person should be identified as an addict, and on the other hand, they should be helped to accept the fact and be ready for treatment. Objective proof should be collected and discussed with the addict. To enhance readiness, rehearsing intervention scenes, discussing with others who have already undergone treatment and increasing reality orientation are essential. Confronting the problem is more important. Detoxification is the next step. It is significant to manage the withdrawal symptoms, as these are very unpleasant and life-threatening. Medical assistance and regular treatment or, sometimes, hospital admission become a must.

Stage 2 is rehabilitation, which includes evaluation, primary care and extended care. The severity and seriousness of the individual's conditions should be evaluated by various screening tests, questionnaires and interviews. Assessment of biochemistry may result in an exact understanding of the condition. Accordingly, medical assistance should be made available. Primary care includes therapeutic activities for attending to higher levels of psychological, social and physical functioning. Extended care is the continuation and consolidation of previous treatment and maintaining its benefits.

In maintenance, that is, Stage 3, there are three types of care. The first is aftercare, which is continuous support and monitoring. Relapse prevention is a precaution that the individual should not regress and start getting involved in addictive behaviour again. As relapse is very common, follow-up becomes a must. Developing the courage to accept reality, understanding self and realizing the ill effects of addiction always help.

Efforts to achieve normal physical functions, psychological and social independence are essential. Most relapses occur due to anxiety and stress. Sometimes, the availability of money increases the possibility. In such a situation, the individual should contact their counsellor and recollect memories of how their life was affected and their conditions had gone bad due to addiction. Imagery should be used for that. Like, for example, the addict should think that they are again experiencing all bizarre things, withdrawal symptoms and pains and stigma, so that the individual can vividly recollect traumatic experiences. Due to that, they may refrain from substance or alcohol abuse.

Bandura's social learning approach explains self-efficacy strategies. It generates competency and self-confidence. Cue therapy and behavioural self-control training are very effective. It enhances coping with any stress. Using other ways to reduce stress is to be taught. Alternate behaviour and thinking strategies are used. Self-monitoring, feedback, coping and record keeping are effective. Extinction is used. A high-risk situation increases the possibility of relapse. One has to practise refusing drinks or substances assertively and firmly. In this case, cues lose their arousal value as there is repeated exposure without reinforcement.

Domiciliary care also becomes essential if the intensity is too much. Independent community living is possible only with the help of a conducive and protective environment.

Self-help groups like Alcoholics Anonymous are very useful for getting a sense of belongingness, and one can share deep-rooted feelings while interacting in such groups. Family and marital counselling and therapy help the family members to manage their stress, to achieve better emotional catharsis and, as a consequence, to understand the addict in a better way. This indirectly helps the addict to get better support. In aversion therapy, electrical aversion and chemical aversion are commonly used. Covert sensitization based on verbal aversion is also used to achieve better results.

Social skills training using role playing and videos and contingency management work to increase self-efficacy and improve interactions with others. Stress management training may be very effective. In that, biofeedback for relaxation and systematic desensitization are mainly recommended. Harm reduction should be the goal, which may require change and improvement in regular routine and drugs also, like in the case of problems with internal organs or accidents. Yoga and regular exercise, lectures and films to increase awareness are the general strategies for boosting the confidence of addicts.

Workplace prevention programmes are also effective, along with deaddiction camps and centres. Motivating the individual, enhancing self-empowerment, modification of attitudes, beliefs and the functioning should be the constant focus of any guidance. The use of motivational enhancement therapy is also recommended.

'Insight is cure,' said Sigmund Freud. Enhanced contact with reality results in diminishing problem. Addiction leads to a lot of psychological pain, disturbed interpersonal relations, poor self-image and low self-confidence. The addict has to overcome a lot of inferiority, hopelessness and overwhelming fear.

While counselling, it should be remembered that addiction is a compulsive-obsessive disorder. It requires lots of empathy and unconditional acceptance. Unconditional support, even in case of relapse, becomes essential. Goal setting should be done in terms of short-term goals.

Willingness to help oneself and motivation to lead a better life are the most significant issues. The counsellor should help the addict to achieve it. Emotional catharsis strengthens an individual's capacity to dissolve emotional blocks and to perceive the situation and problems objectively. Action therapy makes it actually happen, which means a small change may result in better confidence and courage in the addict. So, the counsellor should introduce it and encourage the addict to practise it.

Drug abuse is essentially related to mental and physiological health issues. The government, society at large, and health policies should consider its importance and have all the provisions for prohibition as well as stringent rules for preventing drug trafficking. Public awareness needs to be developed. There is a lot of ignorance regarding the actual impact of drug abuse and the exact ill effects of various drugs on youth. In a way, it directly affects the future of society, at large, and the whole nation. Such awareness may be developed during formative years through the formal education system.

8.6. SUMMARY

Addiction has become a serious problem in India. There are different types of addictions prevalent in India. The ill effects on the physiological and psychological health of an addict cannot be underestimated. Once an individual gets involved in addiction, it becomes difficult to get rid of it. It spoils an addict's life in every sense. That, in turn, affects their families and society at large. Addiction makes an individual more vulnerable to developing a daring for family violence, sex crimes and all other crimes.

There are many common problems and ill effects of different sorts of addictions. These are to be understood with reference to intervention programmes and the roles of family, friends and society, at large, in helping the addict. The most important point is that the individual should objectively accept their condition, problems and effects of addiction, and the counsellor should help them to develop confidence, so that the addict can help themselves. Enhancing awareness and reducing wrong notions about it is essential.

Suicide and Attempts to Suicide

9.1. INTRODUCTION, NATURE AND THEORETICAL PERSPECTIVE

The famous film *3 Idiots* depicts three suicides of students with reference to career-related stress, frustrations and agony. One was indirectly referred to, the other was shown directly and the third was an attempt at suicide. It was a very effective presentation of psychological problems, parental pressures, extremely strict implementations of rules by educational institutes and helplessness and hopelessness of young adults.

In 2009, *3 Idiots* was very well received by the audience. It has shown the psychological distress of Indian students and has become very popular all over the world.

Why does an individual want to end their life? How many individuals want to commit suicide? Can it be prevented (Ahmed, 2013)?

Many such cases of suicide are daily reported by the mass media. On 1 February 2019, Siddharth, a student from IIT Hyderabad, killed himself by jumping off his hostel building. It was reported that he was suffering from depression. This was the third suicide at the institute within one year (*Times of India*, 2019). In January 2019, a medical student, Shramistha, killed herself due to examination stress (News18, 2019). Payal Tadvi, a medical student in Mumbai, killed herself because of harassment by three of her seniors (*India Today*, 2019). Many Indian celebrities from the film industry have committed suicide.

According to one estimate, more than 46,000 individuals from the age group of 15–29 years commit suicide every year. The age group is globally reported to be the most vulnerable. Across the world, one person commits suicide every

40 seconds. Generally, the suicide rate increases with age in most countries. However, in India, suicide among young adults is three times the national average. This country has the highest suicide rate among the youths in the world, that is, 35.5 per 100,000 youths. Suicide attempts are 20 times more than actual suicidal deaths, and lifetime prevalence of suicidal ideation is approximately 14 per cent in the general population.

Sui is self and *cide* is murder. According to WHO, India is one of the leading countries where suicide rate is quite high. 17 per cent of the world's total suicides are committed in India. This rate is gradually increasing every year. In 2015, it was reported that 15 persons killed themselves in one hour. The male–female ratio is 2:1. It is the most serious problem of mental health. More than 90,000 young adults committed suicide in India, according to the National Crime Record Bureau[1] as on 2 September 2020. According to the *Hindu* (2020), students' suicides are increasing substantially. On an average, 28 students commit suicide every day (29 January 2020).

There are numerous definitions of suicide. In all these definitions, the intent to end one's life and self-directed harm are highlighted to be the common factors. It is deliberate self-harm. Suicide is defined as 'death caused by self-directed injurious behaviour with an intent to die as a result of the behaviour' (Crosby, 2011). Suicide is a human act of intentional cessation. It is a consequence of problems that are perceived as impossible to solve and of unbearable anguish and worthlessness. The individual wants to get rid of the situation which has no solution according to them. Shneidman (1973) has focused on ambivalence in the act of suicide. The wish to die and the wish to live are both present in the person. On the one hand, the individual consumes poison and, on the other, they want someone to help them out and save their lives. Such persons commit suicide when the former wish becomes predominant.

Attempted suicide, also called parasuicide or pseudocide, is a nonfatal, self-inflicted, potentially harmful behaviour with an intention of dying. To put it simply, attempted suicide is an unsuccessful suicide attempt. It is like Raju Rastogi's suicide attempt in *3 Idiots*. It

[1] www.indiatoday.in

is reported that approximately 10 per cent of individuals attempting suicide manage to commit suicide in the next few years. Suicidal gesture is overtly an attempted suicide; however, the individual does not have any real intention to die. It means that the individual pretends to commit suicide to achieve some end, but in reality, he/she does not intend to die. In November 2019, due to some conflict between lawyers and police in Delhi, a lawyer stood atop the Rohini Court building in a bid to commit suicide (*Times of India*, 2019). He was just threatening and was trying to attract attention to the issue. Deaths in such cases are almost always accidental, not intentional.

Suicidal ideation is related thoughts, beliefs and other cognitive processes reported by the person regarding intentionally ending their lives. Researchers have reported recently that suicidal ideation, which is serious consideration of suicide, is seen more among females than males. Even suicide attempts are more in females than males in the Western countries. It has been a controversial issue, as there are differential results in different cultures.

In India, the rate of suicide among males is reported to be 25.8 per 100,000; among women, the number is reported to be 16.4 per 100,000 in 2019. Men have more access to availability of firearms and have stronger intent to kill themselves. In India, the most commonly used method of suicide is consumption of poison by women and the use of firearms by men. Marriage may be a protective factor for men but may not be so for women. It means, statistically, the probability that a married man will commit suicide is less. However, the same is not true in the case of women. More married women commit suicide as compared to unmarried ones. In fact, marriage-related issues contribute the most in suicides of women. Doctors and other professionals in medical field may have higher rate of suicide because of higher accessibility to drugs and knowledge about their usage. In India, consumption of pesticides is very common in rural areas, especially in the case of farmers. Contagious suicides are more prevalent in adolescents and young adults. Here, an individual wants to commit suicide as a result of hearing or observing someone else's suicidal act. This may happen because of an intense emotional bond with the person who commits the act of suicide or similarity of problems between both the individuals.

Suicide is a multidimensional and multidisciplinary problem. An individual kills himself/herself as a cumulative effect of and complex and complicated interaction of genetic, biological, social, psychological, environmental, economic, cultural, familial, and/or academic problems. The reasons may also include factors, like mental health disorders and addictions or natural calamities. Actually, suicide is a goal-directed behaviour, where the goal is to get rid of unbearable pain and anguish. When such pain is accompanied by feelings of hopelessness, it results in suicidal ideation. For some time, the individual just thinks about it, then plans about the actual act but may defer it due to the fear of death. If the situations do not improve, they try to gain enough courage and strength to actually kill themselves. They may or may not be successful during the first attempt, but it has been seen, in numerous cases, that those with suicidal tendencies, eventually, manage to achieve the goal. Some of them, for example, start burning a small portion of their body parts, like fingers, toes or cheek, just to increase their tolerance before they set fire to self and kill themselves.

Suicide has been a burning problem for generations. An act of suicide puts a premature end to human life. It negatively affects the whole family, friends, and relatives and acquaintances. Scientific, empirical and theoretical research on suicide can be traced back to the emergence of psychology as an independent discipline. Sociology, medicine, genetics, anthropology and philosophy are some other sciences which have been involved in understanding the reasons behind it and helping the individual before it is too late. Each of these branches of these sciences tries to explain and interpret human thoughts and behaviour regarding suicide.

Sociologists highlight social interactions as the most influential factor responsible for suicide. Durkheim, a famous sociologist, who had done pioneering work on suicide, had classified suicides as:

1. **Egoist suicide:** When a person is completely isolated and thinks that they have no place in society, they commit suicide. This person is self-centred. Alienation is responsible for the idea that individual's death is not going to affect anyone.

2. **Altruistic suicide**: This type of suicide is related to close and intimate relations of the individual with community. Identification with their group with reference to norms, values and interests leads to it. In the case of people like Eskimos, who live in extreme climates, if there is no food, some of them commit suicide for the benefit of the group. Due to social customs, the individual commits suicide like the sati custom.

3. **Anomic suicide**: Due to some sudden breakdown of equilibrium, like bankruptcy, individuals may kill themselves. When there is no stability, belongingness and meaning to life that is provided by society, normless life results in disorientation. Such uncertainty leads to suicide.

4. **Fatalistic suicide**: It results from over regulation by society, like a servant committing suicide (Durkheim, 1897).

There are four types of individuals who commit suicide, according to Scheindman. He is known for his pioneering work on suicide and respected as the father of contemporary suicidology. A number of research articles and books have been published by him (e.g., Leenaars, 2010).

1. **Death seekers:** These are individuals who want to seriously die, and even if they experience ambivalence, their attempt is fatal.

2. **Death initiator:** Most of them are terminally or chronically ill, and it is to speed up the process of death and avoid loss of quality of life and increased dependence due to ill health.

3. **Death ignorer:** These individuals believe that death is not the end and there is a better life after death.

> This type of shocking case is that of the Chundawat family from Burari in North Delhi in 2018 (*Economic Times*, 2018). Eleven members of one family were found dead; 10 were found hanged and one strangled. It was a mass suicide to attain salvation. Is it a case of shared psychosis? Blind faith in possession and the hope of going to heaven after death were the basic ideologies. They also believed that they were not going to die after that act of hanging, as their late grandfather would come and save them.

4. **Death darers:** Betting one's life or taking a chance on whether one dies or not in a given situation may lead to death.

Euthanasia helps an individual to fulfil his or her wish to die. There are two types: the first is voluntary, where a third person behaves in such a way that the individual's life ends. Here, food or medicine or life support systems are discontinued. The other type is physician-assisted suicide, where the physician helps for terminating life of an individual. A physician gives a lethal dose to help an individual to die.

This type of assisted suicide is legal in some countries. There are many legal controversies regarding it. It is related to the right to die with dignity.[2]

It is a multidimensional and multidisciplinary problem. The individual kills themselves as a cumulative effect and complex and complicated interaction of genetic, biological, social, psychological, environmental, economic, cultural, familial and/or academic problems. It may also include factors like mental health disorders and addictions or natural calamities.

There are four types of classification of suicide. They are as follows.

- **Individual suicide and collective suicide:** If it is collective, it is according to the group norms and expectations. If it is individual, it may be against social and cultural expectations and approval.

  Two girls, hardly 13-years old, and an adolescent boy, all three of them killed themselves by hanging from a tree in Rajasthan in April 2018 (Times Now, 2018). They were having relationship with each other. It is socially and culturally unacceptable but acceptable to the group.

- **Planned and impulsive suicide:** Some individuals pre-plan everything about their suicide for months or for years. Some of them are emotionally so labile that, at the spur of the moment, they commit suicide within a few hours. It depends on emotional and cognitive characteristics or general instability and impulsivity of the individual. Intensity of emotional ups and downs determines the exact plan and behaviour of suicide.

- **Active and passive suicide:** In the first type, the individual actively does something which may result in their death. An

[2] htttps://courses.lumenlearning.com

individual who sets fire to their own body is of this sort. Not doing anything to save oneself is a type of suicide in some situations. If an individual does not run away from a house which has caught fire is going to die; that is passive suicide.

- **Attention-getting and sincere suicide:** In case of attention-getting suicide, the person may not be really wanting to kill self but is craving for attention and affection. In November 2019, a young man Rohit Patowal tried to commit suicide in front of a police station in Pune (*Loksatta*, 2019). Obviously, he was saved by the police. Sincere suicide is when an individual wants to commit suicide, irrespective of other things.

The other types of suicides are:

- **Chronic suicide:** This happens when the person is ascetic and avoids all pleasures and is very strict due to religious practices, is disabled or invalid, addicted or has psychopathological disorder.
- **Organic suicide:** It results from organic diseases with psychological difficulties.
- **Focal suicide:** It is related to self-mutilation, malingering, impotence, multiple accidents, etc.

Shneidman (1975) has given three types of suicide—logical, catalogical and paleological. Logical suicide takes place due to extreme physical pain. The individual's thinking is logical, and there are no fallacies in it. Catalogical suicides are linked with distorted thinking, dichotomous ideas and semantic errors. The third type is paleological. These suicides are related to delusional types or primitive reasoning.

Another classification given by the same author is egotic, dyadic and ageneratic. Egotic suicide results from intrapersonal dispute indicating destruction of ego or self. The person is generally confused, surprised and hears inner voice leading to doubt, pain and fear. Dyadic suicides are related to interpersonal interaction. It is a reaction of the individual indicating self-punishment, boldness, revenge, withdrawal and disaffiliation. Ageneratic suicide is related to alienation, void, disengagement, boredom, lethargy and lack of interest.

Generally, the person who commits suicide or wants to commit suicide is emotionally unstable and weak. Most of them, that is, 90 per cent, suffer from some clinical disorders. Researchers have repeatedly proved that in the Western countries. However, the frequency of clinical disorder among those who commit suicide in India is much less, that is, 30 per cent, approximately. There are individuals who commit suicide with full awareness and understanding. They do not suffer from any psychological disorder but want to accomplish something for cultural norms or highest values of society. In Indian culture, there are examples of such sorts from ancient times. Sati, *jauhar*, *samadhi*, *prayopweshan*, or fasting till death, are known for generations. In recent years, immolation or setting fire to self for attracting attention of the authorities to injustice or lovers committing suicide with each other and even suicides to express loyalty to the dead leader are seen.

9.1.1. Psychological Theories of Suicide

As suicide has been a fertile field of theoretical and empirical research for more than 100 years, there are a number of theories explaining psychological reasons and aspects related to it. Let us consider some important theories in brief.

Freud (1923) explained suicide as repressed and internalized hostility towards same-sex parent like in Oedipus complex. Death instinct is related to the desire to escape from tensions. It results from conflict between ego and superego. Jung (1933) gave the idea that over dependence on therapist may lead to negative thinking. This leads to suicidal tendencies. Fenichel (1945) has explained suicidal act as an impact of excess superego. When it is for ideals or values, death is perceived as liberation and the only way to get freedom, or it is counterphobic reaction to death, when the person expects that death may lead to reunion with loved ones who are dead.

Family plays a crucial role in suicide. Adler (1948) has put forth the view that suicide is committed to hurting family members indirectly by hurting oneself. Such persons are dependent, helpless and feel inferior, as they cannot achieve what they want to. Similar ideas are given by Shneidman (1967). Rejection in interpersonal relations and simultaneous dependency lead to negative feelings. Life is perceived as futile and void. Sometimes, inner conflict and some religious and philosophical ideas may lead to suicide. Suicide is perceived as solution to psychological pain. Pretzel (1972) put forth the idea that if adolescents are not capable of fulfilling parental expectations, they feel extremely guilty and ashamed. Feelings of rejection and being unwanted result in suicidal ideation. Most of them have cognitive dissonance. They want people to persuade them not to commit suicide and save their lives. This is like a suicide gesture. Hendin's (1964) theory states the importance of culture, child rearing and the focus of culture on a particular achievement and cultural perspective regarding human relations in deciding causes of suicide. Experiencing intense negative emotions and psychopathological setbacks depend on interpretation and importance given to life events.

West (1965) explains suicide with the help of frustration–aggression model. Hostility is directed inwards. Even the criminals commit suicide immediately after the crime.

Horney's theory (1950) considers various alternatives responsible for suicide. There are three types of expressions. A person may move against people where they become hostile, away from people where they become isolated or towards people, in which case they become helpless. Horney explains suicide as an expression of uncontrollable neurotic urge to destroy others. A hostile person cannot kill others; an isolated person wants to get completely detached, and a helpless person wants to get sympathy, maybe, at least, after death. Disturbances in intrapersonal and interpersonal relations, anxiety and alienation of true self from self-system are the causes of suicide, according to American psychiatrist Sullivan (1953).

Rejection by family members has exactly identical effects to physical pain in terms of biochemical changes. Human brain interprets both in the same way. Grey matter, corpus callosum, frontal lobe, hippocampus and amygdala are affected.

Social interactions are highlighted by some experts. Jecobs (1971) gave a theory based on social isolation and perceived inability to solve problems. Kobler and Stotland (1964) gave a theory based on social interaction coupled with hopelessness and helplessness resulting in suicide. Attempts to commit suicide and verbal expression of having the intention of killing oneself may be related to particular environmental problems. When an individual thinks that there is no other way to solve the problem, they may express it verbally in the hope that the listener will be able to help. If no one is interested in helping, the person becomes even lonelier, and the possibility of suicide increases.

Moreno's (2014) theory is based on role playing and its appropriateness. If an individual cannot play their roles properly, they feel that it is better to play no role or play the role of a dead person. At least, after death, others will praise their contribution; that is the expectation.

Sheldon et al. (2003) have put forth the idea that endomorphic or overweight individuals perceive interpersonal relations as most important. When they are isolated or have disturbed relations with significant others, they try to kill themselves. Mesomorphic or individual having a muscular body build commits suicide due to loss of strength, which leads to loss of control over others. Working under a stronger person is also difficult to tolerate for them. As ectomorphs or individuals having lean and delicate body build do not share things with others, they struggle hard alone and are more prone to suicide.

Beck (1985) is known for his work on basic issues related to suicide and measurement of risk. He has highlighted the role of hopelessness in suicide. The risk of suicide is 11 times greater when one experiences hopelessness. Previous exposure to events of suicide makes individual's thoughts and ideas more active and recurrent. Baumeister (1990) has given an escape theory. When there is substantial negative discrepancy between expectations and reality, it creates negative emotions, and the person concentrates on personal inadequacies. This, in turn, results in sadness, worry and distress. As a consequence, an individual wants to get rid of this negative effect and negative self-awareness. In this case, cognitive deconstruction takes place, which leads to a type of numbness. Meaningful thoughts about self are replaced by lower-level ideas. Reduced impulse control and reduction in inhibition may facilitate suicide-related thoughts.

In 2011, an integrated motivational and volitional model was given by O'Connor. Background factors and triggering events are considered in pre-motivational stage. In motivational phase, ideation and intention formation are taken into account. In the last volitional phase, behavioural execution is included.

The fluid vulnerability model was given by Rudd in 2000. According to it, suicide episodes are time-bound. The risk factors that trigger suicide and determine duration and severity of an episode are fluid. There are individual differences in baseline risk. When acute risk goes beyond a certain level, suicide is committed.

A well-accepted recent theory is given by Joiner (2005), which highlights the importance of interpersonal relations with reference to three things: thwarted belongingness, perceived burdensomeness and acquired capacity for suicide. Thwarted belongingness is a state of isolation and sense of being cut off from others. The person feels that others are not capable of understanding their conditions as they have not experienced it. This results in distorted perceptions and mental illness. The concept of burdensomeness means perception that the person cannot contribute anything to the world, and others' lives will be better if they disappear. The third is acquired capacity for suicide. The person must conquer fear of death and habituate physical pain resulting from harm. These individuals develop absence of pain during repeated self-injury. Witnessing a lot of violence and pain may enhance this capacity.

Some other theorists have highlighted the link between physiological diseases and suicide, like Huntington's chorea. The relation between depressive state of manic depressive disorder, schizoaffective reaction and hostile tension are some examples. Those who try to commit suicide but are not successful are generally neurotic or sociopath.

According to researchers, 75 per cent of depressed individuals have ideas about suicide, 10–15 per cent attempt it.

> Renuka was the only child of her widowed mother, who had been a single parent since Renuka's childhood. When Renuka was about to complete her graduation, her mother expired suddenly due to a fatal accident. Renuka was unable to tolerate that overwhelming grief and was in deep depression. In spite of all attempts by relatives and friends to help her, she cut her vein near her wrist, and that laceration proved to be fatal.

Indian theories of suicide are rarely seen. Geet and Agashe (1995) have given the theory based on idea of revenge. The person wants to teach a lesson to significant others. Some people kill themselves for public issues like for getting a facility or reservation for a particular caste or to attract attention to pollution of the Ganges river. Some others may commit suicide because of unbearable insult, agony, frustration and intense disappointment. Hence, according to this theory, extreme emotional distress is responsible for suicide.

9.2. CAUSES, RISKS AND PHENOMENOLOGICAL CORRELATES

There are numerous causes and risk factors. They are classified in different ways. Researchers have classified causes in different ways. The first type is individual or micro level, which includes poor self-esteem, lack of confidence, low self-efficacy, negative thinking and psychological problems as depression, hopelessness, helplessness and worthlessness. Bereavement, loss in childhood and trauma are related to it. Behavioural issues related to maladjustment, disturbed interpersonal relations and the inability to act according to one's own wish also play an important role.

The second type is social, which is at the macro level and is related to problems associated with social isolation, social discrimination, rejection due to lower caste, creed and community, sexual harassment of ladies by male teachers, bosses or roadside Romeos.

A meso level is complex and complicated by the interaction of personal and social problems. It is psycho-social. Even behavioural and societal issues are interdependent. The impact may cause serious problems in the family, educational institutes and job.

Ultimately, the perception of an individual and their capacity to cope with challenges are the most significant determinants. All these factors merge together into a psychological imbalance. It may be due to psychological disorder, illness, social isolation or natural calamity. The ways in which an individual interprets that experience and copes with it are the most significant issues.

There are different motivations related to suicide. They are as follows:

- Sympathy winning
- Help seeking
- Threatening
- Retaliation
- Sincere wish to kill oneself

The major types are as follows:

1. **Psychological factors:** Psychological impact of:
   - Mental disorders such as depression, bipolar disorder, schizophrenia, personality disorders and mood disorders
   - Rape, physical, verbal, sexual abuse, assault, domestic violence and so on
   - Substance or alcohol abuse
   - Family violence
   - Emotional abuse
   - Problems with social relationships, failure in love affair, marital difficulties such as separation, divorce, widowhood, being single and living alone
   - Break-ups, premarital pregnancy, inability to marry and so on
   - Ragging and bullying
   - Extreme poverty, homelessness, being a refugee and so on
   - Family history of suicide
   - Self-accusation, guilt, worthlessness, agitation, nihilistic ideation, insomnia and hypochondriacal delusions
   - Loss of hope, helplessness and so on
   - Loved one being victimized, feeling of being exploited, taken advantage of and so on
   - Rejection/dejection by family, friends, society and so on
   - Serious disappointment, academic failure, insults and so on
   - Tendency to harm self
   - Traumatic life events such as death of a loved one and intense emotional pain
   - Availability of firearms at home

- Exposure to suicidal behaviour of others, previous attempts of suicide
  In developing countries, substance abuse and post-traumatic stress disorders are more predictive of suicide. Alcohol abuse increases impulsivity and lowers inhibitions related to death.

2. **Social factors:** There are many social factors resulting in suicidal tendencies. Some examples are as follows:
   - Peer pressure/attractions like Blue Whale
   - Incarceration, imprisonment or legal custody
   - Prolonged unemployment, loss of job, money, house, etc.
   - Facing aggression and humiliation, threatening, trapping and blackmailing
   - Demographic factors associated with suicide—retirement and sudden fall in socio-economic status, sudden loss in gambling

3. **Physiological factors:** These factors include the following:
   - Peak age of 15–24 and male gender are more vulnerable.
   - Chronic or terminal diseases such as AIDS, strokes and permanent disability.
   - Major accidents leading to limitations.
   - Chronic pain.
   - Genetic factors like family history of mental disorders have been proved to be a significant correlate of suicide. Genetic factors are responsible for the increased rate of suicide in a given family and blood relatives and twins. It is, generally, accompanied by impulsive aggression and neuroticism in families.
   - Biological explanation—biological problems may be related to imbalances of hormones, neurotransmitters, chronic diseases, impairments, suffering and agony due to treatment having strong side effects.

For example, low level of serotonin is found to be responsible for suicide. A chemical produced by serotonin called 5 hydroxyindoleacetic regulates emotions and moods. It is associated with mental disorders. Severe conflict in the family or on the job, which leads to neurotransmitter imbalance, is also reported to be associated to suicide. Hypothalamic-pituitary-adrenal (HPA) axis abnormalities are also associated to suicide. Use of 17-OH corticosteroids in the form of medicines is related to suicidal behaviour (Pandey, 2013).

Multiple factors and its cumulative effects are seen in most of the cases. Faulty attitudes, negative thinking, broken family, wrong role models, lack of confidence and lack of support also enhance negative effects on an individual.

The basic predisposing factors are:

1. History of depression
2. Vulnerability factors and impulsivity
3. Trigger factors such as schizophrenia, loss and stress
4. Relative risk and ratio of suicide rate in acquaintances

Rape, sexual assault and sexual harassment are the most traumatic experiences leading to suicide.

Fatimah Lateef, a 19-year old bright student, committed suicide by hanging from the fan in her hostel room. According to her suicide note, it is a case of harassment and discrimination.[3]

There are many true stories like this. In case of sexual harassment, sexual exploitation and rape, the victim is subjected to extreme social stigma and guilt. The offenders take it as a pride and there are caste and religion issues in it too.

9.1.1.1. Causes of Suicide in India

Highest contribution is of family-related problems, that is, 27 per cent. In that, marriage-related issues including non-settlement of marriage and husband–wife relations as well as relations with in-laws are most important. Demands regarding dowry are still contributing a lot. Twenty-one dowry deaths were reported every day in India in 2017. Every year it is increasing. Suspected/illicit relations, extramarital affairs, divorce, impotency/infertility are some glaring examples. Love affairs and related issues like illegitimate pregnancy contribute for approximately 25 per cent suicides in India.

---

[3] http://thecognate.com, http://www.hindustantimes.com and many other sites.

'Why Are India's Housewives Killing Themselves?' (Biswas, 2016). Number of suicides by housewives is four times more than that of farmers. However, it is hardly acknowledged by the media. Approximately 20,000 housewives commit suicide every year. Suicide rate is high among married women.[4] About 40 per cent of the women who commit suicide globally are Indian and are mostly married.

Illness either mental or/and prolonged physical illness such as AIDS, cancer, paralysis, sexual and emotional abuse, conflict, trauma or natural disaster, property dispute, unemployment and drug and substance abuse are some common causes. Farmers and students are the groups having the highest suicide rate. Bankruptcy and indebtedness are specially applicable in the case of farmers. Failure in examination is the most common reason in the case of students for suicide. Unrealistic expectations of parents about academic excellence, too harsh discipline and lack of proper communication are the basic issues. Conditional acceptance and no expression of positive regard are basic reasons related to students' suicide. Low self-esteem and confidence, fear of failure, lack of proper guidance, self-blame and inability to face failure result in suicide. Extreme competition and distorted perception add in the risks. In India, the methods used are poison in approximately 40 per cent, hanging in 30 per cent, drowning in 9 per cent and jumping in front of train or vehicle in 3 per cent of the cases. Men use more violent methods than women.

9.3. MEDIA AND SUICIDE: IMPACT OF MEDIA AND WEB

Very effective presentation of subject matter by mass media attracts attention of almost every individual in contemporary world. Within few seconds after one starts watching television, alertness of brain to process information decreases. Brain waves also become passive, and an individual interprets only superficial things, such as sound, colours and emotions. Thinking process is hampered. Left brain's alertness diminishes. It is completely passive relaxation and entertainment. As a consequence, message depicted is easily imbibed and has serious impact.

[4] theprient.in 13 September 2018

Mass media is one of the most significant causes of suicide. According to some researchers, it is the third cause of suicide. Depicting suicide as one of the easiest ways to solve problems in life has proved to be a potentially effective negative impact. Specially teenagers and youth are influenced more due to social media and mass media.

Many students, especially adolescents, committed suicide as 'copycat suicides' immediately after the film *3 Idiots* was released. The message in the film is interpreted as being exactly opposite, that is, 'Suicide is the only way out in case of academic failure.' For example, a student called Sushant Patil from Mumbai, who had failed in four subjects out of six, watched the film twice on Sunday and killed himself on Monday (*Indian Express*, 2010). He was just a 12-year old studying in 7th standard. Researchers and experts in the field have tried to establish the impact of the film when number of students committed suicide in the same way.

Social media platforms and networks result in substantially overwhelming interaction and exposure to varied information. There are billions of users contributing to it. Hence, social media and internet provides huge amount of information on every aspect of life and death. Such information about suicide affects individuals in different ways. Sharing of ideas, intentions behind suicide, expression of distress, easy ways to commit suicide and information about great men who have committed suicide facilitate wide imagination and determination about the exact ways to commit suicide.

Role of internet in enhancing the tendency to attempt suicide has attracted attention of psychologists and researchers. It includes social media platforms and blogs such as Tumblr, Reddit, chats, video sites such as YouTube, Amazon Prime, Hotstar, Netflix and social networking sites such as Google, Twitter, Facebook, Myspace and personal email, messaging, video chats and WhatsApp. It is shocking that live videos of suicide are available on YouTube, Facebook and the like (Dilli Aajtak, 2018; IndiaTV, 2018; *Times of India,* 2018). This type of videos must have devastating impact on youth having suicidal thoughts. Dramatic reporting and portrayal of suicide in the most dignified way and specifying easy means of suicide are more effective.

In Japan, some pro-suicidal sites suggested that hydrogen sulphide gas can be used to kill oneself. Within short duration, 220 persons tried to kill themselves and 208 were killed. There are many pro-suicidal sites, message boards, chat rooms and forums. Discussions regarding various methods to kill oneself, agreement to commit suicide on a particular day and to support a cause, peer pressure to commit suicide, experiencing the thrill of killing oneself are the common themes. There are some cases where two individuals, two lovers decide to commit suicide on the same day, same time by the same method. They may or may not be together. Lot of exposure to universal injustice and grief of mankind, as depicted on mass media, extreme involvement due to extraordinary empathy and feeling hopeless for not being capable of solving such problems may enhance the suicidal ideation.

Hints for parents, teachers and significant adults to protect the youth are available on Google, like 'Forty Seconds to Action' by WHO,[5] which effectively guide the reader regarding ways to prevent suicide. Every 40 seconds, an individual commits suicide; hence, the title itself is very relevant. Similar suicide-prevention help guides[6] are also very useful. There are helplines for suicide prevention like India Suicide Helpline Directory,[7] which gives information of such helplines all over the country. The first expert to approach is a psychologist; however, in case of severe problems, it becomes a must to consult a psychiatrist. It is essential to treat the imbalance of neurotransmitters with drug therapy.

To protect adolescents and youth from such negative impact, it is essential to discuss and disclose real-life orientation and possible alternatives to solve problems. Help should be made available if at all suicidal ideation is experienced. Objective and logical evaluation of causes and consequences of an individual's attempt to suicide on individual, family and society at large should be made clear to the younger generation. Most important is that an individual should not be left alone to interpret the meaning of suicide. Open discussion is a must. Right from the beginning, adolescents should be trained to

---

[5] wwwhealthissuesindia.com>suicide 2019

[6] www.helpguide.org November 2020

[7] www.aasra.info>helpline

develop resilience, hardiness, frustration tolerance, assertiveness and positive thinking to strengthen their personality. Relation of mental health issues to suicide must be made clear to parents and teachers, as well as administrators of various workplaces. The sites showing live suicides and attracting attention of the younger generation to suicidal ideation or, in any way, depicting pro-suicidal matters may be banned completely.[8]

Modelling, learning by imitation and social learning, in case of suicidal tendencies, should be carefully controlled. Along with it, signal against immediate-gratification orientation is given, which is responsible for lack of tolerance of any negative thing or event and delay of gratification. There are logical errors in the thinking process of adolescents, like all-or-none perception of the world. This is due to immature thought processes that are distorted and tilted. They are influenced by temporary and superficial things like identification with the hero in a movie. Due to hedonism, youth want to be a big boss without any efforts, whereas in reality, one has to struggle hard to achieve anything. Contact with reality is a must to maintain proper perspective.

Cyber bullying is a major problem which may result in suicide of the victim. Misuse of advanced technology against women, for example, to prepare mms and blackmailing ladies, modifying their photographs and using these to threaten them, sending vulgar messages and the like may lead to suicide. Let us take an example of the suicide trap on web.

9.3.1. Blue Whale

Blue Whale is a death trap which is labelled as a game just to attract the innocent minds. It has claimed the lives of a number of children and adolescents all over the world. General curiosity, urge to experience some thrill and doing something new for boosting self are the primary motives of starting the game. Lack of awareness leads to further involvement in this deadly game. The present game actually

---

[8] https://suicideprevention.nv.gov/

started in Russia around 2013 and then spread all over the world. It was developed by a 22-year old Russian guy. The initial group was called F57 on the social media website of Russia. In 2015 alone, 130 individuals, mostly adolescents, committed suicide due to Blue Whale. Such groups are called as death groups as the group motivates and compels the participants to end their lives.

One by one, increasingly difficult challenges are expected in this trap (BBC News, 2019; UNICEF, 2019). The players are supposed to watch a very scary horror movie alone at night and abuse self, such as cutting one's lips, carving with a razor some secret number on one's body and tolerate painful activities as suggested. The player is supposed to complete it within a particular stipulated time. This continues for 50 days. The participants are ordered to carve a picture of Blue Whale on their forearm. Not talking to anyone else is also one important task. The last challenge is to commit suicide by jumping from the roof of a multi-storied building. Once the game begins, no one is allowed to withdraw. If the person wants to withdraw, they are threatened that their parents and family will be killed if they leave it halfway. It becomes the scariest thing. Fear to leave the game halfway, thinking that their parents and family will really be killed, results in compulsion of doing very unpleasant and deadly activities.

In India, the incidence is comparatively less. One of the reasons reported for low incidence is the link between individual's death and Blue Whale challenge, which is, sometimes, not clear and cannot be proved legally. The individual does not share their thoughts and experiences regarding Blue Whale with others and keeps it as a secret. Though this stress, anxiety and unbearable fear of the unknown increase after first few days, the individual does not seek any help, and there is no emotional catharsis. The first Indian suicide took place in Mumbai when a teenager Manpreet Singh jumped from the seventh floor for completion of the final stage of Blue Whale. After that, many adolescents ended their lives. There are some cases where the adolescents are saved by parents, teachers and others after completing half of the stages of Blue Whale challenges. Many such cases of both the types are discussed in detail by various mass media. Now, it is completely banned in India. Indian cities such as Kolkata, Kochi and

Thiruvananthapuram are the cities having the highest number of Blue Whale-related searches in the world. Out of the first 50 cities, 32 are Indian (Sharma, 2017).

There are more than 20 such dangerous apps at present. Adolescents should be taught assertiveness, human rights and strategies to cope with various pressures like peer pressure. Parents should have understanding and empathy, support adolescents and youth wholeheartedly, motivate them to practise effective ways of interactions, respect them and suggest various ways to distract mind from worries.

9.3.2. Farmers' Suicide

Seventy per cent of the Indian population, directly or indirectly, depends on agriculture. Farmers' suicide has been a burning problem in India since the last few decades. Every year, thousands of farmers commit suicide. Maharashtra, Karnataka, Chhattisgarh, Orissa and many more states have substantial incidences. For example, 23,000 farmers killed themselves in Maharashtra since 2009 in just seven years.

Despite the loan waiver, 2,761 farmers ended their lives in 2018[9] and 12,021 in three years (NDTV, 2019). As is reported in the Parliament on 18 September 2020, total 10,281 Indian farmers committed suicide in 2019.[10]

Among all suicides, farmers' suicides account for 11 per cent in India. Many of them are young farmers and young family members of farmers also. The basic reasons are economic problems, bad weather conditions affecting farming and not getting expected minimum benefit out of the yield. However, it is a complex and complicated interaction between these issues and mental health issues, family problems, personal issues, distress due to debt and not getting appropriate support.

Payal is 17 and has completed 10th. Her father, who is a poor farmer, now, is worried about her marriage and, especially, the expenditure expected in

[9] http://www.thehindubusinesslin

[10] www. Downtoearth.org.in>

that. Payal has two younger sisters and a youngest brother. Maintenance of the family is difficult. Due to inappropriate rain this time, there is hardly any income, and everyone is extremely worried. Ultimately, Payal decided to commit suicide, so that at least one responsibility will be over.

There are many such adolescents and youth who are giving up due to overwhelming poverty and uncontrollable reasons behind it. Some of them are depressed as they cannot get higher education, do not get employment and cannot think of even a small business due to paucity of money. All the other reasons of suicide become more intense due to poverty and dependence on unpredictable things. Economic and psycho-social support, awareness regarding the possibility of changing lifestyle and generating more options for earning bread and butter are necessary to reduce these suicides.

Illness results in 21 per cent of the total suicides in India. For example, 385,000 individuals killed themselves from 2001 to 2015 only because of illness (National Crime Records Bureau).[11] Cancer, paralysis, HIV/AIDS and mental illness are the major contributors. One in five suicides in India is due to chronic illness.[12] However, in 2019, 17.1 per cent of suicides are found to be linked to illness (*Hindu*, 2020). Only 10 per cent of the patients get proper treatment. Most of them suffer due to paucity of money and availability.

9.4. PSYCHOLOGICAL PROBLEMS: HOPELESSNESS, HELPLESSNESS AND WORTHLESSNESS

When an individual becomes fed up due to complex and complicated problems in their life, they become too preoccupied with their own thoughts to maintain good interpersonal relations. Intrapersonal relations or their relations with themselves are also disturbed substantially. They may blame themselves for not doing something like not utilizing opportunities and time, not studying properly or not behaving properly during a given situation. They may feel extremely guilty, upset or ashamed due to their own problems and perception that they

---

[11] downtoearth.org.in

[12] https://m.timesofindia.com/latest.cms

cannot solve them on their own. All their thoughts are negative and extremely harmful. There is absolutely no motivation, positive thinking or desire to improve interpersonal and intrapersonal relations. As a consequence of all these, the person is isolated, perceived as being apathetic and difficult to deal with. Their interaction with family and friends changes substantially as they are not in a position to share their feelings with them, nor are they interested in enjoying anything with the others. They feel that no one can help them regarding their serious problem. For number of hours, the person may prefer staying alone and seriously thinking of plans to end their life.

WHO reported that India is the most depressed country in the world. Of the total Indian population, 6.5 per cent suffer from some serious mental disorder.[13]

Depression is proved to be a major cause of suicide. If it is not treated properly, it results in suicide. Hopelessness is a very significant correlate of depression and suicidal ideation. Hopelessness has been proven to be one of the most dangerous correlates and warning signs of suicide. It should never be neglected by family and friends. The individual is convinced that things will never improve, and it is impossible to solve any problem. Hence, there is no point in trying. They want to give up. Due to the feeling of emptiness, void and complete absence of hope, they perceive that death is better than life. Helplessness is proven to be associated with attempts to commit suicide. Researchers have proved that history of attempted suicide is best predicted by helplessness. Being helpless is having a feeling of being overwhelmed, trapped and unable to cope with difficulties. It is accompanied by suicidal thoughts either temporary or permanent. Inner psychological weakness results in overwhelming helplessness. Sometimes, it is much more than the actual problem. The individual is, in a way, immobilized and incapable of even trying to solve the problems. This leads to even more inferiority and the feeling that one is a failure. A concept of inner passivity is given by psychoanalysts. The inner critic may continuously generate negative feedback, find faults and keep on nagging the individual.

---

[13] https://www.indiatoday.in/ 1 November 2019

Worthlessness is an overwhelming feeling of personal failure. The person perceives themselves as useless and unimportant. They think that they are insignificant and cannot offer anything good or valuable to anyone in the world. Those who are neglected in childhood or are abused, generally, face this problem in later life. When individuals cannot solve their own problems, they easily succumb to inner passivity. According to psychoanalysis, it generates from unconscious mind and unconscious ego. Due to it, the individual feels that they are against their inner critic or superego, which is authoritarian and persistent.

Learned helplessness, learned hopelessness and learned worthlessness are essentially important concepts which focus on significance of learned responses towards self. Self-concept, self-worth and self-image are products of interaction between an individual and environment. Positive and negative impressions are created in the same way. Shame and criticism result in the feeling of worthlessness and inadequacy. Self-fulfilling prophecy leads to individual's behaviour being similar to their image created by the others, 'as they have been told they are like'. In a way, it is revenge, where the self-talk is 'if that is what you expect me to do, I will definitely do it.' In this case, it is something negative. Harmful criticism results in one's image that 'I am not up to the mark; I am inadequate and inferior.' Some of them try their level best to achieve something and prove that they are capable. Effects of modelling and observational learning directly affect the individual when they observe that parents have poor self-image and low confidence.

These three negative emotions, namely hopelessness, helplessness and worthlessness, are related to clinical depression and suicide. Substantial research has been done and is being done regarding it. Beck et al. (1985) have given a triad of these three emotions as related to depression and suicide.

9.5. INDICATIONS FOR PREDICTING SUICIDE, ATTEMPTS TO SUICIDE AND SUICIDAL IDEATION

There are various warning signs regarding suicidal ideation and plan of suicide. There is a sudden and radical behavioural change, change in interest, attitudes and interpersonal relations of an individual. Less involvement in friends, get-together and parties becomes obvious. Some important issues are as follows.

- Decreased interest in activities which were previously interesting like hobbies becomes obvious. Individual's apathy regarding one's clothes, hairstyle and appearance, and even negative feedback by parents and teachers is vivid. Lower academic achievement and failure without any emotional reactions is seen. The person lacks the ability to concentrate on studies or work, gets too much or too little sleep. The individual experiences restlessness and constantly feels upset. There is an overwhelming feeling of worthlessness, hopelessness and helplessness. Over consumption of cigarettes, alcohol or drugs makes the individual even more careless and asocial. Declaration of plans to commit suicide to close members of the family or friends is a major indication. They are involved in writing stories, poems and drawing pictures regarding one's death. Reckless behaviour becomes obvious, as they are not worried about any loss or damage.

  They start giving away their valued possessions, such as ornaments, art works, books and even pets, to others. The person puts personal affairs in order like closing bank accounts or cancelling admission for the next year. There are repeated wounds such as cuts on wrists and burns. During the final stage, the previous attempt of suicide and collecting material required for it, like buying and collecting many sleeping pills, are the alarming indications.
- **Verbal signs:** Repeated expression that 'everything is getting spoiled and the individual does not want all this now' is a serious sign indicating that the individual is fed up. They neglect messages from parents, classmates and friends. Two more serious indications are:
  o Negative expressions indicating hopelessness, helplessness and worthlessness
  o Expression of idea that people will be happier and having better life without the individual.

Typical verbal expressions are as follows: 'I want to quit ... I don't know how far I will be able to tolerate it.... If some unwanted thing happens, I am prepared; I have the pills …. While driving, I don't bother, as even if some accident takes place, it's okay…. Nothing is going to improve…. I want to end it now.' These words give clear indication of the suicidal intentions of an individual. If such things are taking place after some loss or mishap, special attention is needed.

9.6. PRECAUTIONS AND INTERVENTION, ROLE OF FAMILY, COUNSELLING AND THERAPY

Prevention starts from understanding and recognizing hidden and direct messages the individual is giving. The majority of suicides are preceded by warning signs, though few of them occur without warning signs. It is necessary to understand verbal and behavioural warning signs. People who talk about killing themselves are actually trying to get some help. Hence, these signals should not be neglected. Support from family members is the most significant step towards prevention. If the basic trust that parents are always with the individual is missing and there is no expression of unconditional love, adolescents don't get any psychological support through interaction with parents. Instead of nagging and insulting them, parents should understand, support and console them. For example, they should encourage the individual to try again and should never over evaluate the importance of grades. Parental threat may lead to end of human life. Accepting the individual as a worthy person, understanding their thoughts and feelings without evaluation are the basic requirements. If there is no family and there are no friends or if they are not ready to help, it is very difficult to save the individual.

The family members and friends should:

1. Encourage the individual to talk freely and clearly about their ideas. Listen carefully, and interpret all verbal and non-verbal messages seriously. They should not evaluate the individual's views and emotions and should never make fun of their ideas.
2. Avoid any discussion which may increase guilt in their mind. They should never criticize or blame the individual and should not argue. They should never negotiate or even partially accept that suicide is justified in any given situation.

3. Not to leave the individual alone and supervise them carefully; remove all harmful sharp objects and medicines which may be used for an attempt of suicide.

4. Encourage them to get proper help and contact experts in the field to provide immediate help. They should keep on helping, even if, overtly, it is not needed, as it indicates concern.

5. Try and convince significant others that they should also help and have better understanding and generate support.

Training should be made available to the individual, which may contribute to decrease in suicidal thoughts. This may include positive thinking, proactive thinking, assertiveness, hardiness, resilience and the like.

In suicide prevention, the person should be saved and protected from themselves, and that is why it is especially tactful. The family members of the individual should not become defensive, punitive or outright reject that they need some help. There are two types of prevention: primary and secondary. Primary is related to the family and society. Societal disorganization, weakened family and religious bonds are responsible for disintegration of the individual's personality. The whole socialization, values and general lifestyle are influenced by it. There is a link between antisocial, aggressive behaviour and self-destructive tendencies.

The individual should be identified as having high risk at an early stage. If characteristics of these individuals are similar to those who commit suicide, then it is a must to make every serious attempt to change their mentality, such as unwed adolescent mothers, depressed patients, drug addicts and alcoholics. Marital discord may also be a major reason in a country like India.

ACP Amit Singh, from Noida, committed suicide using his service revolver due to disturbances in family relations. Immediately after that, his wife killed herself by jumping from the 4th floor.[14]

Secondary prevention is basically oriented towards prevention of repeated occurrence of similar harmful behaviour and reducing associated disability. Those who are from high-risk group, generally, avoid going to psychologists and psychiatrists. Those who try to get assistance are, generally, from the low-risk group. General supportive environment and facilities are the basic requirements. Reducing stress by changing the environment and its perception becomes essential. The person should be helped to realize that the way in which they are thinking is not objective, and it is hindering their capacity to see different alternatives. They should be able to realize that the distress is temporary, and they are not the only one suffering like that. Encouraging the individual for strengthening one's self-understanding and self-concept as well as supporting the individual to ego enhancement are essential.

There are four phases—intention to end one's life, decision about the lethality of means, making them available and execution of the plan. Family and friends must be aware of the phase and try their best to protect the individual. If an individual has substantial distress and it becomes unbearable, counselling helps. When the individual actually tries to kill self by doing some actual action, it is necessary to give medical help and save their life. Many experts have recommended that directive counselling is a better way to help them.

Some rare cases are such that the person survives after a sincere attempt to kill themselves. These individuals feel extreme shame, guilt, hatred and other negative emotions such as perplexity and all sorts of cognitive and emotional confusion. Here, postvention is essential to save the individual from negative thoughts and recurrence of the suicidal attempt.

> Shrikant was involved in alcohol abuse to such an extent that he had taken substantial loan from many sources. Due to the addiction, he could not get a job, and even when he got one, he could not maintain it. His wife left him, and his parents were reluctant to support him in any way. One fine morning, he jumped from a high bridge over a river. He fell down into a muddy area where there was no flow of water. Such an unsuccessful attempt at suicide resulted in social stigma, and he started hating social interaction. He was not supported by his family and friends.

Immediately after such an incident, psychological counselling and therapy should be made available to the individual.

Various steps are necessary to identify individuals having serious problems.

- Evaluation of risk factors is essential; irrespective of the expressions of intentions and clues indicating suicidal plan, it is necessary to evaluate the seriousness and risk.
- Case studies regarding past attempts, their seriousness, and effects on the individual and others may help to suggest the nature of care necessary.
- Assessment of strategies is essential. Lethality may be high, moderate or low. In high, there are high risk factors and after-effects. In moderate lethality, the plan is not well thought out, and anticipated consequences are not fatal. Low lethality means low risk factors and vague, indirect mention. For determining lethality of suicide, availability and arrangement of means should be checked thoroughly.
- Implementing appropriate plan to arrest the individual's potential action of committing suicide is the next step.
- The vulnerable individual should be encouraged to seek help, and there should be no social stigma about going to a psychologist or a psychiatrist. Others should respect it as a sign of courage, strength and insight into one's problems.
- Family and friends must keep an eye and be vigilant about emotional responses of the vulnerable individual to life events.
- Treatment for mental disorders should be provided immediately based on the evidence.
- Significant indications including acquired capacity of an individual to tolerate induced pain and easy access to means for killing oneself must be carefully observed and interpreted. Habituation leads to more expertise and less fear of it. More exposure to pain and increasingly getting exposed to more intense pain have to be taken care of.
- Access to various tricks to kill oneself, information about how to collect the necessary material and actually physically getting equipped with the means indicate very dangerous stages of potential for suicide. Family members should immediately take the preventive action.
- Try to attract attention of the affected individual to positive side of their life and traits. Suggesting various possibilities for making life

meaningful may be useful, for example, by helping less fortunate people who are suffering badly.

- Clinics, provision for special wards for indoor patients, telephone services, online counselling and support groups are needed in every urban and rural areas in India. Perspective of the whole society towards such individuals needs to be changed.

There are many non-government organizations in India, such as Roshni, Cooj helpline, Sneha India Foundation, Vandrevala Foundation for mental health, Connecting NGO, https://lbb.in/about-us, Aasra and Suicide Prevention India Foundation. In a book called *Preventing Suicide*, WHO (2014) has considered it from a holistic approach, and it is recommended that suicides are preventable if timely and appropriate action is taken. Crises intervention services may be set up with the help of various medical, paramedical practitioners and psychologists. Training health workers, educators and police for identifying potential suicide attempts may reduce the neglected cases. Enhancing public awareness regarding how everyone can help the individual is essential. Stigma reduction by social support and by positive interaction should be taught to volunteers.

Treatment may differ with reference to intensity of the problem. Some individuals may have suicide potential or suicidal ideation, others may have actually attempted it. Appropriate rapport establishment becomes essential in counselling, because without it, the individual may not feel free to share their innermost feelings and thoughts. Respecting the individual and helping them to maintain their dignity is a must.

Therapy may include supportive therapy to express acceptance and reduce the feeling of being isolated. Family and marital therapy may enhance interpersonal relations and give emotional support. Possible changes in the environment, such as routine and lifestyle, may increase the possibility of reducing distress. It is important to develop insight in the individual's mind about their problems. Group therapy is also useful, as group interaction facilitates many positive things. Meaningful social interaction helps an individual to recover. Cognitive behaviour therapy and rational emotive behaviour therapy are recommended by experts to help vulnerable individuals. All other possible therapies should also be used depending upon age, gender, education, values and socialization of the individual. Providing new opportunities to increase optimism may include something like giving some work or suggesting rearing a pet, whichever works well. Workplace suicide prevention programme and similar programmes in educational institutes may help the most vulnerable population. It is essential to develop these programmes with reference to the Indian culture, socialization practices, values and emotional needs. Including suicidal ideation in .prevention programme may make it more effective. Follow up of the cases once identified should be continued in the long run.

Prevention is always better than cure. Hence, it would be better to enhance awareness among parents, teachers and others to develop conducive environment in the family, educational institutes and workplaces. Everyone is a worthy person and has a right to lead a happy and healthy life.

9.7. SUMMARY

Suicide results in the premature loss of precious human life, which can be prevented and saved. In India, adolescents and youth represent the highest number of suicides. Hopelessness, helplessness and worthlessness are the three extremely negative emotions influencing the human psyche. In a way, it is related to disturbed intrapersonal and interpersonal relations. It is the failure of the family to cater to the emotional needs of these individuals. The younger generation is facing a number of novel challenges and risks. Hence, it is a must to give priority to mental health of offspring. Parents and other significant adults must support the affected person. Child-rearing practices and general socialization may be oriented towards positive attitudes, hardiness, resilience, proactive thinking, assertiveness and frustration tolerance.

Guidance, counselling and therapies such as cognitive behaviour therapy and rational emotive behaviour therapy are effective in improving an individual's psychological balance.

Chronic and Terminal Diseases, and Trauma

10.1. INTRODUCTION, NATURE AND TYPES

There are various unpleasant experiences in human life which are unavoidable. An individual has to bear the pain, physical and psychological, and suffer due to many setbacks in their life. These are the barriers to optimum psycho-social health. Very few individuals can take this as a challenge and can maintain their balance. For most of them, it makes their lives unbearable and extremely devastating. The impact of chronic and terminal diseases makes an individual's life painful, restricted and difficult to cope with. There are some traumatic experiences due to natural calamities or, otherwise, which may temporarily or permanently shatter human life. It may include loss of property, death of a family member, constant threat, extreme environmental conditions such as earthquakes, floods and tsunamis. In contemporary society, an increasing number of traumatic experiences are due to man-made disasters such as violence and war. All these conditions challenge psycho-social health of an individual and substantially affect their well-being. When it is a natural disaster, there are many others who suffer; however, in the case of diseases, disorders, accidents, personal violence and rape, the individual alone has to bear all the pain and devastating consequences. In the case of a natural calamity, the negative consequences are obvious and easy to understand for others. However, in the case of personal suffering, sometimes, even the family members cannot develop empathy towards the patient.

Physical trauma is, by and large, related to injury, resulting in an intensely disturbing and distressing experience. In physical trauma, mainly patients having spinal cord injury, brain injury and amputees are included. It may result in distress which is beyond the capacity of an individual to tolerate. Such serious injuries may also result from burns and falls, acid attacks, violence, poisoning, drowning and intentional self-harm. Intensity of devastating experiences depends on the severity of injury, sensitivity, age and gender of an individual. It initiates the Hypothalamic Pituitary Adrenal (HPA) axis and immunological and metabolic responses that help to regain balance or homeostasis. The effects of physical trauma and their psychological impact are overlapping and interdependent.

Terminal diseases may develop at any age. Even young children are born with congenital anomalies. Terminal diseases are incurable and not treatable. It invariably results in death of the patients within a particular duration. These diseases are progressive, which means that condition of the patients deteriorates day by day. Different types of cancer, including leukaemia, AIDS, heart diseases and infections such as H1N1, Ebola and Nipah are a few glaring examples. Genetic diseases, like Lesch Nyhan syndrome are also equally serious. Myasthenia gravis, muscular dystrophy, multiple sclerosis and many other terminal diseases are equally dangerous. Breast cancer is one of the cancers that can be cured if treated in early stages. Even Huntington's disease, which is inherited, has an onset in youth. Due to the death of brain cells, the patient suffers from problems regarding mental abilities, dementia, lack of motor coordination and involuntary movements. It is a terminal disease. Devastating pain, extreme despair and hopelessness make individual's condition unbearable.

In India, 62 people suffering from terminal illness kill themselves daily (*Times of India*, 2018). Over 800,000 deaths due to cancer were recorded in India in 2018. However, there are more brave individuals who are fighting back the disease. Many Hollywood actors, celebrities and artists are struggling at a young age due to AIDS, cancer and other terminal diseases in India. Manisha Koirala had ovarian cancer; Lisa Ray had multiple myeloma cancer, and Yuvraj Singh had lung cancer.

Chronic diseases are incurable. They are only treatable. It means that the affected individuals have to take due precautions to control them and deal with the limitations and suffering for the whole of their lives. Though there are ups and downs, the disease exists. It is non-contiguous. So only the individual suffers. There are various functional impairments due to chronic diseases. There are different diseases which are chronic by nature. Some prominent ones are diabetes, asthma, epilepsy, polio, arthritis, hypertension, heart disease like arrhythmia, hypothyroidism, trigeminal neuralgia and blood disorders such as thalassemia and sickle cell anaemia. Blood-related disorders result in extreme fatigue, low haemoglobin and less oxygen availability to the brain. This may directly affect cognitive alertness. In this case, special diet, appropriate medicine and limited physical demands are necessary. Intermittent blood transfusions are also essential, which leads to many other problems. In addition to chronic diseases, there are some chronic conditions which are incurable. Cerebral palsy, hemiplegia, quadriplegia and paraplegia are glaring examples. Congenital problems, sensory problems, amputations, strokes and spinal cord injuries due to accidents are also not curable, and the individual has to adjust to the pain, limitations and psycho-social stigma.

10.2. CONSEQUENCES AND IMPACT ON PSYCHO-SOCIAL HEALTH

Jonny was a patient of stroke who was trying to recover wholeheartedly. He started walking and doing his daily activities. However, his perception of himself and his own body was affected in such a way that he could not recognize the left-half part of his own body as his own. The existence of that part was totally denied. This resulted in many misinterpretations. Jonny used to think that his wife had an affair as he could not recognize his own body. He was suspicious that someone else was sleeping between him and his wife.

The impact of trauma and diseases is so intense that sensations, perceptions, attitudes, equilibrium, personality and body image get distorted. When an individual first learns about their limitations and disabilities, it is devastating. The individual and their whole family get extremely upset and helpless. Loss of mobility, inability to use already acquired training and skills, safety issues, adjusting to unusual places and people, unexpected and painful treatment, change in appearance, embarrassment, dependency on others for personal care, such as feeding and bathing, all these things are difficult to tolerate. Especially when an individual is young, all their dreams are shattered. It leads to a complete loss of self-identity and identity crisis. The individual gets involved in self-blame and pessimistic attitude. Such defensive coping results in many more psychological and interpersonal relation problems. Sometimes, illusions also help with maintaining self-concept, as unrealistic optimism may motivate the individual. Uncertainty and lack of predictability of the disease require patience, resilience and flexibility. Otherwise, depression and anxiety emerge. Worthlessness, guilt and despair are the symptoms of depression. Fear and panic terror are symptoms of anxiety.

Unhealthy coping generates more problems. Aggression, self-blame, giving up and learned helplessness are the correlates of unhealthy coping. Disengagement, unattainable goals, low impulse control leading to drug abuse and gambling are very commonly seen in those cases. Sometimes, substitute satisfaction, like internet addiction, attracts the individual.

Defence mechanisms decide general behavioural pattern and adjustment of any individual. Freud, the famous psychoanalyst, gave different ego defence mechanisms which are used by individuals to regain homeostasis in psychological sphere. It is an unconscious psychological mechanism that helps in reducing anxiety, which is generated by unacceptable stimuli which are harmful. Different ego defence mechanisms are used by those who suffer from chronic and terminal diseases and traumatic situations. Ego defence mechanisms such as regression, repression, overcompensation, intellectualization, rationalization and projection are more common among them. Regression results in reversion of ego to an earlier stage of development. It means an adolescent behaves like a child. Repression means preventing unacceptable aspects of phenomenological reality so that they do not come into consciousness. Overcompensation is developing abilities in one area in the case of deficit in the other. Intellectualization focuses on abstract concepts, logic and intellectual reasoning for avoiding emotions that are painful. Rationalization is justifying feelings and behavioural patterns that are more acceptable than those that are not acceptable. Guilt results in rationalization, projection and undoing. Projection is attributing one's unacceptable ideas or impulses to someone else.

An ego defence mechanism called reaction formation results in doing exactly the opposite of what is expected. It is a tendency for a repressed feeling to be expressed in contrasting form. In such cases, it is difficult to manage the individual's behaviour. Inferiority is associated with identification, compensation and fantasy. Personal limitations may lead to denial, fantasy and compensation. Forbidden sexual desires are reported to result in repression, projection as well as rationalization. Rationalization, repression, intellectualization, isolation of affect, undoing and displacement are neurotic types of ego defence mechanisms. Suppression, humour and altruism are mature types of ego defence. Denial is most common in some patients, even after amputation and brain damage. Primitive thinking prevails, and the individual wants to forget about their disability. Some patients become paranoid. They think that they are suffering due to ill will of someone. Some have intermittent euphoria. They have unrealistic goals and think that they are achievable easily.

Organ inferiority is the concept given by pioneering psychologist Adler. Some individuals are born with some physical defects. They develop a feeling of inferiority. Some others feel inferior for psychological reasons. They attempt to take action to compensate for their weakness. They try to achieve excellence in some other areas. For example, if an individual has weak physique or has some chronic disease, they will try to overcome it by showing extraordinary excellence in some other area. There are real-life examples of players, mountaineers or motivational trainers who either have lost their limbs or are suffering from some disease or disorder. In a way, this is a compensation of inferiority feeling for achieving self-actualization.

All sorts of negative emotions are prevalent in these individuals' psyches. Depression, generalized anxiety, post-traumatic stress disorder, intense sadness and panic disorder are reported to be associated with trauma and terminal disease. Symptoms of depression are feelings of loss, sadness, difficulty sleeping and loss of appetite. There are experiences such as fatigue, low energy and pain without clear physiological cause. It is a complex effect of psychological, biological and social distress, which in turn affects neural circuits in the brain. All these things result in poor self-esteem. Researchers have reported that 25 per cent of cancer patients, 34 per cent of HIV patients and 34 per cent of heart attack survivors are severely depressed. Post-traumatic stress disorder and panic attacks are common.

Frustration, anger, irritation, bitterness and feeling disappointed result from uncertainty, insecurity and perceived inability to fulfil dreams. In the case of these individuals, as they lack physical capacity, it is an internal block. Learned helplessness leads to a tendency to give up. Pessimistic attitude is related to external locus of control. Other correlates of learned helplessness are hopelessness, sense of futility, meaninglessness, sadness and a tendency to under evaluate self.

Mood disorders and post-traumatic stress disorder are related to some sudden shocks, such as accidents, rapes and injuries due to natural disasters. The risk of post-traumatic stress disorder after traumatic brain injury or spinal cord injury in urban youth is 24 per cent.

Suicide is essentially the most intense problem. Restlessness and agitation are extreme in the case of terminal patients. Self-harm is predominant. Hence, some individuals do not want to take medicines and submit themselves to the progress of disease and accept death as it comes.

In the case of terminal diseases, depression, anxiety, loneliness and death anxiety are the most prominent psychological effects. Everything revolves around pain, progressing disease, anticipated deterioration and unfulfilled dreams of the patient, especially when the patient is young. Due to discrepancy between ideal self and real self, low self-efficacy and cognitive dissonance emerge. Forced dropping out, loss of job, separation from family and rejection by loved ones result in further despair.

Delusions, hallucinations, obsessions, phobia and hypochondriasis lead to more complications. Hostility towards other normal individuals and emotionally blackmailing parents are very common. Insisting on exaggerated independence is even more frustrating. Individual's frustration tolerance decreases due to suffering. It is also reported that the individual may get involved in attention-seeking and interrupt others' activities. Hopelessness results from unavoidable suffering. Lack of motivation becomes a major problem. Due to despair and giving up, the individual does not want to do anything to help themselves.

There are no goals. This leads to self-blame, self-devaluation and self-hatred. Ultimately, intraindividual relations are spoiled. Such individuals do not accept and love themselves. There is self-doubt, and the individuals become a third person of their own selves. Mostly, male members start abusing alcohol or drugs. It gives them temporary relief from all their negative experiences.

The affected individuals become so much involved in their own problems that they cannot even think about others' feelings, difficulties and so on. Hence, their behaviour is interpreted as bizarre by others. The individual becomes even lonelier at night when others sleep. They keep on thinking about their misfortune and future disasters. As a consequence, they cannot sleep properly and develop insomnia.

Chronic illness is a never-ending, dark, suffocating tunnel for patients. They have to face same problems, same limitations, same suffering, same despair, same awkward feelings, same disappointments year after year. Similar concerns, worries, medicines, timetable of treatment, doctors, testing and so on continue for the whole of their lives. It is a vicious circle, and a lot of psychological energy of the individual is wasted due to it. It leads to apathy, boredom, irritability and bitterness in general personality.

General reactions to chronic illness are anger, anxiety, insecurity, depression, frustration, pessimism, uncertainty, inferiority, fear, dejection and shame. Rejection by self and others results in burnout. It is a lifelong series of adjustment and compromises.

> Manpreet has been suffering from asthma for the last few years. He is studying in the 11th standard and his whole class is going on a study tour. Since it is a rainy session, he is suffering badly and has to take many precautions. He is not capable of travelling and tolerating cold weather. The tour is compulsory, still he has to submit a medical certificate for exemption from it. He has become apathetic regarding every special activity.

Chronic illness may become intermittently mild or severe. One has to adjust not only medicines but daily routine, precautions and bear limitations accordingly. Constant tension, distress and generalized anxiety result in depression. The individual feels frustrated due to the lack of possibility of enjoying life, even leading a normal life and getting benefit of available opportunities. For every minor change in routine, one has to plan in advance and make a provision regarding necessary arrangements.

In 2019, it is reported that prevalence of Type 2 diabetes, only among the Indian youth, is about 10 per cent. Additional 15 per cent are in prediabetic state.[1]

These young patients, sometimes, interpret others' messages and communications in a distorted manner. Indian researchers have found that in chronic diseases, most of the patients have external health locus of control. Neuroticism is also related to chronic diseases. Eccentric views, peculiar behavioural patterns and expecting that everything will take place according to their own wish are some common things in chronic diseases. Pain can be organic or psychogenic. Daily living is affected such as maintaining hygiene, eating, sleeping, work and even entertainment. Social isolation, financial burden, poor performance on the job or in academic field and loss of job are the consequences. If the nature of disease is unpredictable, like epilepsy, the individual experiences lot of uncertainty about future. Helplessness increases. All the roles related to every sphere of life change and the individual's self-worth, self-efficacy and self-confidence deteriorate.

10.3. LIMITATIONS AND DISAPPOINTMENTS

Self-image, self-esteem, self-efficacy and self-confidence are hampered due to various limitations. Poor achievements in spite of excellent intellectual capacities and no participation in extracurricular and co-curricular activities lead to low self-worth Quality of life and general well-being are hampered. For example, a youth cannot drive a two-wheeler or a car and cannot travel alone. This makes them feel inferior, dependent and invalid. Not only in terminal but in chronic diseases also, one has to plan every small thing, pace activities and bear embarrassment and awkwardness. In front of many students appearing for examination, an asthmatic patient has to use nasal spray, if needed, and so on.

[1] https://www.ijmr.org.in

In case intermittent or periodic treatment is necessary, such as blood transfusion, iron injections, dialysis and chemotherapy, one has to adjust to the pain, side effects and cancel all other activities. Malnutrition, deficiencies such as vitamin deficiency, decreased strength, overwhelming fatigue and physical limitations with inability to perform some activities are major issues. All these things result in strained family relations, poor acceptance by friends and others, prejudices, stigma, discrimination, isolation, outcasting or being ostracized and even divorce, if at all the individual gets a chance to marry. Many times, it may result in divorce of parents as mother is more involved in welfare of the affected individual and that leads to conflicts.

Occupational life of an individual is also equally affected. Though they are well qualified, they may not get any opportunity to serve. There is poor employability. Considering their disabilities, either they are rejected or they do not have the stamina to fulfil the job requirements. As there is less reservation, less awareness, lack of facilities, less provisions for convenient jobs such as part-time jobs and work from home, many of them cannot serve. They have to depend on others economically. There are no schemes where these individuals get some economic support by the government or society at large. This, again, hampers their self-concept, and they feel inferior, though they are otherwise capable.

Marriage is another very salient developmental task during this age. The affected individual does not get a life partner or has to compromise, as the partner they get is equally or more affected. They have to face many rejections, denials and people may openly insult them due to their disability and disease. Most of these individuals face sexual problems due to psychological issues. Some medicines have side effects due to which sex drive and libido decreases. Due to suffering and lack of involvement, they become apathetic regarding sexual pleasures. This may increase the problems with their life partner. It is proven that prolonged uncontrolled diabetes leads to sexual inability among men. As a cumulative effect of all these, married life becomes unsatisfactory. As a consequence of all these limitations, it is difficult to maintain good relations with the life partner. In addition to that, if a young lady is suffering from the heart condition or similar other aliment, she cannot take a risk of being pregnant. Depending on the family's pressure, this can lead to marital discord. So in short, it is difficult to get a life partner due to compromising quality of life and economic status. If at all one could get, it is difficult to maintain satisfactory relations with the partner. Due to various difficulties and emotional complications, divorce takes place.

Interpersonal relations with family members are affected by these diseases. The family members have to support the individual in every sense: emotional, economic, social and in terms of time and energy. They have to accept various limitations with reference to their own activities. For example, if an individual is suffering from some serious disease, his mother leaves her job and stay back at home to take care of that individual. Their fathers have to take them to the doctor as per the schedule, and their sisters must learn mature behaviour to adjust to their mood swings. Some family members may not be able to develop a proper perspective and empathy and they show resistance, think that parents are showing favouritism and may not be willing to sacrifice. In a way, they also suffer.

Akhilesh is suffering from motor neuron disease. He has been wheelchair bound for the last two years. He was a pilot. He lost his job, his fiancé left him, his friends hardly get any time to visit him and he is totally isolated. Only his mother consistently helps him with routine activities. Other family members are too busy to spend time with him. His sister-in-law hates and avoids him. She blames him openly as he is a burden on her husband's economic resources. He is completely shattered and depressed. It is impossible to get a job, a companion and there is no possibility of improving the condition.

Psychological and cognitive limitations may be related to memory deficits, concentration problems, psychological fatigue, deterioration in attention span and problems with activities of daily living. Sometimes, behavioural problems are also present. In rare conditions, lesions in the brain due to neurocysticercosis may result in various problems, including extreme headaches and fits.

10.4. COPING WITH SUFFERINGS, LIMITATIONS AND LOSS

Post-traumatic growth is a positive change after experiencing adversity for higher level of functioning. It is not as achieving the same level of satisfaction as was before disease or trauma but making life much more meaningful. Reactivity of an individual decreases and one can cope with similar distress in the future. The term was given by Tedeschi and Calhounin (1996). The individual can understand the new meaning of life, interpret every experience from a new perspective and there is a renewed appreciation of life. It is thriving, which goes much beyond resilience. The individual finds benefits in challenges. After trauma, the individual tries to adjust to the new reality with added efforts.

There are five domains of post-traumatic growth. They are as follows.

1. **Personal strength:** The person becomes more confident, mature, humble and even more creative. The individual is more oriented towards humanity.
2. **Relating to others:** Improving relationships with others, empathy and ability to forgive.
3. **Appreciation of life:** Understanding the meaning and purpose of life, development of a philosophy of life.
4. **New possibilities:** Changed goals, skills and subjects and mindfulness.
5. **Spiritual life:** A sense of gratitude and prayer.

> 'However difficult life may seem, there is always something you can do, and succeed at. It matters that you don't just give up.'
>
> —Stephen Hawking

Stephen Hawking, a great cosmologist, suffered from motor neuron disease due to which he was completely paralyzed. With all his problems, he continued his research till his last breath and became a very well-known scientist.

There are examples of individuals dancing with one leg, painting without hands and swimming without all four limbs. People are capable of coping with the disabilities and performing extraordinary things. However, it is essential to have a realistic orientation, a positive attitude, intrinsic motivation and the capacity to bear pain necessary to go ahead in spite of limitations and disabilities. For example, Sudha Chandran always wanted to practise Bharatanatyam dance. Her leg was amputated when she was just 16. According to medical professionals, it was difficult to even walk, but with her artificial Jaipur foot, she has been dancing for the whole of her life. Music director Ravindra Jain is visually challenged, but he still achieved success in his field. Badminton champion Girish Sharma lost his leg when he was a kid. He plays with one leg.

It is proven that there is a positive correlation between post-traumatic growth, psychological development and physical well-being (Park & Helgeson, 2006). Optimism, self-motivation, self-appreciation and gratitude are also related to post-traumatic growth. Pain can be utilized for self enhancement. Late adolescents and young adults experience more post-traumatic growth. More women than men can achieve it. One has to focus on what one can still do, strengths, potential and ways to learn more about various useful skills. This results in new strength and concentration on ways to improve one's health conditions. The affected individual should be as independent as they can be and should not aspire to special attention. This is the most effective way of gaining self-confidence and self-management skills. Rational thoughts lead to optimum adjustment. Pain can be managed with love and intimacy within the family.

To cope with the situation in a better way, knowing more about it is essential. Scientific knowledge helps to understand what improvement can be expected, side effects of medicine and the general range of illnesses with probable risks and dangers. It helps to plan future activities. The individual should mix with other similar patients, talk openly and share problems, as this may enhance emotional catharsis. Online groups are equally effective. Healthy coping is constructive coping. Here, an affected individual tries to overcome the problems as far as possible. Different roles, new adjustments and inferior quality of life are tackled efficiently. Effective coping with distress requires flexibility. It is the adaptive value of coping that is most significant. Coping may be problem focused, emotion focused, meaning focused, proactivity focused and engagement versus disengagement focused.

Though the individual may lose friends, it is time to find out who the true friends are. However, if the conversation is only about the illness and trauma, even the kind friends may lose interest. Some take undue advantage and may take the chance to spoil their psychological health further.

To manage unstructured time and thoughts about pain, misfortune and uncertain future, one may take up activities that are possible to pursue with all the limitations. For example, a wheelchair-bound man will take up training in computer skills; a young woman of the same sort may start learning embroidery and take classes for the same.

Every patient has to face the side effects of drugs. In a terminal disease like cancer, the side effects are severe that the patient has to suffer a lot. Some affected adolescents and youth are overwhelmingly upset, and they do not stick to the prescribed schedule of medicine and do not keep away from the things that they are advised to avoid. This may include alcohol, smoking, eating sweets or particular types of activities. Maintaining motivation for further education, exercise, trying to improve one's physical and psychological health and keeping good interpersonal relations help a lot.

Very few individuals can achieve post-traumatic growth. It depends on general personality of an individual, their optimistic outlook, confidence and maturity. As a consequence of post-traumatic growth, quality of life and psychological adjustment improve. Negative things such as distress and post-traumatic stress disorder decrease. Some experts think that there is cognitive dissonance in post-traumatic growth. It may also include rationalization. Positive illusions present in post-traumatic growth are useful for positive or less-negative appraisal of disease. The correlates of post-traumatic growth are extroversion and openness to experience. Those who are young, educated, have social support, better coping style and come from high socio-economic status are mostly capable of achieving post-traumatic growth. It is worth noting that pain in the case of chronic diseases like arthritis also diminishes. Even so life expectancy increases.

Kalpana, a well-educated and motivated lady, was diagnosed as breast cancer patient at the age of 32. After necessary treatment and suffering, she was completely cured. Since then, she enjoys everything in her life: her family relations, her job, her friends' circle and so on. Every day, she is well dressed, pleasant, enthusiastic and ready to help others. She devotes her time to counselling cancer patients in various hospitals and is known for her work.

There are different models of post-traumatic growth. Some important ones are as follows.

1. **Shattered assumption theory by Bulman 1992:** Due to trauma, individual's inner world and safety assumptions are shattered. Feelings of security diminish. Hence, the individual has to reconstruct everything again around the experience of trauma.

2. **Optimistic valuing theory:** Given by Joseph and Linley in 2005, the theory says that the individual must overcome obstacles and regain their confidence with the help of social environment. If no reordering is done and old views are maintained, it leads to negative attitudes and self-blame. If an individual can use accommodation and modify previous schemas positively, it facilitates post-traumatic growth.

3. **Transformational model:** It was put forth by Tedeschi and Calhoun in 2006. It says that because of excessively negative thoughts, effects of trauma increase. Emotional management means one has to learn disengagement from negative thoughts, which leads to decrease in distress, changes in perception and leads to post-traumatic growth.

In 2016, Tandon and Mehrotra found that in India, most of the cancer patients studied demonstrated post-traumatic growth. Patients in early stages reported more growth. Self-efficacy, social support and seeking support and information were positively related to growth. Some other researchers found that religious practices enhance post-traumatic growth.

10.4.1. Self-actualization

Maslow, the famous psychologist, included this concept of self-actualization in the theory of motivation. It is the ultimate stage one can achieve by utilizing all their hidden capacities. Self-actualization is a natural tendency to strive to fulfil one's potential. Autonomy, self-realization and psychological empowerment are the predictors of self-actualization among affected individuals. Independence, good interpersonal relations, motivation to face challenges, willingness to put in efforts for new roles, self-discipline and emotional management are the pillars of self-actualization among the affected individuals. There are examples of affected individuals achieving self-actualization in its ultimate sense.

> Károly Takács was the winner of the Olympic gold medal in the shooting competition. He was serving in defence and a hand grenade burst in his right hand due to which it was amputated. He started practising shooting with his left hand as his aspiration was to get a gold medal. Two Olympic competitions were cancelled. Still, he continued practising and won a gold medal at the 1948 Olympics. Consistently putting in a lot of effort in spite of severe problems may lead to such actualization. India has received 19 medals in paralympics in September 2021.

Recently, Arunima Sinha, a national-level volleyball player, was pushed by some robbers from the railway, due to which her leg was amputated. With all her extraordinary determination and motivation, she has conquered Mount Everest and is planning to conquer other similar highest peaks in the world.

There are different strategies to enhance an individual's journey towards self-actualization. Art therapy, dance therapy and such other strategies also work very well. Self-actualization takes place when an individual can exploit all their talents while considering all their limitations.

Self-actualization is accompanied by the following.

- **Accepting self and others:** It is a challenge for the affected individual. Interpersonal relations depend on accepting others as they are. Individuals expect others to have special consideration for them, which may or may not materialize. They should remember that one cannot change others' behaviour but can change reaction to their behaviour. It is better to understand others' limitations.
- **Being autonomous:** In the case of diseased and disabled individuals, achieving complete autonomy is difficult. However, the individual should try to gain as much autonomy as they can.
- **Having a sense of purpose** and interrelating various activities with it. Leading life without a purpose becomes futile. The individual should develop an achievable goal and a meaningful purpose to

their activities and life. Sometimes, the individual feels so lonely and isolated that they cannot relate to others. If they have a purpose, their lives become more meaningful.

As Alisha was suffering from anaemia, she could not work or do any hectic activities. However, as she sings very well, she sings as a commercial activity. Whatever money she gets, she devotes to the welfare of cancer patients. She has been donating lakhs of rupees for years. She is known for her sacrifices. She gets a lot of satisfaction, fame and meaning in life due to this activity.

- **Perceiving reality from one's own perspective and from others' perspective:** Distorted perception leads to undue expectations from self and others. If an individual perceives oneself as more disabled than what they actually are, they may not help themselves and expect others to do everything for them.
- **Maintaining meaningful interpersonal relationships:** Communicating only negative things, complaining about limitations and pain, criticizing and blaming others are the ways that are detrimental to interpersonal relations. Developing socially acceptable pleasant style of communication works well.
- **Demonstrating empathy for others and having compassion for them:** There are individuals who take it for granted that their sufferings are the only sufferings. They do not think about others and their problems. Even their family members have their personal difficulties, and an individual should be able to show empathy and compassion for them.
  - o **Experiencing happiness:** Whatever activities generate happiness in life of an individual should be repeated. Affected individuals should be able to experience positive emotions and intentionally generate such things.
- **Having appreciation for goodness of life:** One should be grateful regarding whatever positive things are available and whatever progress is possible.
- **Capacity to accept one's mistakes in a lighter mood:** Humour and self-correction help to keep a proper perspective. The individual may use their mistakes for generating good atmosphere and maintain better relations.

10.4.2. Gratitude

Gratitude development plays a major role in maintaining mental health. It is prosocial behaviour which develops interpersonal connectedness, forgiveness, motivation for self-improvement, reciprocity and humility. One has to be grateful for every good relationship, every help and every pleasant experience in life. It is perceived that life is a gift. Moral emotions are associated with gratitude. Such individuals enjoy life, have less envy and less depression and anxiety. They experience more empathy, hope and life satisfaction.

The sense of well-being is more. They can cope with stress in a better way. Gratitude generates resilience. Coping with disasters is better in case of these patients. In a way, it is protection against psychiatric disorders. Gratitude also maintains physiological indicators in normal range such as heart rhythm, respiration, brain rhythm and blood pressure rhythm, which leads to capacity for optimum experience of life. Fewer aches and pains and improved immunity are reported to be present with gratitude. Those who cannot understand and accept one's shortcomings are materialists, have victim feelings, narcissistic, have envy and resentment and cannot develop gratitude. Gratitude enhances coping with illness. High neuroticism and low extroversion result in difficulty expressing gratitude.

10.4.3. Resilience

Resilience is one of the important skills essential for overcoming trauma or diseases. It is related to realistic optimism. Flexibility, adaptability and perseverance are the pillars of resilience. It is the capacity to recover from difficult situation. Mindfulness or consciously living in the present, remaining calm, considering bodily feedback, enhancing positive social relationship and finding purpose of life play an important role. Self-awareness, maintaining positive emotions, having flexible and stable attention are essential. Gratitude, compassion, forgiveness, acceptance and finding meaning enhance resilience. It is the ability to be successful and happy after trauma or disease.

Physical resilience is capacity of one's body to recover quickly and adapt to challenges.

Resilience training can be given from childhood. Resilience is related to availability and accessibility of culturally relevant resources. Strengthening social relations and overcoming financial problems are important achievements. Emotional intelligence is positively correlated to resilience. Positive perception about environment is also a correlate of resilience. Resilience may lead to confidence and motivation.

Those who lack resilience become overwhelmingly helpless; their coping styles are unhealthy. It is worth noting that patients who attempt suicide have low resilience score. American Psychological Association has also published *The Road to Resilience* for helping people to learn ways to cope with difficult situations.[2]

10.4.4. Hardiness

Hardiness is an individual's ability to endure difficult conditions. Hardiness is the capacity of an individual to face limitations and pain. Maddi and Khoshaba are the pioneer workers (2005). It is an individual's ability to manage stress and properly respond to stress with such coping mechanisms that potentially harmful and unpleasant situation can be converted into learning opportunities. The individuals who have hardiness can remain healthy even when they are under stress. Their bio-physiological symptoms also indicate the same. Reactivity of sympathetic nervous system decreases. Commitment, control and challenge are the three things in hardiness. Involvement in task, interest and curiosity constitute commitment. The second aspect, control, is similar to internal locus of control. The individual thinks, believes and acts with a firm idea that they can influence the events in their life with their efforts. Challenge is the belief that change is a normal process, which generates motivating opportunities for personal growth. In this way, with all these three things, the individual can convert the potential calamities into opportunities.

Hardiness influences the way in which an individual perceives the world and self.

It improves coping, performance and social support, which in turn leads to effective self-care and other health-related practices.

Perception regarding self improves and one thinks that they are capable of handling the situation. Change in the situation is perceived with reference to the whole and becomes less threatening. It is converted into opportunity to develop some new skills and better understanding. This is called transformational coping. Hardiness is related to health-protective behaviour like exercise and reduced risk of alcohol and drug abuse. Hence, the affected individual may get number of benefits of hardiness to overcome the ill effects of disease and disability.

On 10 December 1914, a massive explosion took place in Edison's laboratory. The sight of the huge fire was devastating. However, Thomas Edison was calmly watching. He said, 'It's all right, we just got rid of lot rubbish ... although I am 67 years old, I will start all over again tomorrow' (*New York Times*). It was a tremendous loss; approximately 23 million dollars in contemporary conditions. All his records of painstaking research vanished. At 5:30 in the morning, he immediately started rebuilding it. Thomas Edison, who invented the light bulb, could not get any opportunity for formal education. He was labelled as 'too stupid to learn anything' by teachers. He was hearing impaired since childhood. He also had diabetes mellitus. He was continuously trying even after 1,000 unsuccessful attempts, and finally, he was able to achieve what he wanted.

10.4.5. Positive Thinking

Positive thinking is the faith that positive attitude towards life results in positive output. Positive thinking is a personality characteristic. Positive thinking is related to the general well-being. Even when an individual is experiencing a lot of distress, positive thinking helps. It is proved that women suffering from breast cancer recover early if they think positively. They start their routine earlier than others having the same problem. Positive thinkers, generally, have problem-focused coping style. This is the style which takes for granted that something can be done to solve the problem. The positive thinker looks at the good things, benefits and facilities available to them. They are ready to put in efforts for improving the condition. They do not blame others.

They never avoid ways to adjust with the disability or disease and do not passively depend on others. It helps to decrease anxiety, hostility, helplessness, dissatisfaction, inactivity and depression. The strategies necessary are self-acceptance, self-love, unconditional regard for self and self-grooming. Intraindividual relations should be properly maintained. Self-respect is a basic support for positive thinking. Positive thinking results in better general health, resistance to common infections, decrease in distress and better coping at the time of disaster. As far as serious diseases are concerned, it leads to reduced risk of coronary heart disease, easier breathing in lung disease and better coping in case of various medical conditions.

10.5. INTERVENTION AND MANAGEMENT

The role of family is the most significant in improving psycho-social health of the patient or victim. Adjustment regarding routine of the patient and evaluation of improvement impacts adjustment of an individual and their family. The family is affected by the patient and patient is affected by the family. If parents are overprotective and devoted only to the individual, it leads to more dependency. This leads to exaggeration of concern and doing things for the patient that they can do. The person may also use their ailment for exploiting others and for leading more convenient and comfortable life. More attention should be attracted to what the individual is capable of doing than what they cannot.

Parents should have achievable expectations; the individual should not be treated as the centre of attention; over worrying and over protection should be avoided. Parents should not have the perfectionist expectations. There is always scope for improvement. One should be encouraged to try to do the best that they can. Even if the individual has irrational fears, others should not make fun of him. They should have empathy and try to understand the individual's problems and psychological as well as physiological condition and limitations. Parental counselling and family therapy are very effective from that perspective.

In case of chronic diseases and trauma, premarital counselling and genetic counselling become essential. Accepting the partner with all of their limitations becomes a major issue. They have to help each other and compensate for each other's limitations. To make life more meaningful and satisfactory, they should develop lot of maturity and understanding regarding each other's life and sufferings. Counselling helps them to do so.

> Genetic counselling is for the couples to enhance their understanding regarding the contribution of genetic factors to their problem and its implications for the next generation. It includes, in detail, scientific information about testing, management, prevention and resources. Considering family history and inheritance pattern, one can predict the possibility of recurrence.[3] For example, if both of them have diabetes, their progeny may develop diabetes. The probability of such suffering depends on the exact nature, intensity of the disease, age of the mother, other health problems of the parents and sex of the infant.

For family members also, counselling and therapies should be used, as they have a lot of stress, grief, worry, financial burden and extreme physical and psychological fatigue.

The role of family cohesion cannot be underestimated in it. Communication skills, community support and emotional regulation are required for achieving that. Kenneth Ginsburg has given competence, confidence, connection, character, contribution, coping and control as the 7 Cs which are the keys to learn resilience for young individuals. Resilient people have self-awareness, self-care, internal locus of control, optimism, problem-solving skills and coping skills. It is scientifically proved that resilience influences progression and outcome of the illness. It helps patients of all sorts like rheumatoid arthritis or even cancer.

There is a direct relation between psychological disorders and daily life with reference to attitudes, behaviour and satisfaction. Some glaring examples are worth considering.

Depression results in affective, somatic and cognitive symptoms, loss of energy and interest, worthlessness, suicidal thoughts, depressed mood and insomnia. Depression after stroke or myocardial infraction leads to more mortality. Insomnia leads to more restlessness and more health problems. Anxiety, depression, distress due to immobility,

---

[3] http://en.m.wikipedia.org; http://www.cdc.gov

restrictions and weak respiratory muscles lead to lack of sleep. Post stroke and head injuries lead to loss of control over various body parts and severe disability, which is permanent. That also leads to depression. The individual cannot think of any self-help. Sometimes, deterioration in language and communication with cognitive impairment are seen. Sexual problems result from many conditions like heart problems, including pots, stoke, paraplegia and quadriplegia. Due to medical problems, there is decreased frequency of expression of sexual interests. As a consequence, attitude of the partner changes and it affects the whole interaction and motivation to please the partner. These difficulties result in emotional problems, fear, anxiety, guilt and feeling of rejection. Both of them may be attracted to sex perversions and unhealthy satisfaction. That generates shame and guilt. The affected individual may have doubts about infidelity of the partner. Spinal cord injury or injury to sex organ leads to inability regarding sex and lack of attractiveness. Not only is the attractiveness goes down, but fertility may also be impaired. Depending on the intensity of the disease, bladder and bowel control are hampered. Impotency may become a root cause of discord between husband and wife and even divorce.

Counselling gives a chance for emotional catharsis. It helps to understand the exact problem. Giving objective information and conducting programmes for improving general psychological and physical health are also necessary.

Anger and depression management, knowledge of legal rights, disability rights, as well as participation in support groups and workshops are the basic and essential issues in intervention. It is difficult to interpret psychological tests, as there is no comparison group having similar problems. Hence, it is necessary for the psychologists to use their own discretion. Adjustment to illness, needs, expectations, fears and concerns need to be evaluated and improved. Phenomenological understanding is more important than objective evaluation of the condition. Hence, the family members, caregivers and counsellors should develop sensitivity necessary to deal with such a situation.

Palliative care centres and support groups and death counsellors for terminal patients and their relatives are working all over India, like AIIMS hospital, Delhi, but rural areas hardly get the benefit.[4] Pain-related adjustments and pain management depend on irrational thoughts. If thoughts are irrational, there is more pain. Cognitive restructuring assists the individual for reducing pain. Cognitive evaluation of life with pain and emotions related to pain are related to threat to comfort and future activities. Cognitive barriers should be taken care of. It is a never-ending pattern of failure, awkwardness, guilt and worthlessness.

10.6. THERAPIES

Professional help always boosts morale and motivation. Activity participation, altering environmental factors, optimized living, opportunities of work, treatment of mental problems like depression, strengthening self-image, self-management including emotional management, gratitude therapy, educational facilities, group therapy, family therapy, concentration and memory improvement and positive reinforcement generate substantial enhancement in the quality of life.

The most important thing for counselling, in dealing with individuals suffering from chronic and terminal diseases as well as those who are facing traumatic situation, is developing empathy. It is a difficult job, but dealing with emotional problems of the patient is impossible without it. Counselling, psychoeducation, relaxation, individual therapy, safety training, hobbies, occupational rehabilitation, cognitive behaviour therapy and rational emotive behaviour therapy may help the individual.

- Existential therapy, client-centred counselling and, above all, unconditional acceptance and positive regard expressed by not only therapist but by near and dear ones may prove to generate substantial support and feeling of security. Insight therapy and supportive psychotherapy, also, are very effective. Antidepressant drugs are given to these patients. Side effects of drugs, especially of antidepressant, should be taken care of.

[4] livemint.com, 2 January 2020

- Cognitive behaviour therapy has proved to be effective for such affected individuals. Crisis counselling helps the counselee to a substantial extent.

Some therapies accepted to be effective by the experts all over the world are:

- Relaxation and progressive muscle relaxation, guided imagery, systematic desensitization
- Biofeedback gives a sense of increase in perceived control. It may help facing surgery
- Group therapy generates a sense of social support and belongingness. Giving exact scientific information, training regarding necessary skills, meaningful social interaction including catharsis are the major issues. Encouragement for self-help and developing self-efficacy are also effective programmes
- Training about altruism, stress reduction and gratitude are thinking styles that lead to positive attitude
- Modification of health-related attitudes helps a lot. Prevention of risky behaviour such as smoking, malnutrition, lack of exercise, alcohol and drug abuse and unprotected sex may multiply individual's problems
- Health-related locus of control—it is proved that chronic patients have greater internal locus of control. External locus of control results in less efforts to help oneself. Those who have internal locus of control have positive attitude, better achievements and take care of themselves. External locus of health control results in more dependency. In this case, restoring the pre-morbid physical functions and psychological moods should be the goal
- Yoga and meditation are always useful for enhancing psychological and physical health
- Accepting reality—to combat depression and anxiety, one has to accept one's disability, current abilities and limitations. It is essential to accept new roles in family and workplace.

Instead of avoiding social interaction and get together, they should mix with people and regenerate their relations with relatives and friends.

Though all of them may not be very cooperative, some may be ready to help for the betterment of their lives.

Family intervention is a must as family support is as important as medication.

10.7. INDIAN SCENARIO, CULTURAL VIEWS AND PRACTICES

As far as the Indian scenario is concerned, there is hardly any awareness regarding psychological impact of chronic and terminal diseases and trauma. Many Indian religious and philosophical perspectives explain these things as a consequence of God's wish or nature's rule.

Indian situation, its specific perspective and cultural interpretations, everything affect the individual in every sense. In India, there are different therapies such as allopathy, homeopathy, ayurveda and god-man therapies. Some educated people also have blind faith. They give some treatment which is completely illogical and redundant. Some cultures teach hiding pain; some cultures interpret that an individual must have done some sin due to which they are suffering. Some perform religious activities; some keep prolonged fasts, and many primitive people depend on medicines available in jungle in the form of trees and fruits. Fake quakes are also abundant in India.

In India, there are different types of specific shortcomings with reference to supporting the affected individual. First, there is hardly any awareness and scientific knowledge about various diseases and disabilities and effects of trauma. There is lot of social rejection, social stigma, direct ridicule, banter and disrespect that the individual has to tolerate. People keep on asking insulting questions even during travel, social functions and day-to-day interactions. They expect that they should get the complete information and should get an opportunity to stare at the individual, show sympathy and so on. Many affected individuals even have to apply and beg for simple things like change in sitting arrangement at the time of examination. Illiterate and semi-educated individuals are even not aware that their reactions are causing irritation to the individual and their family. Generally, no one is interested in making friends, spending time and helping these individuals. If an individual is suffering from a terminal disease, some religions expect that they life should be humbly submitted to the wish of the utmost power.

As far as chronic diseases are concerned, illiterate, semi-educated youth do not care for their health and recklessly continue their routine activities which are detrimental to their life. There are people who are afraid of facing even a patient with unbearable suffering. If any empathy is generated, they will have to suffer due to unpleasant emotions. So, they avoid the affected individual.

In almost all Indian families, mother is supposed to take care of the affected offspring. It is expected that the mother should not go anywhere if the individual is home bound. She is expected to devote all her psychological and physical energy and time for the welfare of the offspring. Possibility of divorce increases as the husband is dissatisfied about her devotion to her child. By and large, the individual is perceived as being a burden by their own family. Especially in case if the daughter is affected, it is for 24 hours that the mother has to devote. It is difficult to get anyone else so trustworthy to take care of an immobilized young lady.

In India, institutional care is costly, rare and, mostly, not satisfactory. Some institutes are not ready to shoulder any responsibility of even sexual exploitation, and it is compulsory to give a written consent that even if that happens, the parents would not go against the institute legally.

In very traditional and uneducated families, the parents still depend on some illogical and blind faith-oriented treatment. They either depend on uneducated gurus and practise some threatening things or sacrifice some animals or birds in the name of God. Poverty is also one important reason for not treating the patient properly. Lack of availability of medical facilities and no proper conveyance easily available from rural area are also some obvious reasons. Lack of awareness on the part of the general public leads to delays in the treatment.

In India, there are an inadequate number of institutes for helping terminal patients and long-term rehabilitation of these individuals. Even when trauma takes place, there is hardly any provision for advanced treatment, especially in rural areas. Long-term rehabilitation, both psychological and social, of trauma victims is also, generally, neglected.

The paucity of qualified psychological counsellors, various availabilities and social groups is a very significant issue. Increased social awareness, developing non-government organizations, improved attitude and better hiring practices to support the disabled are essential. Though there are hardly any special institutes for their rehabilitation, every institute should accommodate disabled persons in appropriate positions.

For terminal patients, irrespective of the type of treatment, palliative care is necessary. It is aimed at reducing pain, giving emotional support and improving the quality of life. Hospice care is provided at home to give emotional and spiritual support for the patient and their family. In hospice care, the patient spends maximum time with their loved ones. Terminal patients need care regarding daily routine activities, hygiene, food, medicine and psychological support.

Terminal patients need psychotherapy and psycho-social intervention. One has to appreciate patient's strengths. For extreme suffering, some sedatives are used. In the last few days, similar provision has been made. A lot of provisions are necessary to make their lives bearable.

10.8. SUMMARY

The present chapter tries to encompass various psycho-social effects on an individual's life due to trauma, terminal and chronic diseases. The setback may substantially deteriorate an individual's psychological health. It may lead to frustration, anxiety, depression and many other problems leading to severe maladjustment. Increased dependency, loss of valued roles, and pain and suffering add to a sense of futility. It leads to overwhelming unhappiness, loneliness, hopelessness, learned helplessness and worthlessness.

The individual and their family should be helped to accept the limitations and disabilities of the affected individual. The individual should be helped to enhance their self-worth, self-confidence and readjustment to life.

Clinical Disorders

11.1. INTRODUCTION

According to one recent estimate, by the next year, approximately 20 per cent of Indians will suffer from some mental illness.[1]

Many individuals, who are leading a superficially normal life, may be suffering from psychological health problems and are identified only if their symptoms are analysed properly by an expert. In India, there is hardly any awareness regarding psycho-social health problems and, hence, guessing the exact incidence is difficult. People hide their family members' problematic behaviour and avoid going to a psychologist or a psychiatrist. It is associated with a social stigma. So unless and until the condition becomes worse, a patient is not taken to any of them. In an advanced country like the USA, 26.2 per cent of adults suffer from some mental health problem and 6 per cent suffer from serious disorders. On the basis of this, we will be able to imagine what must be the real scenario in India.

WHO has reported that India is facing serious problems regarding mental health. Approximately 38 million individuals are suffering from an anxiety disorder and 56 million from depression.[2] In a survey, it was found that 47 per cent of the normal population is highly judgemental and thinks that any interaction with mental patients would affect their own mental health. Approximately 26 per cent are afraid of mentally ill patients. By 2020, 20 per cent of Indians were expected to suffer from some mental disease.[3]

[1] https://economictimes.com

[2] https://qz.com/india/

[3] mictimes.com

Many mental health problems emerge during adolescence. It is known as a period of storm and stress. Due to overwhelming changes, there is a substantial risk of psycho-social health problems. During this period, an individual is confused and stressed. It affects social roles and increases ambiguity in interpersonal and intrapersonal relations. A lot of problems regarding behaviour and immaturity affecting understanding of realities about self and others are common. There is a complex and complicated interaction of cognitive, emotional and behavioural problems. Such distress is associated with eccentric behaviour and negative ideas and attitudes. This, in turn, affects the mental health of an individual. It affects the capacity to function effectively in every sphere of life. In these circumstances, any failure, discord, break-up, insult or serious issues like sexual abuse lead to intense psychological health problems. Mental illness affects the whole lives of such individuals negatively. In such cases, culturally and socially unacceptable patterns of behaviour, thoughts and general personality of an individual are seen. The most important sign is that the individual's contact with reality deteriorates. In the case of all serious disorders, the person gets some more stimuli from within and responds to them. The actual stimuli that are there in the physical environment may or may not be interpreted properly or are distorted by the concerned person. An individual screaming with fear due to the sight of a snake which does not exist is an example of an abnormal distorted perception.

11.2. MODELS OF MENTAL HEALTH

The biopsychosocial model proposes that all three, that is biological, psychological and social, factors contribute to mental disorders. The model of sociocultural influence highlights factors such as gender, socio-economic status, religion and spirituality and race and ethnicity, as all of them affect mental health. A holistic view is given by the multipath model, which highlights complex and complicated interactions between various factors affecting mental health.

Genetic endowment, epigenetics, normalcy of structure and functions of the central nervous system, brain anatomy, biochemical processes, interactions and imbalances, hormonal balance, functions of the autonomic nervous system and reactivity are the basic aspects included in biological dimensions.

In the social dimension, social support, family and other interpersonal relationships, marital status, community interactions and emotional experiences related to belongingness and love are considered as contributing factors to mental disorders.

The third is the sociocultural dimension which includes gender, sexual orientation, race, religion, caste, socio-economic status, culture and ethnicity. The psychological dimension takes into consideration cognitive, emotional and personality dimensions, coping strategies and skills, childhood experiences, self-esteem, self-efficacy and values.

There are gender differences in how one can deal with psychological stress and tensions. All over the world, even in developed countries like the USA, women mostly internalize their conflicts, which results in anxiety and depression. Men, generally, act out and externalize, which results in drug and alcohol abuse. It is necessary to consider general cultural background, expected and accepted behavioural pattern for the given age, education, socio-economic status, gender, urban or rural background and so on before labelling an individual.

If one's behaviour is not within the acceptable range, it indicates that there is some problem. Most of the time, it is difficult to understand the link to deep-rooted and hidden psychological complex problems. Hence, it is necessary to know at least the outward symptoms which indicate that it needs intervention.

DSM-5 is the recent revision of classification of mental disorders which is followed all over the world. It includes some core intense psychological disorders leading to substantial disturbances in human life. Some common ones are discussed below.

11.3. SCHIZOPHRENIA AND DELUSIONAL DISORDERS

11.3.1. Schizophrenia

It is one of the most serious psychological disorders. It is a chronic disorder, in the sense, it cannot be cured completely. It is treatable but not curable.

As far as schizophrenia is concerned, age group from 16 to 25 years is the most vulnerable population. Boys and men are more prone than girls and ladies.

Global incidence is 1 per cent. Its causes are genetic, biological and psycho-social. Contact with reality is comparatively poor. There are problems with distorted perception and thinking. In such patients, there is decreased motivation or complete loss of motivation, decline in social interest, less mixing with others and detachment along with isolation. Bizarre expressions of emotions and clumsy physical movements are very common. Emotions are incongruent. Being expressionless or unnecessarily crying is also seen. By and large, these patients are detached, withdrawn and aggressive and think illogically and incoherently. They experience delusions and hallucinations, which are thoughts inconsistent with reality and perceptions of things that are not physically present. Hallucinations about auditory stimuli are common, but visual-, taste-, touch- and smell-related are rarely experienced. Abnormal physical movements are also reported.

> Sunil is a 23-year old dropout from a low socio-economic status. He is not doing any work and spends the whole day either relaxing or doing pastime activities. He is not interested in doing any meaningful activities despite repeated opportunities created by his family. He threatens his family members that he is capable of doing anything, can kill an international don, be a political leader or a famous actor. He claims that they cannot understand his worth. Generally, he perceives some ghosts that appear for a moment and then disappear. More than half of his speech is incoherent and inconsistent.

Schizophrenia is seen among all types of races, cultures and socio-economic strata in all nations and across genders. In India, the incidence is approximately 1 per cent, and men suffer at an early age. Loganathan and Murthy reported in 2011 that more Indian male patients are unmarried; they hide their problems and experience guilt and shame. Such males experience social stigma at the workplace, and women experience it during marital relations, pregnancy and childbirth.

The major symptoms of schizophrenia are hallucinations, delusions, passivity and thought alienation.

There are several sub-types in each one. In hallucination, thoughts echo or loud voices as if speaking out thoughts are heard. Some comments or even arguments are heard.

Shephali has completed her BPharm. She is a bright student. However, nowadays she stays alone in her room and avoids any interactions with her family members. She says that someone tells her that her father is not her biological father and gives her some instructions about how to behave. Sometimes, she complains that someone comes at night and rapes her, when everyone knows that nobody is around.

This is auditory hallucination and command hallucination.

A delusion is a false belief or reality interpreted in an unrealistic way. This is held persistently, though there is contrary evidence. There are two types of delusions: primary and secondary. Primary delusions are seen in early stages and are inconsistent with perceptions and experiences. Secondary delusion is, in a way, related to other abnormal experiences. In passivity, the individual thinks that their thoughts, feelings and even actions are controlled by someone else. Sensations are interpreted as being imposed by someone. Thought alienation is addition or subtraction of thoughts and is interpreted as being governed by some external force. Sometimes, the patient thinks that others are getting the knowledge of what they think. All these things affect every cognitive process of the individual. Negativism and affect disturbances are the correlates of these symptoms.

Amir is a 22-year old dropout. He is always preoccupied and thinks that there is a chip in his head. That chip delivers some messages from the American president and he has to work on some international anti-terrorists activities. Amir considers himself the commander-in-chief of these activities and plans various things. He is so convinced about it that he behaves as if he is one.

What type of delusion is it?

Common delusions in schizophrenic patients are as follows:

1. **Delusion of grandeur:** Exaggerated self-importance and self-image are seen.

2. **Delusion of persecution:** The patients think that some people are against them and they are trying to manage everything in such a way that the patients will have to suffer.
3. **Delusion of reference:** If some individuals are talking to each other, the patients invariably think that they are talking ill about them and they become restless.
4. **Delusion of control:** Such patients think that their whole life is being controlled by some external power. Sometimes, they claim that they know it.
5. **Hypochondriacal delusion:** It is also known as somatic delusion. In this case, the individual has various doubts about their health and is worried about it, though there is no evidence.

Delusional jealousy and delusion of love are also seen in some patients.

Schizophrenia is diagnosed with the help of the following characteristics.

1. **Disturbances in thought and speech:** These include:
   a. **Inconsistent speech pattern:** There are different styles of speech which are easily recognized by others as being incoherent and abnormal. It is a spontaneous speech where things discussed are not related to each other. From one subject to another, from one reference to another, the conversation shifts very often. It becomes difficult to comprehend.
   b. **Blocking of thoughts:** While talking, before the idea is completely expressed, the individual forgets what they were talking about. They may stop even in the middle of a sentence.
   c. **Neologism:** The patient constructs new words and, sometimes, uses common words in a distorted manner. This results in difficulty understanding what they want to express.
   d. **Other speech problems:** Complete lack of speech, limited speech, poor content of speech, echolalia or repeated speech are some common speech problems.
2. **Problems regarding perception:** These include:
   a. **Hallucinations:** Auditory and visual hallucinations are generally reported. Other sensory modalities are rarely involved.
3. **Disorders of emotions:** Emotional expressions are inconsistent and reduced. The patient is not capable of establishing emotional contact

with others. There are symptoms such as apathy, emotional shallowness, inappropriate emotional response and emotional blunting.

4. **Problems with motor activities:** Either increased or decreased activities are seen in the case of these patients. Aggressiveness, excitement, agitation and restlessness increase and spontaneous activities, grooming and self-care decrease.

There are more than eight sub-types of schizophrenia and the symptoms vary accordingly.

11.3.2. Theories

1. Biological theories
   a. **Genetic factors:** If both the parents have schizophrenia, the possibility that an individual will be affected is very high, that is, 40 per cent. It is proved that the occurrence of disease is 46 per cent in identical twins and, approximately 14 per cent in fraternal twins. Generally, relatives from extended family are more affected by schizophrenia and the percentage is 10.
   b. **Biochemical theories:** Disturbances in some neurotransmitters such as dopamine, serotonin, acetylcholine and GABA are associated with schizophrenia.
   c. **Studies regarding brain imaging have proved some specific facts:** Enlarged ventricles, mild cortical atrophy and so on are reported in MRI, CT scan. PET scan shows hypofrontality and decreased glucose utilization in temporal lobe.
2. **Theories dealing with information processing:** Problems regarding attention, difficulty in maintaining a set and poor integration of perceptions are reported in schizophrenics.
   Psychological theories are based on the impact of distress, inappropriate information processing, wrong parenting and various concepts of psychoanalytic theory.
3. **Family-related causes:** Mothers who are schizophrenic and anxious, dependency on the mother, parental marital conflict and lack of parental affection are some common causes of schizophrenia.
4. **Psychosexual theory:** It assumes regressions to oral stage and the use of various, specific ego defence mechanisms are related to schizophrenia.

11.3.3. Treatment and Intervention

- **Drug treatment:** Drugs are essential to treat the patient. Electroconvulsive therapy becomes essential if the intensity is substantial.
- **Psycho-social intervention:** Family therapy, psychoeducation, individual and group psychotherapy are effective for treating schizophrenic patients. Enhancing rehabilitation requires halfway homes. Vocational skills, guidance and sheltered employment workshops help the individual.

11.3.4. Persistent Delusional Disorders

There are other psychotic disorders related to delusions.

All the disorders where delusions are persistent are grouped together. They are discussed in brief below.

Delusional disorder was known as paranoid disorder. It is worth remembering that there is no hallucination present; however, specific delusions are prevalent. Contact with reality is poor. The individual does not have insight into their problem. Personality disturbances are substantial. This, in turn, affects general performance. Some important ones are—delusion of grandeur, delusion of persecution, hypochondriacal delusion and delusion of jealousy and infidelity.

Erotomanic delusion is also seen in some cases. It is the delusion of love. This is included in DSM-5. Shy, sexually inexperienced and emotionally dependent women suffer the most. The individual thinks that someone loves him or her irrespective of exactly the opposite evidence. The person may come from a high status, may be a famous person, married and, hence, not interested or even a dead individual or completely imaginary individual. The patient tries to prove that what he or she is thinking is true. This may become chronic. The whole life of such patient gets affected because of this delusion. However, depending on intensity, some of them can lead approximately normal life.

There are examples where a young lady thinks that a well-known actor loves her, and he wants to meet her. In that delusion, she waits for hours in front of his gate and tries to wave her hand when he goes in his car.

Madhoshi (2004) was a film showing that the heroine (Bipasha Basu) was in love with a young man (John Abraham), who did not exist. This is a clearly depicted picture of erotomania.

There are some more delusions in the present disorder. Otherwise, there is no organic mental disorder. It is different from schizophrenia and mood disorders.

11.3.5. Other Persistent Delusional Disorders

The basic characteristic is that in this type there are auditory hallucinations and delusions. It is, generally, for short duration like a few months. One more variation is induced or shared in delusional disorder where the delusion is shared between two or more individuals who are close to each other emotionally. There are acute and transient psychotic disorders.

11.3.6. Schizoaffective Disorders

It is a more complex and complicated type of disorder. In that, symptoms of both schizophrenia and mood disorders are present simultaneously. Three main types are given by experts: manic type, depressive type and mixed type.

In one more type called Capgras syndrome, the patient perceives that others are not their real self but their duplicate or are replaced.

11.4. MOOD DISORDERS: BIPOLAR DISORDER, MANIA, DEPRESSIVE DISORDERS

Swaroopachary reported in June 2018 that the prevalence of bipolar disorder in India is about 0.5 per cent. However, the lifetime prevalence is 7.8 per cent.[4]

A mood is a sustained and comparatively stable emotional response or state of an individual. Mood disorders are of various types, such

[4] www.amhonline.org

as mania, depression, bipolar disorder, recurrent depressive disorder, persistent depressive disorder and other disorders related to mood.

11.4.1. Mania

Aman was very happy and active. He was spontaneously welcoming the guests who were coming and was eagerly interacting with them with great pleasure. While making them comfortable, he switched on the tape recorder. As soon as his favourite song started, he was so excited that he started dancing. The day before yesterday, Aman's mother had expired.

An individual who is suffering from mania is full of vigour and energy, wants to do many things simultaneously, can produce more creative ideas and their general productivity increases. Due to their overactivity, they get attracted to risky behaviour. Their appetite and sleep decrease. They get involved in excessively interacting with even unknown people. Their inhibition about sexual activity also decreases. They can become hypersexual or even promiscuous.

Manic episodes are temporary for a few days or months. The typical symptoms are elevated mood and irritability. The exact nature depends on the intensity of the manic episode. There are the following four stages.

- **Hypomania:** In this stage, the individual's mood is slightly elevated. They become happier and their sense of well-being increases. However, it has nothing to do with real-life circumstances.
- **Elation:** Along with moderate elevation of mood, the person's sense of enjoyment increases. Activity level increases and a lot of confidence is seen in their actions.
- **Exaltation:** The degree of elation increases and a delusion of grandeur is experienced. As a consequence, the individual feels that they are capable of doing anything and solving all their problems.
- **Ecstasy:** Here, extreme elation of mood is seen. Blissfulness is also part and parcel of psychological status of the individual. A lot of enthusiasm in interpersonal interaction is seen. If someone prevents the individual from doing what they want to do, they become very irritable.

The person affected speaks loudly and speedily, teases others and tells jokes. A sudden change of subject and incoherent speech are seen. A minor environmental stimulus can change their activities and thoughts. Such an individual experiences hallucinations and delusions. Restlessness and excess activity are also essential features.

11.4.2. Depression

Depression is found more among women than in men. The risk of depression is 12 per cent among men and is approximately double among women. Approximately 5 per cent adolescents suffer from depression, and some of them also suffer from self-harming behaviour like suicide. A global estimate says that there are 350 million reported cases of depression in the world.

Deepika Padukone's interview regarding depression (2018) on YouTube may give a fair idea of the suffering of a patient having depression.

11.4.2.1. Signs and Symptoms of Depression

Such a patient is persistently sad, upset, apathetic and depressed. The individual is constantly involved in self-criticism and experiences generalized weakness. As a consequence, they are not interested in new experiences, spontaneous reactions or any excitement. Symptoms include depressed mood which interferes with daily routine activities and basic functions for more than 15 days. There is a sudden change in routine, like a loss of appetite. The person affected eats very little and experiences digestive problems. Agitated or slow movements are seen. Inability to sleep or insomnia, or excess sleep, low-energy level resulting in fatigue, irritability, inactivity and trouble with daily routine activities, sudden weight loss or weight gain and generalized pain are the prominent physiological symptoms.

Psychological symptoms include inability to concentrate on any activity or work or even entertainment like watching television, lack of interest in activities which are otherwise important for the individual and interactions with others, general inability to enjoy, feeling of worthlessness and guilt, indecisiveness, hopelessness and frustration. The individual may think of committing suicide and constantly think that their family will be better off without them.

As a consequence, social withdrawal, decreased productivity, poor interpersonal relations and anhedonia—which means no interest and no pleasure in any activity—becomes their way of life.

They feel that they are worthless. They perceive themselves to be inferior and inadequate. They feel helpless. They have no hopes for the future. Hence, these three conditions, namely hopelessness, helplessness and worthlessness, make their lives difficult. These effects are shown in Figure 11.1.

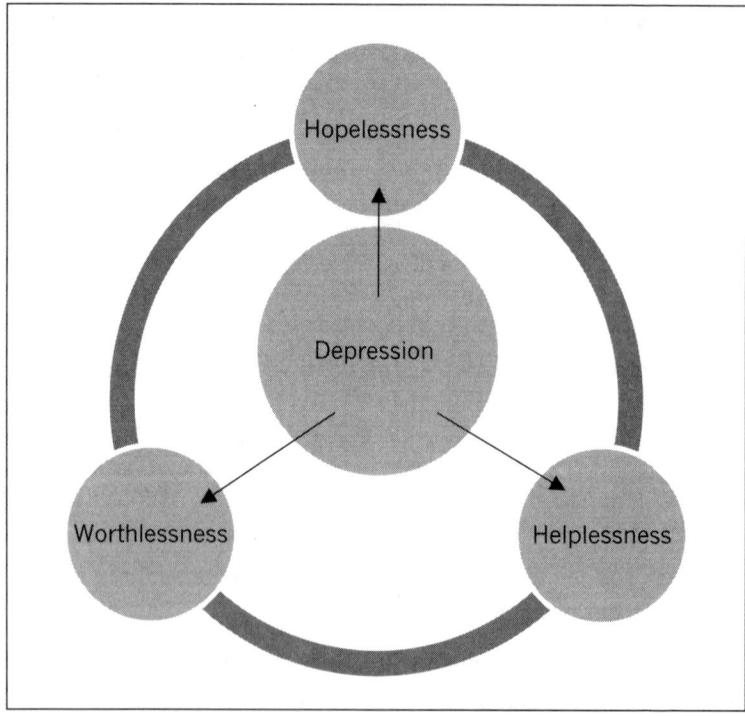

Figure 11.1 *Effects of Depression*

It generates poor self-worth, underestimating self and many other negative feelings. In some cases, the delusions are such that they enhance these depressive thoughts. They are regarding death, void of life or ideas that one's brain or body is ruined or has vanished.

The risk of suicide is higher during these phases.

11.4.3. Bipolar Mood Disorder

'Living with Bipolar Disorder' (Napiorkowska, 2019) is a short film depicting experiences, doubts and agony of a patient suffering from bipolar.

In bipolar disorder, severe mood swings from manic phase, where the individual has a lot of energy and vigour and extreme positive feelings, to depressive phase, where there is no vigour and energy and the individual faces problems due to apathy and negative thoughts, are common. In manic phase, there are extreme mood swings, continued activity without sleep, speedy speech, excessive overconfidence and casual risk taking.

There are other variations like in the case of bipolar type 2; the manic stage is comparatively less severe, which is called hypomanic stage. So in this stage, social and occupational functions are maintained.

These recurrent manic and depressive attacks come in any sequence, intensity and as a combination of both. Unipolar depression and persistent mood disorders are equally disturbing. These changes may take place rapidly or gradually. The affected individual may get some time between two episodes where their behaviour is approximately normal. Women experience rapid cycles of changing moods. Unipolar depression lasts longer than bipolar. Generally, manic episodes last for four months and depressive for six months. Chronic depression is comparatively less intense and is accompanied by personality disorders, hypochondriacal symptoms and the like. Disturbances in immune system are correlated with depression. Post-partum depression is a form of depression among women after delivery, and it adversely affects their lives in every sense.

11.4.3.1. Theories Regarding Mood Disorder

1. Biological theories include the following.
   - **Genetic basis of mood disorder:** Researchers have found that incidence is 25 per cent in first-degree relatives and 65 per cent monozygotic identical twins.
   - **Biochemical theories:** Many neurotransmitters are involved in mood disorder. Disturbances in dopamine, norepinephrine, serotonin, acetylcholine and GABA are related to it. Neuroendocrine system is also correlated to mood disorders. It includes hypothyroidism, Addison's disease and Cushing's disease.
   - **Abnormal brain imaging:** Changes in blood flow and metabolism in some areas of brain such as the prefrontal cortex and anterior cingulate, white matter hyper intensities and ventricular dilatation are reported.
2. Psycho-social theories include the following.
   - **Psychoanalytical theory:** explains it as fixation in oral sadistic phase, intense craving for self- love or narcissistic tendencies, mania is as reaction formation to depression.
   - **Distress:** Overwhelming stress in developmental period is capable of generating and enhancing symptoms of mood disorder.
   - **Cognitive theories:** Learned helplessness, anger directed towards self or anger in, negative and depressive cognition are significant correlates of mood disorders according to this theory.

11.4.3.2. Intervention

It is essential to give drug therapy. Along with it, psychological therapies should be made available.

Cognitive behaviour therapy, psychoanalytic therapy, behavioural therapy, interpersonal therapy and other therapies such as family therapy and group therapies are also effective.

11.4.3.3. Self-help for Sub-clinical Depression

Every day, some meaningful activities should be done for some time. Some activity in which the individual is interested and experiences enjoyment should be given priority. It should give a sense of achievement. It is also recommended that individuals should be involved in social activities for some time every day. It reduces negative self-talk. Encouraging self and giving rewards for even small achievements, using relaxation methods, emotional catharsis and discussing openly with someone who is supportive help.

It is worth remembering that recent research has demonstrated that young people who are inactive for substantial time of the day suffer from depression by the age of 18 (Indo Asian News Service, 2010).

11.5. ANXIETY DISORDERS

How many of us think that we are calm and focused while appearing for an interview?

Psychiatrists from Delhi, Bhatia and Goyal (2018), have stated that anxiety disorders range from 4 per cent to 20 per cent among children and adolescents. Girls experience more problems. As the age increases, anxiety increases in this age group in India.

Anxiety and depression among adolescents are common but overlooked by adults as general irritation. Intense, persistent and out of proportion anxiety is detrimental to cognitive functions and affects social interactions and emotional state. Approximately 10 per cent of adolescents are suffering from anxiety even in developed countries. Worry, which is the primary stage of anxiety, can be divided into two types—micro and macro. Micro worries focus on self and dear ones; it can be about losing a job or failure in examination. They are negatively correlated with mental health. Macro worry is about someone else or even the universe. They are related to positive well-being.

Anxiety is a very common disorder, where the apprehension is not in response to and in proportion of the actual external danger. It is related to the unknown and internal cause. In case of some individuals, there is a tendency to be anxious, in general, which is a trait of anxiety. The state of anxiety is feeling anxious at a particular moment. The signs are fatigue, palpitations, sweating, shortness of breath, muscle tension, hyper-vigilant reflexes, abdominal pain, back pain, shakiness, numbness, feeling of fear, dread and impaired sleep, concentration and sexual desire.

Sunita is a housewife who has to shoulder all the responsibilities, as her husband has been out of India for two years. Her daughter, Sara, is now four and goes to school. When Sara leaves for school, Sunita is worried about her. She keeps on thinking about the potential risks of sending Sara alone on the school bus, such as the possibility of an accident to the bus and sexual harassment by anyone on the bus or school and impatiently waits for her arrival. She experiences extreme uneasiness, palpitations, headaches and backaches and cannot even complete her routine activities.

Social anxiety leads to presentation anxiety, even avoiding social situation and, in extreme case, avoiding schools and college also.

Do you know?
Prevalence of anxiety disorder in India is reported to be 20.7 per cent (Reddy & Chandrashekhar 1998). More Indian women suffer from anxiety and depression and out of the patients of depression and anxiety, more women commit suicide. Every sixth victim of suicide in India is a housewife (Prasad, 2020).

Generalized anxiety leads to uncontrollable worry regarding various aspects of life. It results in the inability to follow conversation or complete a task, fear of daily activities such as crossing a bridge, social anxiety resulting in avoiding gatherings and get together, feeling awkward in a crowd and thinking that people are talking ill about them, looking at them for judging them.

Symptoms of anxiety disorder are basically of two types:

1. **Physical:** In physical symptoms, again, there are the following two types:
   a. **Autonomic and visceral symptoms:** Dry mouth, sweating, palpitation, hyperventilation, flushes, dyspnoea, dizziness, frequent micturition, diarrhoea, etc.
   b. **Motoric:** Restlessness, muscular twitches, tremors, facial expressions and side remarks indicating feeling of being afraid.
2. **Psychological:** These symptoms are cognitive, affective and of other types.

a. **Cognitive symptoms:** Hyperarousal and distractibility, lack of appropriate concentration, negative thinking, derealization and depersonalization.
b. **Affective symptoms:** Inability to relax, feeling of apprehension, fearfulness, irritability and cursing one's luck.
c. **Other symptoms:** Sleeplessness, startled reaction and exaggerated sensitivity to auditory stimuli or noise.

Anxiety disorder has two variations. One is generalized anxiety disorder and the other is panic disorder. Generalized anxiety disorder is chronic anxiety. This type of anxiety is part and parcel of many other disorders. By and large, anxiety is more prevalent in the early 30s.

Panic disorder is characterized by panic attacks where an individual experiences intense fear of death. There are physiological symptoms such as very rapid heart rate, dizziness, cold or hot flushes, chest pain and extreme uneasiness. There may or may not be any precipitating factor. Sometimes, it resembles phobic reaction.

There are different theories regarding anxiety disorder. Genetic theory is based on the fact that anxiety disorder is generally seen among 20 per cent of relatives of the patient. In case of identical twins, the probability that both of them will suffer is 80 per cent. Biochemical theories focus on imbalance in neurotransmitters like GABA, which may result in anxiety disorder. The imbalance of other neurotransmitters such as serotonin, dopamine and norepinephrine may also cause anxiety disorder. Chemically induced anxiety results from inhaling 5 per cent carbon dioxide and some chemicals like caffeine; sodium lactate may increase the possibility of panic disorder.

Extreme air pollution like that in Delhi may develop anxiety symptoms in larger public without any other causative factor.

Neuroanatomical theories explain that some areas of brain such as prefrontal cortex, limbic system and some other areas are sometimes affected as regional cerebral blood flow becomes abnormal. This produces anxiety. Organic anxiety disorder shows correlation of anxiety and hyperthyroidism, coronary heart disease or similar conditions.

11.5.1. Treatment

11.5.1.1. Psychotherapy

Supportive psychotherapy is used with drugs as per requirement. Cognitive behaviour therapy is generally used for panic disorder and generalized anxiety. Relaxation techniques are commonly used for managing anxiety, for example, muscle relaxation and breathing exercise. Biofeedback is also used to control the symptoms as the individual gets direct feedback of their own bodily functions.

11.5.2. Phobia

Phobia is an intense irrational fear of an object, activity or situation, which results in avoiding that situation and various limitations in human life. The fear is overwhelmingly disturbing and is not proportionate to the actual danger. The individual also understands that such extreme fear reaction is not justified. However, they cannot control the reaction. They are always preoccupied by the thoughts of that stimulus and finds out various ways to avoid the situation. There are clear gender differences in phobia. More girls and women are affected by phobia than boys and men. It mostly develops around the age of 17–32 years. Suddenly, the patient develops phobia without any obvious reason. It increases gradually, and as it grows, the restrictions in patient's life increase. In case of some patients, ups and downs are also seen.

'The Top 7 Most Common Phobias' a short film on you tube (Psych2Go, 2020) gives scientific information of common phobias.

There are various types of phobias which are hampering human life in different ways.

Some common forms of phobia are as follows.

1. **Agoraphobia:** It is the irrational fear of being away from familiar setting. This may include crowded places, open places or places from where it is difficult to escape and, sometimes, any public place. There are youth who are compelled to leave their

job also because of this. The patient thinks that they will not be able to get any help if they experience any sudden serious symptoms due to which they may feel helpless. Actually, these are panic reactions. In severe cases, the individual perceives the whole world as being risky and never wants to leave their residence. For 24 hours, the person prefers to be at home and, irrespective of their knowledge, wish to work and need, is not capable of working or interacting with the world directly. They avoid regular educational routine, job, social functions, daily responsibilities outside home and so on.

There are two types of agoraphobia, one is with panic reaction and the other is without it.

2. **Social phobia:** In this case, the irrational fear is concentrated on all social interactions: public speaking, group interactions, public performance, talking to unknown people, talking to authority figures, even eating in a group or using public washroom.

3. **Phobia regarding objects or situation:** Here, the individual experiences panic attack as a particular object or situation generates extreme anticipatory anxiety. This results in distress and avoidance situation. Some common types are as follows.

   • **Claustrophobia:** This indicates fear of closed places. The patient becomes restless and feels very uncomfortable in closed places such as lifts, theatre and other closed places.

   Savita was suffering from severe headache for more than eight months. Finally, the doctors advised that she should get MRI of head done. As she was having severe anxiety of closed places, she was reluctant to do that. She was afraid of the machine that requires her to be inside completely closed, very compact environment for at least half an hour. The family members, however, compelled her to go for that. When she was inside the machine she started screaming loudly. Before she was set free, she became unconscious.

   • **Acrophobia or fear of high places:** If a student gets a hostel room on 7th floor and they cannot even think of going to 7th floor, they have to miss the opportunity to stay there and it may lead to many problems. These individuals feel giddiness and cannot stand the perception of reduced size of articles down on the earth. There are feelings of being very much frightened and threatened.

- **Algophobia:** It is an irrational fear about pain. Most of the normal individuals also intermittently have to face pain. However, those who have algophobia cannot tolerate pain and are scared that they will have to tolerate pain if they have to undergo any surgery or any other similar treatment, even taking an injection. This may affect their health adversely.

  Think of an individual who is injured due to some sharp rusted object and is reluctant to take tetanus injection. What will be the impact on their health?

- **Zoophobia:** It is the fear of animals. There are individuals who are afraid of animals who may be harmful and also of those who are harmless. Abida is afraid of even a small kitten and gets upset if it is around.

  The individual is so much frightened that he or she is not capable of staying back in the room or premises where these animals are present.

- **Xenophobia:** This is fear of strangers. The individual avoids interacting with strangers in any case. This is a major restriction in their life.

  Recently, researchers have given a variety of more phobias. The basic problem is same—debilitating fear. There are phobias even of dirt and germs.

  There are many celebrities who are suffering from different types of phobias (Smoky Evening, 2019). Alia Bhatt is afraid of darkness; Deepika Padukone has a phobia of snakes; Shah Rukh Khan cannot tolerate horses and Ranbir Kapoor is afraid of cockroaches and spiders.

There are different theories of phobia, which are as follows:

1. **Behavioural theories:** These are based on the basic principle of classical conditioning. The first response of fear is related to some dangerous stimulus. That reaction is associated to some other neutral stimulus. After that, the neutral stimulus is enough to generate extreme fear.

   Well-known psychologist Watson has demonstrated this approximately 100 years ago. An 11-month old child Albert was previously very comfortable with all sorts of white objects. Then, a loud noise was paired with white stimulation several times. Soon, Albert started developing fear and avoiding white stimuli.

Guddi is 4-years old and has zoophobia. She starts screaming loudly as soon as she comes across a cockroach. Actually, it is not so harmful and scary. Once when she was playing in kitchen, her mother suddenly started screaming and running in dreadful scared condition. Then she realized that her mother was scared of a cockroach. Her mother, who is just 24, cannot even understand the consequences of her action.

This principle of conditioning is very useful to plan effective treatment for phobia. They are flooding, exposure and response prevention, systematic desensitization and realization.

2. **Psychodynamic theories:** Anxiety is generally managed by repression. The individual wants to forget about it and avoids the situation so that they can live peacefully.

   Traumatic experiences in childhood affect the psychological state and brain in such a way that the individual becomes vulnerable to anxiety. This theory explains agoraphobia and connects it with separation anxiety in childhood. Sometimes, loss of parents in childhood is directly linked to it. Displacement takes place as the individual associates the fear to some neutral stimulus. This neutral stimulus is selected in such a way that it can be avoided easily in daily activities.

3. **Biological theories:** These theories assume that the biological factors that are responsible for panic disorder may be related to some phobias causing panic disorder.

The patients having phobia become comfortable after avoiding the scary stimulus—either object or environment. With all the limitations, they feel no anxiety. However, it may also affect the life of others like the family members, if the individual is dependent on them for several activities. The patient will continue to rely on others for years if not treated.

Systematic desensitization is useful for phobias. Gradual exposure of the fearful object and associating it with some pleasant thing or experience works very well. Conditioning principles are very effective and systematic desensitization depends on conditioning principles.

This technique developed by Wolpe in 1961 is the most useful behavioural therapy for all age groups including young children. This is based on counterconditioning. Understanding perceived anxiety–stimulus hierarchy is essentially the first stage. What is the environmental stimulus provoking anxiety with reference to intensity of anxiety is studied, for example, if an individual has a phobia of cockroaches, hierarchy may be rating about various experiences regarding cockroach. Systematic pairing of some pleasant stimulus with fear-producing stimulus is to be done. Ice cream, pleasing and relaxing music, praise or any other reward should be associated with the stimulus. Increasing hierarchy of fear should be dealt with by gradually increasing the pleasant experiences. The exact procedure depends on age, gender, actual intensity of the problem, etc. The individual can face the situation without any fear after some trials. Relaxation, cognitive reappraisal and counterconditioning are the stages involved. Even test anxiety also can be treated with this technique.

Drug therapy is essential, depending on the intensity of the problem. Psychotherapy helps a lot like cognitive behaviour therapy.

11.5.3. Obsessive–compulsive Disorder

It is reported by researchers that 2–3 per cent of the general population is affected by obsessive–compulsive disorder. It is seen that obsessive–compulsive disorder is more in unmarried male members in India. Especially those who are from high socio-economic strata and are intelligent suffer more. Depression is significantly related to it.

There are three types in it: obsessive thoughts, compulsive acts and both obsessive thoughts and compulsive acts.

Obsessive–compulsive disorder is characterized by the following symptoms:

- Repetitive and intrusive thoughts, images or impulses which are irrational and illogical. It is also recognized as being absurd and the individual tries to resist it. As they cannot, this leads to severe distress.

- Compulsive behaviour is repetitive behaviour to deal with repetitive thoughts. Typical behaviour such as washing hands for more than 30 times a day, checking whether the door is locked again and again, spending hours in it, bathing again and again or solve problems repeatedly to ensure accuracy.

Due to overwhelming obsessions and compulsion, these individuals suffer from slowness in their daily activities. There is no overt expression of anxiety.

There are many very interesting short films depicting the impact of obsessive–compulsive disorder on an individual's life. Some are: 'Living with OCD', (Napiorkowska, 2016) and 'Recognizing OCD' (Health, 2017). It is discussed in detail that obsessive–compulsive disorder can be recognized by six years.

Many celebrities in India suffer from different types of obsessive–compulsive disorder. Many film stars are reported to be suffering from obsessive–compulsive disorder. Still, they are very successful and leading a happy life.

11.5.3.1. Theories Regarding Obsessive–compulsive Disorder

There are three major types of theories. Biological theories explain brain pathology and problems related to this disorder such as basal ganglia lesion, specific encephalitis, hypothalamic and third ventricle lesions. Contribution of genetic factors is also highlighted in these theories. Psychodynamic theories explain that obsessive–compulsive disorder is related to childhood disturbances leading to fixation, overuse of specific ego defence mechanisms such as reaction formation, regression to anal–sadistic phase, displacement and undoing, which is associated to isolation of affect. This, in turn, is responsible for linking fear to neutral stimuli. Behavioural theories explain obsession as a product of conditioning and compulsion as a learned behaviour. These ideas are useful for treatment.

There are some measures of obsessive–compulsive disorder. Experts have included different forms of obsession such as sexual, perfectionistic, contamination-related cleaning and the like. The compulsions evaluated are washing, cleaning, checking, counting, repeating, compulsive hoarding and the like.

Psychotherapy, behavioural therapy and cognitive behaviour therapy are commonly used. Behaviour modification techniques are very effective. Systematic desensitization, response prevention, modelling and thought stopping also work well. Drug treatment is given as per the requirement.

11.5.3.2. Trauma and Stressor-related Disorder: Post-traumatic Stress Disorder

Post-traumatic stress disorder is also a type of manifestation of anxiety. It is a response to life-threatening catastrophic life experiences. It is delayed and repeated response. It is, generally, seen in case of rape, severe abuse, natural disaster, traumatic accident and so on. Sometimes, even witnessing the event may result in such a disorder. The impact is so severe that symptoms may develop after some time. It is re-experiencing the event in terms of flashback memories, thoughts, perceptions and images. Even dreams may precipitate the symptoms. Partial amnesia and emotional numbness are some symptoms which are obvious. Anger, despair, difficulty in concentration and emotional numbness are common. A condition called anhedonia results, which means that the individual cannot experience pleasure in any activity. This leads to apathy and enhances negative thoughts and depressive mood.

Panic disorder includes physiological symptoms, as if some calamity is going to take place. It results in debilitating fear with shaking, sweating and palpitations. In recent research, it is seen that if the group morale is strong in a situation like combat-related stress and an individual is committed to a job, post-traumatic stress symptoms are less common and less severe. Even after a traumatic experience, if an individual is placed in a supportive and socially conducive environment, symptoms may be less severe. It is worth considering that the whole society supports if a soldier suffers and shows sympathy, as they are related with a noble cause. This advantage is completely missing in case of a rape victim, though the victim is not to be blamed. This directly increases the symptoms and sufferings.

Intervention includes psychotherapy and drug therapy as per requirement.

11.6. DISSOCIATIVE DISORDERS

It may be associated to any mental disorder or even malingering. Malingering is pretending that one is sick. It is more prevalent among ladies. Behaviour of these patients is uncontrolled and impulsive. They may get involved in hypochondriasis or ideas that they are suffering from a serious disease and need urgent medical attention. They keep on collecting information about different diseases and going from one expert to another. Such patients have vague somatic symptoms. They are manipulative, and their personality is dramatic. Though they are involved in seductive behaviour, they suffer from psychosexual dysfunction. There are different types of dissociative disorder.

They are as follows.

1. **Conversion disorder:** Unbearable distress may cause conversion disorder. There is no physical abnormality associated with it. It affects motor or sensory functions.
   - **Sensory disorder with dissociative anaesthesia:** The patient may complain about loss of senses in specific area like till wrists and ankles. There are no physical evidences for that. These sensory disturbances are not consistent with any disease. Sometimes, vision and hearing are also affected in a specific way. Often, all the sense modalities are affected in the same manner. Combination of motor limitations and sensory limitations are also seen.
   - **Dissociative motor disorder:** Paralysis-like symptoms involving one limb, two or even four limbs are experienced by the patient. Tremors, unusual tone, disturbances in gait not withstanding any disease are seen. Symptoms may decrease when the patient thinks no one is observing them.
   - **Dissociative convulsions:** This is very commonly reported in India. It is a pseudo seizure. Partial loss of consciousness and some convulsive movements are seen. It is purposive and occurs in a safe place. Symptoms of epileptic seizure are

not seen such as urinary and faeces incontinence, injury and tongue bite. Speech and head movements are seen with partial awareness. Even electroencephalogram is normal. In communication, there are lapses, long pauses, gaps and discrete thoughts.

2. **Dissociative disorder:** Loss of identity, consciousness and memory disturbances are the major characteristics. Stress is followed by such problems. The condition may improve suddenly.

   • **Dissociative amnesia:** It is loss of memory regarding personal information and traumatic life events. There is no biological cause behind it. Adolescents and young adults suffer more due to dissociative amnesia. Incidence is more among girls and young ladies. There are four types of dissociative amnesia.

     o Memory loss about all the personal events in a specific period of stress.
     o Selective amnesia is the loss of some memories of specific events, while others are intact.
     o Continuous memory loss after some traumatic experience.
     o Inability to recall all personal events while experiencing overwhelming stress.

   • **Trance and possession disorder:** It is more common in India due to blind faith. A spirit is supposed to control an individual's personality, thought and behaviour. The individual is aware of that.

   Spirit possession is control of human behaviour and thoughts by gods, spirits, aliens or demons. It is seen all over the world in various communities and religions. Women suffer more due to it than men (Asia Calling, 2014; Wikipedia). 'Demonic possession on an Indian girl' depicts the actual interaction of the patient with the so-called god-man (Samachar Nama, 2017).

   • **Fugue:** The individual forgets one's identity, earlier life and adopts new identity. The individual is completely unaware of that.

   • **Multiple personality disorder or dissociative identity disorder:** Two personalities are present in an individual, and one of them operates at a time. They are different from each other, have completely different mental functions and behaviour patterns. The individual suddenly shifts from one to the other. Both of them are unaware of the existence of the other.

Such condition may be associated with depression, post-traumatic stress disorder, anxiety, self-harm, etc.

Rehan et al. (2018) have reported a case having seven personalities of a 55-year old drug addict lady. These variations include a seven-year old child and a male adult as well.

In 10 famous cases of dissociative identity disorder, Frater gives amazing cases of such condition having 46 personalities.[5]

There are some dissociative disorders which are rare and comparatively mild.

Biological theories explain this disorder in terms of abnormal functions of brain such as epilepsy, hidden diseases and problems in the cerebral cortex region. According to behavioural theories, dissociative responses are learned responses for avoiding overwhelming stress like war. Getting rid of that stress is the reinforcement which strengthens that response. Psychodynamic theory focuses on secondary defence mechanism to protect self from the anxiety generated by fixation at Oedipus complex.

11.6.1. Intervention

Along with drug therapy, behavioural therapy is also used. There is every possibility that the patient's behaviour is for attention seeking. Hence, if excess attention is given to them, the symptoms may increase. They should be treated as normal individuals. Aversion therapy may be effective to control the symptoms. Strong suggestions with some medicines and hypnosis become more useful. In psychotherapy, efforts to bring the conflict into the consciousness are done. Then, memories, thoughts and emotions can be changed. Supportive psychotherapy and psychoanalysis may be helpful.

---

[5] http://listverse.com

11.7. SOMATIC SYMPTOM DISORDER

Approximately 7 per cent adults suffer from this disorder.

The patient suffers from multiple physical complaints without any evidence—physical or biochemical. The person becomes extremely anxious about physical symptoms. Thinking, feeling and behaving, everything is about the symptoms, due to which daily activities are hampered. Here, the individual experiences physical symptoms due to psychological problems or emotional distress. Constant anxiety about somatic problem is seen. Sufferings are exaggerated and constantly emphasized. The individual spends a lot of money, time and energy for relief from symptoms, though no diagnostic test proves that there is anything wrong.

Two variations are seen in it.

1. **Somatization disorder:** Adolescents and young adults are affected by it. Women are more vulnerable than men. Vague somatic symptoms involving different organs are present without any disease at least for two years. The patient tries to consult different doctors.
2. **Hypochondriacal disorder:** The individual is afraid of having some serious disease on the basis of their own interpretation of some minor dysfunction which persists, though there is no evidence. This is not a delusion.

Problems like premenstrual syndrome among young ladies are very common.

In intervention, it is a must to accept that the complaints are true or real. The individual should be helped to understand the causes and their real relation with negative emotional experiences like stress. After some insight is generated, changes in routine activities and intermittently giving some rewards and pleasurable activities help. The most common therapy is cognitive behaviour therapy.

11.8. EATING DISORDERS

There are different types of eating disorders which are generally neglected. However, these disorders may become a serious problem.

1. **Anorexia nervosa:** Adolescents and young adults are more affected by this disorder. Onset is from 13 to 19 years. More females are affected. Their self-esteem is low. They have self-imposed dietary restrictions. At the same time, they are involved in a lot of exercise. Some patients vomit intentionally or take laxative. In spite of actual weight or body mass index, the individual is afraid of becoming obese. The individual's perception regarding his or her own body is distorted. The individuals are depressed and may have obsessive–compulsive disorder. The individual is underweight, though there is no disease. Gynaecological problems like amenorrhea, that is, lack of menstruation or delayed menstruation, are reported among females. These females hate being a female, have fear of pregnancy and their sexual adjustment is poor.

   It is really shocking to see the extremely thin individuals affected by anorexia as depicted in '5 Most Extreme Cases of Anorexia' (MindChop, 2015). Due to food deprivation, 10 per cent of the patients get killed. (CBS, 2007).

2. **Bulimia nervosa:** It occurs in adolescence or teenage.
   Half of the patients have bulimic episodes. When they are alone, they keep on eating even when they are not hungry. This is called binge eating. Then the person realizes what they have done and wants to get rid of it by self-induced vomiting, taking laxative and the like.
   Behaviour therapy is effective. The goal is to motivate the individual to maintain normal weight. Group therapy and family therapy enhances the effectiveness of intervention.

3. **Obesity:** Morbid obesity affects 5 per cent of the Indian population (Obesity in India, n.d.). Ahirwar et al. (2019) reported that in India, more than 135 million individuals are obese. The range is 11.8–36.3 per cent in different populations. More women are obese than men.
   Obesity may take place due to biochemical disturbances, drugs or other physiological reasons. However, it can result due to psychological causes also. It is a reaction to extreme distress. Extremely obese women, sometimes, have unpleasant experiences in the past such as child sexual abuse, parental neglect and emotional deprivation. As a compensation, they start eating more than required, basically junk food. It is similar to binge eating. Some of

them also aspire to be the most obese person or break some similar record. They keep on eating despite medical advice.

4. **Binge eating:** In binge eating, there is no control over eating, and the individual keeps on eating throughout the day. There is no proper time for lunch and dinner. The patient prefers to eat when he or she is alone, as they are ashamed of overeating. Here also, depression and guilt are reported to be the cause.

5. **Psychogenic vomiting:** Without any substantial physiological cause, the individual suffers from vomiting after or in the beginning of meals. There is no nausea which compels the patient to vomit, but he can control and suppress it. Though it is a chronic disease, there is hardly any weight loss.

6. **Kleine–Levin syndrome:** It is a rare condition, but basically youth are affected. Hypersomnia, hypersexuality and excess appetite or hyperphagia are the three symptoms. Hyperphagia is the condition where excess eating is related to an increased appetite. Only male members are affected in this syndrome. Delusion, hallucination, psychotic symptoms, bizarre behaviour, general confusion and social withdrawal are associated with it.

Hyperphagia can be easily misinterpreted as improvement in health and increased appetite as its indicator. It is essential to carefully distinguish between the two.

Stress management techniques and better coping strategies help.

11.9. SLEEP DISORDERS

There are two types of sleep disorders.

1. **Dyssomnia:** These are disturbances regarding quality, amount and time of sleep. It further is divided into insomnia, hypersomnia and disorders regarding sleep–wake schedule. Insomnia is difficulty in going to sleep and maintaining it. Some physical or mental illnesses, idiopathic insomnia, addictions or side effects of medicine are responsible for that. Watching television or smartphone for number of hours at night may also cause insomnia.

Hypersomnia results in sleep attacks, excessive sleep and excess time to awaken. The individual is confused and disoriented during that period. Similar causes are responsible for that. In addition, narcolepsy is reported to be associated with it. It affects individuals between 15 and 25 years of age. Due to narcolepsy, sleep disturbances in night-time and excess sleep during daytime occurs. There is a condition called sleep paralysis. During this rare condition, the person is unable to move their body just before or after sleep. Sleep apnoea is the condition in which the person cannot breathe properly for 10 seconds or so.

2. **Sleep–wake schedule disorders:** These are caused by jet lag, changing shifts of work and unusual sleep–wake cycle.

3. **Parasomnia:** Sleep walking or somnambulism is when the patient is involved in automatic walking during sleep or any other motor activity.

You may find this type of depiction of somnambulism in some popular Hindi movies like *Housefull* in 2010, in the song 'Papa Jag Jayega.'

Sleep terror is the condition where the individual wakes up screaming loudly during sleep, has tachycardia, sweating and hyperventilation. Sleep talking is also seen in some patients where they cannot remember it.

Other sleep disorders include some serious issues such as nocturnal angina, asthma, seizures, head banging and sleep paralysis. Drug therapy and psychotherapy are generally given.

11.10. SEXUAL DISORDERS

Sex-related health is the most neglected area, which is of immense importance in human life. Individual's physical, psychological and social, all sorts of life are affected due to it. Others also suffer due to it. Sexual disorders are classified under four categories.

1. **Sexual dysfunction disorder:** Without any organic problem, the individual suffers from it and cannot respond to sexual interactions in a normal way. There are sub-types of the present disorder.

a. **Sexual desire disorder:** There is a poor desire for sex and absence of fantasies. It is common among females. The causes may be fatigue, fear of pregnancy, marital disharmony and unpleasant past experiences.

b. **Sexual aversion disorder and lack of sexual enjoyment:** Sexual activities cause anxiety and negative emotions, in general. Most of the time, it is related to sexual abuse and history of molestation, especially in childhood. In India, the culture has taught a lot of taboos and bias about sex. That may generate guilt, shame and awkwardness about sex.

Lack of enjoyment in sex or sexual anhedonia is common among women. It can be linked to regular practice of marital rapes in many marriages.

2. **Sexual arousal disorder:** It includes erectile function disorder, impotence and psychological impotence. Both physiological and psychological factors are responsible for that. Genital pathology, neurological, endocrine and cardiovascular disorders are the basic causes. Psychological factors are anxiety, mood disorder, lack of knowledge, lack of privacy, poor interpersonal relations with the spouse, child marriage, sexual abuse in childhood and socially unaccepted ways of sexual interaction as premarital and extramarital sex may result in sexual arousal disorder.

3. **Orgasmic disorders:** Marital discord, endocrine problems and local surgery may enhance such problems.

There are some other problems such as sexual pain disorder and sexual problems due to medical conditions.

4. **Sexual preference disorder or paraphilias:** In this case, sexual pleasure is related to some object, child or person who is non-consenting. It may include suffering or humiliation of self or partner. There are ten different types in it.

- **Sexual sadism:** Without humiliating and harming the partner, such individual does not get the sense of sexual arousal. The actual act depends on severity from beating and tying to burning, raping and even killing the partner.
- **Sexual masochism:** An individual is not sexually aroused without experiencing humiliation, injury or suffering and expects

the partner to fulfil that expectation. Sometimes, both sadism and masochism are present simultaneously.

- **Fetishism:** By and large, it is seen in male members. The individual gets aroused by some object used by the opposite sex such as dresses, shoes and undergarments.
- **Fetishistic transvestism:** Only after wearing a women's dress, a male member is aroused sexually.
- **Exhibitionism:** Exposure of one's private parts to a stranger of opposite sex who gets a shock, as they may not expect it to happen. Male members are involved in it.
- **Voyeurism:** Again male members are affected by this disorder. The patient is interested in watching a female undressing or involved in sex, especially when she is completely unaware.
- **Frotteurism:** It is getting sexual pleasure by touching and rubbing against a person of the opposite sex when they are not expecting it and not interested in it.
- **Paedophilia:** Here, an adult gets sexual satisfaction by having sex with children.
- **Zoophilia:** Sexual activity with animals gives sexual satisfaction to the affected male.

There are some more forms where sexual arousal is achieved by even excreta and urine of the opposite sex.

Intervention for these disorders include psychoanalytic psychotherapy, behaviour therapy, hypnosis, group psychotherapy, dual-sex therapy/master and Johnson's relaxation technique.

11.11. PERSONALITY DISORDERS

Personality disorders affect about 10–13 per cent of the world's population. Hence, there are many individuals who can be easily identified as having these problems. Adolescence and early adulthood are the periods when these problems emerge.

If personality traits become abnormal, they may result in maladaptive behaviour and impairment in efficiency in social, occupational and personal life. However, in this type of disorder, the changes are ego syntonic, meaning the individual accepts them as being consistent with their whole personality and, hence, does not seek any help. There are three major types, and each one is divided into sub-types. The individual projects their own ideas on others and misinterprets their intentions in every minor act. It is associated with detached and neglected parenting.

1. First cluster is on schizophrenic continuum—odd and eccentric type. The three major sub-types are paranoid, schizoid and schizotypal.

   a. **Paranoid personality:** It is common in men. Important symptoms are:

      - Suspiciousness in interpreting others' actions in a negative way, being hostile and contemptuous
      - Serious doubts about infidelity of life partner, though there is no evidence about it

   A very well-known English movie *Sleeping with the Enemy* (1991) and nine remakes based on it in various languages like *Agni Sakshi* are the best depictions of this type of abnormal personality.

      - Excessive self-importance
      - Persistently involved in grudges as the patient cannot forget and forgive
      - Over-sensitivity to insults and setbacks
      - Excessive awareness of personal rights in combative way
      - Tendency to explain everything in a conspiratorial way

   b. **Schizoid personality:** This disorder is reported to be more common among male members. It has a direct link between cold and neglecting parenting experienced in childhood.

      The basic features of the individual's personality are emotional detachment and coldness, preference of being and working alone, lack of experience of pleasure and limited expression of emotions like anger or warmth. There is hardly any consideration of social norms, praise or criticism. These individuals have no close friends.

   c. **Schizotypal personality disorder:** The symptoms are social withdrawal, no interest in interacting with others, cold and aloof emotions, doubts others and vague thinking with odd speech patterns. These patients do not pay any heed to cultural norms; hence, their behaviour is eccentric and appearance is bizarre. More serious symptoms are transient delusions and hallucinations, obsession by sexual or aggressive thoughts and the most serious is depersonalization and derealization.

d. **Antisocial personality disorder:** Impulsive, inconsistent parenting, affected father, attention deficit and some physiological abnormalities are reported in these patients. It is more common among men. The impact decreases after late adulthood.

The basic symptoms are low frustration tolerance, aggression and violence in response to minor disagreements, no guilt and no impact of punishment. These individuals hurt others without concern, do not maintain relationships and blame others for disagreement with the society.

Four types antisocial personality disorders are given by experts: creative, aggressive, sexual and inadequate.

e. **Histrionic personality disorder:** It is more common among women. Acting out and dissociation are the basic ego defence mechanisms underlying. There is an intense dependency need.

They have over concern about appearance, attention seeking behaviour and attitude, exaggerated need for approval and excess expressions of emotions in a dramatic way. They are more suggestible, oriented to immediate gratification and show seductive behaviour and style. They have shallow and labile affect, ego-centric and manipulative behaviour. Mild exhibitionism is seen in some cases. They cannot maintain interpersonal relations

f. **Narcissistic personality:** This disorder was given by Freud. Delusion of grandeur and inflated self-importance are the most salient symptoms. More male members are affected by it. These patients have poor self-esteem, inferiority complex, with haughty and arrogant ways of interaction. They need constant praise, have fantasies of unlimited success and constantly exploit others.

Attention seeking ways of behaviour, lack of empathy for others, lack of interest in external world and a tendency to get depressed by minor events are associated with it. Inadequate parenting is the major cause behind it. Over-indulging parents, extreme pampering, unreliable parenting, excess praise, unempathetic mother, emptiness and worthlessness, neglect, abuse and trauma may be the deep-rooted causes.

g. **Anxious/avoidant personality disorder:** Here, the individual is extremely sensitive to critical evaluations and negative feedback. It leads to fear of rejection, criticism, disapproval, inferiority, feeling of inadequacy and belief that one's personality is not appealing. There is an excess need of physical security along with a constant tension and apprehension. They need assurance that one will be appreciated. They tend to avoid activities related to interpersonal interaction.

h. **Dependent personality disorder:** The individual does not have any confidence to make decisions about one's life. He or she is cognitively dependent on others. By and large, many Indian housewives are of this sort. Such individuals are submissive and have responsive behaviour pattern and 'I am not okay, you are okay' type of attitude.

They allow others to make decisions about one's life. They perceive themselves as being weak, helpless and incompetent. They think that they are unable to take care of self and feel helpless when alone. They have a fear of being abandoned.

i. **Emotionally unstable personality disorder:** There are two types of this disorder: impulsive and borderline. In impulsive type, lack of impulse control and emotional instability are reported. Outbursts of violence and threatening are common in response to criticism.

Borderline personality also carries emotional instability. Such individuals are confused about their self-image, aims and sexual preferences. There is a void in their life along with boredom and emptiness. They give unstable and changing transient emotional responses. Relationships are also unstable and intense. All these things result in suicide attempts. The inability to stay alone is seen.

There are some more types, like a perfectionist may have obsessive–compulsive personality disorder. Extreme involvement in rules, systems, rigidity stubbornness and expectation that others should follow their style are the major characteristics.

Passive aggressive personality disorder is seen when there is passive resistance to demands for proper performance and behaviour, and the individual pretends to be inefficient. They may pretend to forget things, postpone or delay things to achieve their goal.

11.11.1. Intervention

All these disorders are comparatively mild, and the individual is capable of leading approximately normal life. Most of the time, no help to improve their conditions is made available. Generally, individual and group therapies, family therapy, and if the intensity increases, drug therapy are used.

These are some major mental disorders. There are some other types, and the exact expression depends on physiological, biochemical and psycho-social conditions. Culture also plays an important role in it.

Neurotic disorders are comparatively less serious, and the individual otherwise leads a normal life.

For example, unexplained bodily pains and aches, fatigue, dizziness, headaches and sleeplessness are typically seen among educated housewives when they are dependent on someone they hate. Adjustment problems and stress reactions are also included in it.

Stress management training, supportive psychotherapy and crisis intervention are generally suggested.

Emotional catharsis, normal mourning according to social tradition, enhancing understanding that it is a part and parcel of life and others also suffer, help the individual. Positive thinking and positive memories are useful.

11.12. SUMMARY

The present chapter describes major psychological disorders briefly. There is hardly any awareness in India regarding many conditions, and no help is made available to the individual who is affected.

If the symptoms are comparatively mild, the patient may be taken to a clinical psychologist. If the symptoms are severe and it is difficult to lead a normal life with them, it is essential to take the patient to a psychiatrist.

Family members also need to understand that the individual is not misbehaving intentionally, but it is due to the disorder that they are compelled to act accordingly. Psychological support, empathy, endurance and unconditional acceptance are necessary for improving the patient's condition.

COVID-19 and Psycho-social Health

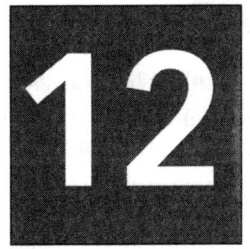

12.1. COVID-19: GENERAL THREAT, EXPOSURE AND INFECTION

Sonam is a single mother of a one-year old baby and is managing everything on her own. Her mother is hospitalized due to cancer treatment. However, since lockdown due to COVID-19, her routine has been disturbed, and she is worried about everything. The day care is shut down. When she leaves for her job, she has to depend on her maid to look after the baby. Is it safe to leave the baby with the maid? If she does not go to her job, she will lose her temporary job. Is it recommended to travel and work outside for the whole day? Who will look after her mother if she cannot visit the hospital? If she gets infected, who will look after the baby? How to manage if there is extra expenditure due to ill health?

Sometimes, there are unexpected threats to human life, communities or even nations. It may be an earthquake, flood or war. However, it is restricted to a particular area, state or nation. Recently, the whole world was stunned and frightened: young and old, males and females, all human beings on earth are shattered due to a pandemic. Devastating threats and fear of death are engrossing human life. It came as a sudden blow to everyone. Currently, COVID-19 is making human life difficult to cope with. It affects every sphere of life every moment, either directly or indirectly. India became the global epicentre of COVID in August 2020. Approximately, half of the Indian population is completely or partially vaccinated by August 2021. A new strain of coronavirus has already spread in 41 countries as of 6 January 2021 (*Maharashtra Times*, 2021). India was the second worst hit country in the world.[1] New mutations like Delta variant, Mu variant, C.1.2

[1] science.thewire.in

are breakthrough infections leading to greater transmission in spite of vaccination. (*The Economic Times*, 26 July 2021, bbc.com 23 June 2021). The total daily cases were 2.34 lakh in India.[2] Brazil had advised women to avoid pregnancy due to the risk of corona.[3]

> Globally on 25th August 2021 there have been 213,050,725 confirmed cases of COVID-19, and 4,448,352 deaths as reported by WHO.

Coronaviruses are a group of RNA viruses. It causes respiratory tract infections ranging from ordinary common colds to severe acute respiratory syndrome (SARS), Middle East respiratory syndrome or COVID-19 in human beings. The strong varieties may kill approximately 30 per cent of the infected individuals. It may cause pneumonia, bronchitis or SARS (Wikipedia). It affects important organs such as the kidney, the brain and the heart. Kidney failure, heart attack or stroke due to brain damage are reported in the cases of serious patients. Blood clots are formed which create hindrance regarding blood supply to these organs, and their functions are disrupted. Anticoagulants are not effective in treating these clots. The drug commonly given in the initial stages has side effects such as arrhythmia, heart problems and a negative impact on vision. Especially those patients who have other pre-existing health problems, like chronic diseases, suffer a lot. This type of comorbidity includes diabetes, hypertension, asthma, arthritis, epilepsy, any autoimmune disorder or cancer. In short, those who are continuously under treatment for a substantial duration have poor immunity and they cannot fight back. The death rate is higher in the case of such patients. WHO has stated that 40 per cent of COVID-19 transmissions may take place through asymptomatic people.[4] Hence, it is difficult to manage. The persons infected are also not aware of the fact that they are infected.

The lockdown was an experience that was unexpected and resulted in many problems: personal, economic, social, interpersonal, work-related and regarding maintaining routine. People from all age groups,

[2] www.ndtv.com

[3] news18.com 18 April

[4] https://www.livemint.com/ 9 June 2020

genders and different socio-economic status and different educational levels are suffering in the same way. Most people are staying back at home with their families. In the initial stages of lockdown, some individuals developed euphoria. They were enjoying the situation because there was no work, no routine studies, no exams and no stress. However, after a few days, they realized that it is extremely boring, there are a number of restrictions, one cannot go out, meet friends and there is no social support even in case of difficulty.

Some people are quarantined, that is, isolated due to the exposure of patients or journeys, which makes them vulnerable. Such potential patients are to stay in quarantine for 14 days. They are required to stay detached from their family and friends. There is a possibility that they might develop a corona infection. Hence, they are under constant stress. They are tested repeatedly. The arrangements for stay are, sometimes, compromising. There is nothing that they can do to engage their minds. They also face problems such as depression, boredom, anxiety and constant unbearable stress. When family members are quarantined or affected, there is unbearable stress.

Japan has appointed the first ever minister of loneliness to tackle the increasing suicide rate due to the pandemic on 19 February 2021.[5] In India also, due to financial problems during the lockdown and stress due to the threat of coronavirus, many suicides are reported. Students, nurses, small businessmen, unemployed youth and such other groups are more affected.

In AIIMS hospital, Nagpur, a lady COVID patient killed herself due to unbearable shock and extreme stress. She jumped from the fifth floor. She was 45-years old.[6] On 30 May 2020, a young man committed suicide in a quarantine centre in Chandrapur, Maharashtra; another young man, a suspected patient of coronavirus, committed suicide (PTI, 2020). A young lady committed suicide near Lucknow, as her husband could not return home from a foreign country due to COVID-19 (News18 Lokmat, 2020). In Kanpur, a young man, Mukesh, killed himself immediately after his wife died due to COVID-19 (2020). He has three children.

[5] www.businesstoday.in>story

[6] maharashtratimes.com

A number of patients being treated for COVID-19 in various hospitals and who are struggling hard for survival also committed suicide. There is a dreadful unavailability of beds, oxygen and ventilators. The idea that one will suffer dreadfully is so threatening that before the actual diagnosis also, individuals are extremely upset and frozen with fear. Although the recovery rate fluctuates (e.g., from 34% in May 2020 to 95% in March 2021), the intensity of suffering is traumatic, such as high fever and especially breathing difficulties. According to some experts, the corona will not vanish and may last 10 years.

12.2. EFFECTS ON VARIOUS SPHERES OF LIFE: LIMITATIONS AND DISAPPOINTMENTS DUE TO COVID-19

Educational institutes are oriented towards the all-sided development of students. It includes not only cognitive but also emotional, social, physical and ethical and all sorts of development of students. In India, 320 million students are affected educationally due to educational institutes being closed. Most schools are opting for online education. Very young children are also supposed to sit in front of computers for hours. However, only 23.8 per cent of Indian households have internet access. Even if it is available, like a smartphone, only male members use it. All the teachers from primary, secondary and higher education are not well-equipped with the training necessary for online teaching (Sahni, 2020). After one year, they are in a better position to deal with the situation.

In the case of online education, the basic issue is that of a complete lack of proximity and deprivation of spontaneous interaction. It affects the expression of emotions, support, enjoying each other's company and the development of social skills among young children. Sharing physical settings means a lot, which is missing completely in online education. It is a tedious job to constantly concentrate on some devices without any company. It is an artificial environment which may adversely affect the teaching–learning process. The government is thinking about cutting down the syllabus for next year. The basic question is how to give them the cognitive stimulation which is necessary for learning.

Many families have lost their livelihood and cannot provide any new facilities at present. Many students and employees are staying alone, though there is no work as they cannot travel during the lockdown. Those who are in the final year of their degree examinations and are aspiring to higher education are confused and worried. Every day, new decisions are being declared by different state governments, which are controversial. Even if examinations are conducted online, there are many compromises regarding practical experiments and the nature of examinations. Malpractices during online examinations are very common. An uncertain future makes the youth disoriented, aimless and there is a void in their lives. Some students were selected for placement and scholarships. Now, they are either withdrawn or postponed.

Among the major problems of youth during the lockdown, the loss of employment and economic crisis are especially important. During lockdown, most business organizations are closed completely. It affected, for example, hotels and restaurants, tourism, all sorts of travel—even air travel, saloons and beauty parlours, businesses regarding gold, diamond and similar ornaments, and even marriage-related businesses such as halls, decorations and the like. Ola, Uber, Swiggy, Zomato and even the clothing business, book sellers and many others have completely lost their business. No work, no income, family crisis, depression, frustration are the direct effects. Television and film artists and drama-related companies have stopped working. A very well-known company, Atlas Cycles, has given lay-off to all 1,000 employees in Sahibabad for an indefinite period of time in January 2020.[7] Even well-educated youth work as labourers. The loss of a job, salary cut and no other option to earn money make an individual awkward, dependent and helpless, which results in low self-esteem. Job and salary compromise, standstill business, hopelessness and breakdown of roles lead to confusion and sadness. Every pleasure is lost in various activities and a state like anhedonia prevails.

---

[7] https://www.zeebiz.com/

Manmeet Grewal and Preksha Mehta, 25-year-old TV actors, committed suicide due to unemployment and financial problems (*Maharashtra Times, 2020*).[8] The well-known Tamil actor Sridhar and his sister, who was also an actor, committed suicide due to lack of work and income in June 2020.[9]

In a single city like Pune, 68,000 employees are under constant threat that they might lose their jobs in the information technology sector.[10] Due to unemployment, lakhs of workers were trying to reach their hometown with their families even if they had to walk thousands of kilometres. Ladies and young children, pregnant women and patients suffered a lot. There are examples where, even after such a difficult journey, family members do not allow them to enter their home due to the fear of coronavirus.

There is hardly any support that one gets, even from the family. The meaning of relationships and family are changing. There are dead bodies lying in the hospital, and family members are not even showing up to sign the form to submit the body for disposal.

In Aurangabad, Maharashtra, a man who was corona negative died due to other problems. However, his son denied shouldering the responsibility of the last rituals and requested the health administration to take care of it (*Maharashtra Times, 2020*). Even if a person dies on the road, nobody helps to shift the dead body. There are examples where dead bodies are thrown into garbage trucks or just thrown on the roadside. The Supreme Court has remarked that COVID-19 patients and their dead bodies are treated worse than animals (*Hindustan Times, 2020*).

Doctors, nurses, other paramedical staff and ward boys are directly exposed to the patients. Many of them are infected and some have lost their lives. Burnout in healthcare workers is common. Policemen and women are trying to maintain discipline and find hidden patients. They are also experiencing a lot of stress. A number of policemen suffered. In December 2020, it was reported that 28,500 police were

[8] https://www.news18.com/

[9] india.com

[10] https://www.saamtv.com/

infected and 312 lost their lives. They cannot take care of their own families. Even mothers cannot meet their young children. Till May end in Maharashtra, 21 policemen lost their lives and 1,964 were infected (*Maharashtra Times*, 2020)

Till 6 May, 548 doctors, nurses and paramedical staff members were infected in India (*Hindustan Times*, 2020).

12.3. IMPACT ON PSYCHO-SOCIAL HEALTH

It is essential to understand that there are some positive effects of the lockdown also. On an environmental level, pollution has been reduced to a large extent. Industries are shutting down and vehicles are standing still. Water, air and noise pollution are at a minimum, and there are better results regarding even the ozone layer. A calm, clear and healthy atmosphere exists as never before.

Shekhar stays in London with his wife, who is expecting. Due to the lockdown, their parents or even friends staying in other localities in London expressed their inability to be with them and help them, even for a while. Shekhar never knew how to cook or take care of an infant. Now, every day he is trying to learn different recipes and enjoy them. They are taking online training programmes regarding how to take care of an infant from the first day. The bond between the two is becoming strong, and they are feeling ready to face the challenges.

There are many new things that one has to learn. Now, new software, such as Zoom, Google Meet, Microsoft Teams, Cisco, Webex and GoToMeeting, are being used for online lectures and attending webinars. Not only students but teachers are also learning new skills in online presentations, making voice PowerPoint presentations, using Google Classroom and so on. There are new challenges in every field. There is a lot of creativity that is required. Let us take an example from the hotel industry. Now, there is an approximately 80 per cent loss. Some hotels located in remote places known for sightseeing are combining both quarantine and sightseeing with due care taken. This way, their business is flourishing. Organizations working for needy ladies are stitching masks on a large scale and surviving.

Marriages are being celebrated with a minimum of people around and minimum of expenditure. A young lady travelled some 24 kilometres alone, driving a two-wheeler, to her in-law's place where she got married without the presence of her parents and other relatives. Recently, in Utter Pradesh, a man travelled 100 kilometres alone on his bicycle to marry and brought his wife a double seat while coming back (*Hindu*, 2020). It may lead to some long-awaited changes in social attitudes and traditions.

As many things are not available on the market, everyone has to compromise and wait for some more time. As a consequence, every child, adolescent and even young person is required to learn delay of gratification. This may make them more mature and ready for future challenges. Everyone is getting lots of time to interact with and understand their own family members and help them in this demanding situation to maintain good psycho-social health. A young man may get time to emotionally support and serve his old parents, understand the problems of his siblings and enhance trust and compassion in their minds. Nurturing hobbies, contacting extended family members, learning new things regarding house maintenance, learning and helping others to learn essential skills, like net banking, are meaningful and fruitful activities. Preparing for the next entrance examination, getting information regarding educational institutes in and out of India and finding out various options for career opportunities are useful for further planning. Students are getting enough time for all these. They can share their thoughts and ideas with their parents and seek their advice, as everyone is at home.

> Meeta is a postgraduate student, and next year she has to conduct some research. She has been thinking of reading research methods, statistics and learning software for statistical analysis, like Statistical Package for the Social Sciences. Now, due to the lockdown, she could achieve some of these goals.

> Salil has been suffering from diabetes for the last two years. He is just 24 and finds it difficult to control his sugar levels due to long hours in the office, travelling and binge eating. After the lockdown, he has been working from home and eating homemade food as per the expected schedule. It is boring for him; however, eating out is impossible. Within two months, his sugar levels dropped, and he had to reduce the daily dose.

However, there are more negative effects as everyone is tense and stressed. There is a lot of cognitive dissonance that is experienced due to complete change in thinking and behavioural patterns. All the social norms, ways of interaction and manners to express emotions have completely changed. Social distancing is advisable even at home, eating is restricted, going out is banned and so on.

There are different effects on a personal level. Some very common are boredom, restricted routine activities, difficulties controlling anger, loss of self-control, lack of empathy and coping problems. A sense of helplessness and hopelessness emerge due to suffocating uncertainty regarding one's own health status and that of loved ones. Every now and then, one has to be very alert and cautious. Although an individual is healthy, there is no guarantee that they will be healthy the next morning. Money, status, education—nothing is useful to save the individual from infection, unless they take proper care of themselves. As a consequence, money, authority and achievements all become worthless. For example, during the lockdown, one may or may not get a particular commodity or even grocery, though they are very rich. Even getting admission or treatment in a hospital becomes difficult due to overcrowding. Those who have some disability or comorbidity are especially worried. Some of them are developing phobia-like symptoms and panic, as they keep on thinking that if they face any problem, they may not get any vehicle and may not even get admission to any hospital.

A 35-year-old doctor working in the COVID ward, Max Hospital, Delhi, committed suicide on 2 May 2021.[11] A doctor from Kasturba hospital, also, admits that he suffers from panic experiences and his family members are constantly under tension (Curly Tales, 2020).

A very well-known music director Wajid Khan was just 42 when he died due to the corona infection. He had many other health problems, but still, he was very active and creative until that infection.[12]

As a consequence, it becomes difficult to maintain an internal locus of control. It results in the idea that one cannot control their own life, and that their health, sufferings and life expectancy do not depend on their own behaviour.

---

[11] India.com

[12] maharashtratimes.com

Realization that the whole mankind is vulnerable and cannot control such a pandemic may completely change values, faith and priorities. It may lead to a lack of structure and purpose in life. Self-worth, self-efficacy and identity may become distorted. Constant stress and unpredictability may lead to amotivation and apathy. For example, if a student does not know when the final examination will be conducted, they may stop studying and lose interest in academic work. As a consequence, an individual may experience a void in their life.

In particular, adolescents and young adults, generally, spend a lot of time with their friends, celebrating various things and enjoying different outdoor activities. Due to the pandemic, their routine is completely distorted. Panic for a specific type of food is also very common. During lockdown, there are no malls, no online purchases, no pubs, no parties, no contact with friends and girlfriends or boyfriends, which leads to a sense of isolation and disconnectedness. This leads to more boredom, aggression and conflicts between generations. As they are forced to stay at home, they are confused, irritated and lose their self-control. It is like a nightmare for them. Very young children and the elderly can be managed in a better way. In particular, those who have some addiction and depend on some substances or alcohol face problems like withdrawal symptoms due to non-availability of them. Their self-control diminishes and extreme emotional difficulties like nervous breakdown are seen. Some of them may even get involved in redundant activities, resulting in dropout from college or absconding from work. They are not available to work from home. Some organizations depend on very few employees, and they are supposed to carry out all the work. As a consequence, they feel burned out and being exploited.

Everyone has a lot of stress, and anyone may experience physical symptoms such as headaches, sleeping and eating problems, apathy, low motivation, more abuse of alcohol and drugs, a break in religious practices, fear, sadness and anger.

As both of her offspring are abroad, Swati is extremely worried about them. She cannot get proper sleep and for the whole night keeps on thinking about the risk they have. She wanted them to leave their jobs and return to India immediately. However, that is impossible due to the non-availability of flights. She gets nervous, anxious and, for hours, negative thoughts engross her mind. She cannot even fulfil her regular responsibilities.

Mental health and wellness are badly affected by worries, anxieties and fear regarding the infection. For example, one has to wash their hands again and again for the whole day. Generally, it is not done by normal, healthy individuals. However, if an individual is suffering from obsessive–compulsive disorder, they will do the same activity like washing their hands many times without any reason. This awareness may lead to a weird feeling. During the last few months, cases of obsessive–compulsive disorders have been increasing. Some young people may have fake confidence that nothing will happen to them and they are strong enough to save themselves. This is called defensive optimism. Let us take an example of the duration for which one has to wash one's hands, that is, at least 20 seconds. Very few individuals strictly follow this. It is worth noting that such individuals try to justify their behaviour and link unscientific and illogical reasons for it. A mask is essential for protecting an individual from corona. However, some of them are reluctant to wear it. In particular, more male members think that it is a sign of femininity and weakness (*Psychology Today*, 2020). It was found in the United Kingdom based survey that women are more compliant with preventive behaviour. Men find wearing masks shameful, not cool and a sign of weakness (US Survey, 2020).

After the lockdown was terminated, people were completely relaxed and were not taking due care of their health. There are crowds of young individuals on the playgrounds, people in the market and on the road without masks and social distancing. Marriages and funerals are taking place as usual, where many people attend it, as if everything were alright. As a consequence, the number of new patients is increasing tremendously every minute. Festivals, like Ganesh festival in Maharashtra, result in a lot of social interaction with extended families, friends and others even, when no public celebration is allowed.

Some individuals may store medicines unnecessarily. It is also seen that some may get involved in self-medication, which may prove harmful. Continuously watching the news from different sources may increase anxiety and panic. Most reliable news should be watched once or twice. Not only the global but local scenarios also should be known. Some channels may give half-truths about, say, how to protect ourselves from COVID with the help of medicine or their product. If such advertisements are capable of convincing an individual, they may take some unnecessary tonic or medicine without knowing its effects and ill effects. A man was staying at an airport for three months due to the threat of corona (*Maharashtra Times*, 2021).

Worry is associated with apprehension and anxiety. Uncontrollable worry is thinking about a catastrophe. It leads to restlessness, muscle tension, fatigue, difficulty sleeping and concentrating. It is generated because of unexpected, novel, ambiguous and unpredictable issues. Excessive worry generates a feeling of being demoralized, upset or exhausted. It can be related to factual or hypothetical issues. It leads to feeling exhausted.

In a patient guide regarding post-traumatic stress disorder by 'Psychology Tools', the problems of patients who were treated in ICU are considered (Psychology Tools, 2020). The very common experiences of such patients are fatigue, physical weakness, hoarse voice, breathlessness, numbness, change in appearance and poor cognitive processes. It is a traumatic experience to be admitted to the hospital. One feels intense hopelessness and helplessness. Treatment is invasive and painful. Nobody from the medical staff knows the patient; life support machinery gives a constant reminder of fear of death. Delirium, hallucinations and physical discomfort are common. Staff wearing personal protection equipment and masks cannot communicate non-verbally. Other patients may be more serious or may die. An individual is confused, afraid, upset, uneasy and anxious. After getting normal reports, an individual takes time to settle down again. Some patients may develop post-traumatic stress disorder. Approximately 20 per cent of intensive care patients develop post-traumatic stress disorder.

It is reported that during 2020, missing complaints increased substantially in Thane, Mumbai. A total of 1,364 male members and 1,870 women are missing (TV9 Marathi, 2021).

Those who have lost their dear ones suffer a lot and think that they were not capable of serving the patient during their suffering and last days. The patients are left alone since the moment they are suspected of having COVID-19. No one can control anything as to which hospital they will be admitted, when and after how much time, beds will be available, what medicines will be given and as if they suffer from respiratory problems, whether a ventilator will be available and so on. In the case of the demise of the patient, the family and friends cannot even get an opportunity to be at the bedside and pray. It is as if an individual disappears suddenly for ever. In addition, they have to stay at a quarantine centre and adjust to an unknown environment and an uncertain future with extreme fear and anxiety.

Fifteen epidemiological studies about psychiatric illnesses showed that depression, anxiety and such other psychological disorders increased substantially (Ganguli, 2000). WHO has also published similar results in 'Facing Mental Health Fallout from the Coronavirus Pandemic' in May 2020. Stress creates immunodepression and vasospasm among corona patients.

According to News18, from March to August 2020, a total of 43 per cent of people were depressed. It is reported that 20 per cent increase in mental illness is seen among the general public due to COVID. The quality of life is affected substantially. Psychosomatic problems are increasing. Rechecking the past, repeatedly remembering the lost pleasures, guilt and worries about work are very common. Obsessive–compulsive disorder and even hallucinations are reported by some individuals. Prejudice and discrimination, lack of motivation, low energy, apathy and collective trauma are seen very often. By and large, almost everyone suffers at least for some time due to extreme negative thoughts and distorted ideas. Death anxiety is, generally, experienced by old individuals, but during this pandemic, some young individuals may also face that problem. Even separation anxiety may result from constant worry about the health of dear ones. Serious mental health problems such as psychosis, depression, panic, insomnia, somatoform disorders and apprehension are possible consequences. Those who are or were infected or even isolated as a precautionary measure undergo devastating traumatic experiences. Intense death anxiety, pain, physiological and psychological struggle, complete lack of family support, new place, different food, all patients around and continuous negative thinking about the test result in problems such as nightmares, cognitive disturbances, insomnia, lack of appetite, anhedonia and unbearable anxiety. An individual cannot maintain calm and, due to it also, the ailment may increase. Suicidal thoughts are also common due to all these disturbances. Anxiety and depression resulting from corona are found in 28 per cent of the general population (Rajkumar, 2020). Experts have given alarming predictions that, due to economic crises and the deaths of dear ones, confusion and intense despair and the incidence of suicide are going to increase at a galloping rate even after the pandemic is over.

Many patients are committing suicide. Those who are addicted may not get alcohol and suffer from delirium tremens, which is fatal if not treated within time. Suicide rate increases in addicts. COVID-19 is resulting in more still births.

It is reported that in Pune, every day two people commit suicide. Within 14 days, 28 suicides were reported. Depression, anxiety of the future calamity, break-up of relationships and discord in the family are the basic reasons. Most of them are young, 3 are below 20 years of age. Among the total suicides, males are more than females. Males are 79 per cent and females are 21 per cent.[13]

The only easily available pastime activity is gadgets such as smartphones, personal computers, televisions and the like. Ludo, Subway Surfers, Candy Crush Saga and PUBG are played extensively by youth. There is a substantial increase in the consumption of pornography (CBS News, 2020). Male members are more involved in sex and domestic violence. The National Commission for Women has recorded a two-fold rise in complaints of domestic violence in India. Even WHO has reported that there is an increase of 60 per cent in emergency calls by women facing violence from their partners (*Hindu*, 2020).

Demand for child porn increased during lockdown (*New Indian Express*, 2020). It is reported that Chennai has the highest demand. Searches such as 'child porn', 'sexy child', 'teen sex videos' and data from Porn Hub show that traffic from India has increased by 95 per

[13] esakal.com

cent due to lockdown. There has been a 200 per cent increase in demand for violent content like 'torturing children' or 'children bleeding' or 'being harassed' and 'choking'. This indicates that children are at risk during lockdown. According to NBC news, 23 April 2020, child sexual abuse images and online exploitation also increased during the lockdown. In addition to special sites, YouTube, Instagram, Twitter and Facebook are also used for that. At the same time, the Childline India helpline stated that it received more than 92,000 calls asking for protection only in 11 days during the lockdown. Similar situations are reported globally.

Here again, it is worth considering that there are gender-specific problems. Crime against women, in and out of family, has increased substantially. It includes family violence, sexual harassment, online sexual advances, marital rape and rapes in the family. In India, the highest incidences are reported in Uttar Pradesh, Bihar, Punjab and Haryana. The men are at home and frustrated. They do not want to share household jobs and want to vent their frustration. The victims could leave their house and no one else could come to their rescue. Hence, the victims are afraid of complaining, as it may increase the possibility of more intense abuse. Women who are working from home have to manage household jobs, extra work due to the non-availability of domestic help, keep children meaningfully occupied and complete their jobs. It is difficult to manage without some help. It is reported that most of the male members are not ready to contribute anything and expect many things. Such women are overwhelmingly tired, frustrated, fed up and upset. This spoils their mental health. They are becoming impatient and cannot tolerate any discord. The idea of helping in household jobs is still not palatable to most men as it hurts their male ego.

In 15 days of the lockdown, Delhi has reported 21 rapes and 31 cases of molestation (Print, 2020).

On 24 July 2020, in a COVID centre, a 14-year-old girl was raped. Both the victim and rapist were corona patients.[14] A 65 per cent increase in the purchase of sex toys was recorded during lockdown.[15]

---

[14] maharashtra.com

[15] maharashtratimes.com

Non-governmental organizations warn that due to the lockdown, there is a possibility of lakhs of unwanted pregnancies, unsafe abortions and maternal deaths. The Foundation for Reproductive Health Services estimated that due to non-availability of contraceptives, 2.56 crore couples may not be able to use any. Till September 2020, a minimum of 23 lakh unwanted pregnancies must have occured. Such increased risk of sexual abuse, marital rape and unwanted pregnancies are also reported by researchers all over the world. The United Nations has estimated seven million unwanted pregnancies.[16]

In low socio-economic strata, alcohol addiction of male members is so common that, now, as they cannot get money and alcohol, they become extremely aggressive (Roy, 2020).

Social stigma not only affects the status of dead bodies but patients and their family members also. Due to COVID-19 infection, some private hospitals are denying admissions even to serious patients who are suffering from corona.

12.4. COPING WITH RESTRICTIONS, SUFFERINGS AND LOSS

Due to COVID-19, taking care of one's health and saving one's life, primarily, become the individual's own responsibility. Every single individual should contribute to the well-being of the community by religiously following health guidelines. Underestimating the risk and careless behaviour may result in serious health problems. It may affect not only the individual but the whole family or friends. Whosoever is in close contact with such individuals will be dragged to disaster.

There are many other less common symptoms of corona. It is essential to remember those also. They are sore throat, pains and aches, rash on skin, discoloration of fingers and toes, loss of taste and smell, diarrhoea, headache and conjunctivitis. New mutations are producing some more symptoms. Due to the new mutations, several other symptoms were recorded in mid-2021.

Equally important is maintaining one's psycho-social health and that of the family members. It is also one's own responsibility. It is essential to keep proper contact with reality. Even otherwise, contact with reality is

[16] https://www.thehindu.com/

the most relevant indication of the mental health of an individual. One has to accept the situation as it is. It requires a lot of maturity, courage and understanding. One has to change one's mindset from 'I can't tolerate' to 'I can' and 'I will have to'. As far as COVID-19 is concerned, that is the only way to keep oneself safe. It is boring and tedious to wash hands so frequently or to use the mask without fail, but there is no other trick or shortcut to save one's life. A change in attitude and behaviour will follow this acceptance of reality. Replacing inflexible demands with strong desires by compromising with whatever best is available becomes essential. Developing frustration tolerance capacity is essential for everyone.

> Vinny is a 19-year-old student who stays in a hostel at an international institute. Here, there was ample choice of delicious food in the canteen and mess too. However, after the outbreak of COVID-19, these two outlets got closed, and she had to cook on her own. Now, she has to survive on very simple food, which she never likes. She hates cooking too. In such a situation, one may become sad and wish to somehow get what one wants. This may lead to an extreme risk of infection.

It becomes essential to take safety measures, eat nutritious food, practice emotional catharsis, help others and take others' assistance. Everyone should have gratitude regarding every facility, service and opportunity that they get. In particular, the youth should try to help those who are afraid, staying in quarantine, disabled, old or staying in refugee camps.

For dealing with worry, identifying the cause of worry becomes essential. Postponing worrying, mindfulness and being kind to self lead to a balanced view. One has to stay meaningfully occupied. If worry is about something which one cannot alter, one has to accept it without resistance. One has to think of something else. If one can do something to alter, one has to decide what can be done right now. If nothing can be done right now, one has to concentrate on other important things. If some corrective measure can be taken immediately, one has to do it and get rid of the worry. Introspect how much time you worry and when. Limit the time and select a time when you do not do anything important. Challenge thoughts compassionately. Illogical thoughts should be analysed and evaluated. Worthless and far-fetched negative ideas should be discarded. It is very common to worry about loved ones. Hence, any individual should not be harsh while evaluating one's own irrational thoughts and should respect one's own emotional involvement.

It is necessary to increase resilience and apply self-management skills. One must maintain self-respect and respect for others. To achieve emotional stability, patience, self-confidence and maturity are required. One should remember the previous hardships one has successfully faced and the victories one has achieved. Techniques such as thought stopping, relaxation, imagery techniques and mindfulness can be successfully used for that. Therapies such as rational emotive behaviour therapy, cognitive behaviour therapy and similar other techniques can be used by professional counsellors. Irrational self-talk should be avoided. For better sleep, no stimulation like phone or videos should be available while sleeping. If an individual feels better after reading or reciting any religious material, it should be done before sleep. To get rid of post-traumatic stress disorder, professional help has become a must. Cognitive processing therapy, cognitive therapy for post-traumatic stress disorder, learning different coping strategies and reinterpreting trauma memories are recommended. Cognitive processing therapy teaches the skills necessary for challenging recurring negative thoughts and controlling their impact on one's life. Limiting worry triggers and setting a routine help. Being connected with others, pleasure and achievements overlap to produce well-being. If there is any imbalance, the individual's mood will be negatively affected. If a student just plays on their mobile phone for the whole day or watches pornography, there is no achievement, no social contact. If someone is only attending webinars for the whole day and busy studying, they will not get any other pleasure and the lack of being connected may affect the mood. Like that, a balance is needed between all these types of activities.

During the current pandemic, anyone may encounter different unexpected problems. One should be prepared to cope with an unexpected situation.

For example, Shaila is a 24-year-old talented lady who is studying in New York. She was engaged to her American classmate and had planned to get married in

India in the month of April. Shaila had been staying with her parents in India, as she came one month before the date of marriage. He was to come to India with his family and friends. However, the marriage had to be suddenly postponed due to the lockdown. All the reservations for halls and hotel bookings were cancelled. Shaila is frustrated, depressed and helpless. After two–three months now, she thinks that he is dating another girlfriend.

To handle loneliness resulting from lockdown, one has to keep oneself busy, enjoy reading, painting, music and other hobbies. It is essential to do indoor exercise. To combat anxiety and fear, deep breathing is very effective. The most important issue is to fight back irrational thinking and not to entertain negative thinking. However, in a country like India, the general population is attracted to simple shortcuts to deal with any tension. There is a woman called 'Corona devi' or Corona goddess, who claims that she can cure corona and can drive away the ghost causing corona. Many people worship her. In Kerala, Bihar, Assam, Jharkhand, West Bengal and Chhattisgarh, the model of the coronavirus is being worshipped as a god. There are many short films on YouTube regarding the same.

The ultimate use of free time is done by some people.

A couple in Maharashtra utilized a lockdown period to dig a well and solve a water crisis (*Indian Express*, 2020). In Kerala also, a family used free time to dig a well in 17 days. (TNIE Videos, 2020). In Aurangabad, Maharashtra, money collected for celebrating Ganesh festival was used to build a building for using it as a quarantine facility.

'Daily Life during COVID' are the articles provided on Google every day which include psycho-social well-being. The 'new normal' is the concept introduced with COVID-19 (Medvarsity Online Limited, 2020; TGF—The Guiding Factor, 2020). These are new ways of interacting, working and new habits regarding hygiene necessary for protecting oneself and others. New technologies, new roles and new ways of doing routine activities are to be practised. 'Welcome to the New Normal Innovative Lifestyle' (Siam Paragon, 2020) shows how one should operate any door or lift without touching it by hand, how to keep social distance in the office and so on.

For well-being, the first and most important thing is appropriate healthcare facilities. In Maharashtra, a doctor was not given admission and any treatment, as he was a suspected coronavirus patient, though it was not proved so.[17] In Mumbai, a doctor died of corona infection as he was denied admission to any hospital. The non-availability of ambulances and hospital beds resulted in a waste of critical time (Mojo Story, 2020).

Maintaining good interpersonal relations becomes essential for getting emotional support. Religious activities are useful for maintaining peace of mind. Economic management needs alternative ways of earning bread and butter. Thinking of various educational options and readiness to accept compromises regarding jobs prepares one to cope with the challenges of tomorrow. The most significant things are finding meaningful activities and helping others while taking due precautions.

It is completely an individual's responsibility to find out appropriate ways to take care of their own physiological and psycho-social health. It is essential to remember that everyone is facing some kind of problem, and one should not expect too much from others. Developing empathy for others and helping family members make the atmosphere supportive. Self-acceptance, self-determination, emotional regulation and controlled emotional involvement are recommended. Proper medication and related facilities, of course, for patients and due care for others is a must.

One has to remain connected to sanity, maintain basic discipline and avoid excess information which may create emotional imbalance. It may be useful for reducing frustration, anxiety, depression, anger and other negative emotions. Giving priorities to relevant roles, connecting to groups, proper planning and learning skills for online transactions are also required.

As all sorts of abuse, that is, psychological, physical and sexual, have increased during COVID, it is worth noting that 80 per cent of the abuse is done by males while abusing wives. Verbal and emotional abuse has become very common in Indian families. It has increased during COVID-19 due to unexpected workload and a discrepancy

---

[17] indianexpress.com 20 March 2020

in expectations. Insecurities, fears, biases, distorted judgments, trust issues and cognitive blocks result in an increased proportion of divorces. During this stressful period of COVID-19, both husband and wife should try to support each other and contribute to the welfare of the family. One has to respect others and cordially cooperate.

Maintaining optimum self-esteem, self-efficacy, optimism, self-discipline, character strength and modifying habits are basic and significant issues. Finding better options for addictions, treating withdrawal symptoms and reducing screen time may enhance motivation to lead a normal and happy life.

Not only the elderly but youth also have to deal with frustration, depression, loneliness, cognitive impairment, phobias, paranoia and the like. As there is no fixed duration of the COVID-19 pandemic, one has to learn to survive with it. It becomes difficult to cope with this situation. As far as psychological problems are concerned, such as anxiety and depression, an individual has to introspect and write down why they are so upset. Is it fear of one's own death or that of dear ones or both? Is it due to the potential overwhelming pain that the infection causes, worries about family, old and young ones, money that one may need during treatment and the probability that one may survive but with some internal organ damage? One has to list all the negative thoughts that are disturbing them. After that, one has to classify the ideas as those that have a logical basis and those that do not have any. Is it due to over-generalization or extremely far-fetched ideas? Modifying such ideas works well. As already mentioned, the first significant strategy for maintaining mental health is accepting the reality of things that cannot be altered. This solves most intense emotional problems. Hence, one has to concentrate on the things that one can change, even with great efforts. Coping and problem-solving should be problem focused. One has to compromise even if the option available is not perfect. One has to be prepared to deal with long-term issues. One has to manage emotions and practise relaxation and generate substantial social support. One has to stay connected; though there are different styles and perceptions, nobody should judge others. One should never compare and judge oneself and others. Empathetic support and offering realistic hope, undivided attention, unconditional positive regard and encouragement for enhancing resilience are the ultimate strategies to support each other.

If there is loss or grief, one has to help the individual to accept reality and feelings associated with the loss. Emotional catharsis plays a very important role. Let them understand that they have to reinvest their mental energy in life. It is essential to save them from depression and suicidal tendencies. Both social and emotional support should be given. Let them express their despair through reading, writing, drawing or singing, whichever way they choose.

If a client is facing problems such as anger and aggression, a professional counsellor may train them regarding relaxation, calmness, non-threatening bodily postures, emotional catharsis, and protect them from self-harm and hurting others.

In case of cognitive impairment, repeating instructions, giving clear and explicit directions and practising routine and step-by-step problem-solving help. Sometimes, using a memory aid helps.

During this global pandemic, psycho-social support is essential for everyone. A family of two children and their mother were suffering badly. The Gaikwad family from Osmanabad in Maharashtra adopted them (AM News, 2020). On the other hand, some people are leaving their pets due to fear of corona.

To identify one's own state of mind, one can use these ideas. If one watches news about COVID-19 again and again, keeps on repeatedly complaining and indicating lack of patience, unnecessarily keeps on buying and hoarding extra things of daily requirement such as food grains, biscuits and the like, it indicates that one is anxious, worried, afraid, frustrated and angry. During such conditions, one is upset and shares all the negative information one experiences. After that, essentially, one has to learn how to deal with one's emotions and manage routines effectively. Realization and acceptance of the fact that one cannot control these things is the next stage. One devotes less time to acquiring and sharing information on social media. They filter the information. One starts to realize that changes in daily activities are essential and tries to accommodate them. Managing one's emotional upsets becomes essential. Yoga and art therapy can be regularly practised to balance the mind and body. For example, music has a lot of therapeutic use if done wholeheartedly. One has to focus on the type of music which is most useful for calming one's mind and can generate peace of mind. In a similar way, play therapy can be used for young children for emotional catharsis and expression without language.

After achieving this, an individual tries to develop mindfulness and live in the present moment. They develop empathy, understanding and concern for self and others. They also try to enhance positive thoughts in others, such as family and friends. They help them with catharsis. One tries to be positive and optimistic. This is the optimum functioning where an individual learns creative ways, patience and enterprise while facing enormous challenges. One can learn web banking, card payment and purchase commodities such as vegetables and milk online. From panic purchases and getting disturbed by the idea of non-availability, one progresses to helping others and living in the present moment. One becomes grateful for all they have and for the support of family and friends. Spreading hope, adapting to new situations, developing an understanding that one has to take care of self not only for self but for others and having patience are things of utmost importance.

Academicians are contributing by enhancing awareness, like many psychologists are delivering lectures in various webinars that are being conducted about psycho-social health during the corona pandemic. There are many short videos available on YouTube giving details of the conditions of various places regarding corona spread, precautions to be taken and other scientific information regarding the survival of the virus under different conditions. Examples of corona heroes and those who show extraordinary courage to help others and use creative ideas for the welfare of others are also depicted in such short films and news.

'MPower 1 on 1' is a newly launched helpline in Mumbai for domestic violence to help vulnerable and helpless women. The Government of India launched 'Manodarpan' to give psychological support to students and teachers.[18]

---

[18] https://www.hindustantimes.com/

As substantial research is being done about it, more insight will be generated within a few months. More than 200 countries are suffering from the pandemic. However, New Zealand has achieved complete freedom from corona (*Maharashtra Times*, 2020). Even Germany and Finland have been effectively controlling the spread of corona. They are the three countries where there are female leaders. India should also aspire to the same control over corona, and for that, self-discipline is essential for every Indian.

12.5. SUMMARY

Sudden impact of global pandemic COVID-19 has resulted in a stunning, devastating impact on human beings. Everyone is upset, confused and afraid of the disease. Lakhs of people are affected and dying every day, all over the world. Adjustment becomes difficult in such a situation. The nature of problems and the causes of stress are different for everyone. However, the resulting distress, frustration, depression and anxiety are unbearable for some. Those who are safe are also facing problems due to various limitations and restrictions. There is no direct interaction with anyone. Colleges and offices are closed down completely or partially. Loneliness, fear, changing demands of the environment and boring household jobs are making life difficult. Those who are quarantined are under extreme threat. Various unknown treatments, sharing residences with potential patients and isolation from family make them depressed. Serious patients undergoing treatment feel completely shattered and out of their senses. They feel hopeless and helpless due to extreme pain and breathing difficulties.

From a confused state of mind, where fear is predominant, one has to achieve a mature and calm condition. Being careful does not mean being constantly disturbed and anxious. It is essential to develop psycho-social support and help each other. A traumatic situation while in ICU needs a lot of courage and professional help to maintain mental health. Those who face the loss of dear ones need to tolerate calamities on two levels: one about the loss of a dear one and the other about their own health. There is an urgent requirement for services to help all these groups.

BIBLIOGRAPHY

ABP Sanjha. (2016, March 20). Newly married couple shot dead in Amritsar. https://www.youtube.com/watch?v=X3A5Atb9RIw

Adler, A. (1948). *What life should mean to you* (5th impression). George Allen and Unwin Ltd.

Ahirwar, R., & Mondal, P. R. (2019). Prevalence of obesity in India: A systematic review. *Diabetes and Metabolic Syndrome, 13*(1), 318–321.

Ahmed, A. (2013, March 17). I've watched 3 Idiots thrice, admits Steven Spielberg. *Hindustan Times.*

Ahuja, N. (1993). *A short textbook of psychiatry* (6th ed.). Jaypee Brothers.

Anderson, P., & Savage, J. (2005). Social, legal, and institutional context of heterosexual aggression by college women. *Trauma, Violence & Abuse, 6*(2), 130–140.

Asia Calling. (2014, April 1). *India's ghost fair: Banishing evil spirits* [YouTube channel]. YouTube. https://www.youtube.com/watch?v=6UNKXgCfeSQ

Aware. (2017). Depression and Child Sexual Abuse: Dr Rosaleen McElvaney. https://www.youtube.com/watch?v=q8zaFkusDd0

Bandura, A. (1973). *Aggression: A social learning analysis.* Prentice-Hall.

Bandura, A. (1997). *Self-efficacy: The exercise of control.* W. H. Freeman and Company.

Basu, M. (2012). U.S. broadens archaic definition of rape. https://edition.cnn.com/2012/01/06/justice/rape-definition-revised/index.html

Basu, S., Zou, X., Lou, C., Acharya, R., & Lindgren, R. (2017). Learning to be gendered: Gender socialization in early adolescence among urban poor in Delhi, India, and Shanghai, China. *Journal of Adolescent Health, 61*(4), S24–S29.

Baumeister R. F. (1990). Suicide as escape from self. *Psychological Review, 97*(1), 90–113.

Baumeister, R. F., & Leary, M. R. (1995). The need to belong: Desire for interpersonal attachments as a fundamental human motivation. *Psychological Bulletin, 117*(3), 497–529. https://doi.org/10.1037/0033-2909.117.3.497

BBC News. (2018). Indian national jailed over sex assault on US flight. https://www.bbc.com/news/world-asia-india-46563084

BBC News. (2019, July 6). Webcam sex tourism.

Beautybythelady. (2014, December 4). The burning bed (1984) movie clip. https://www.youtube.com/watch?v=q-5y0_M8mNY

Beck, A. T., Steer, R. A., Kovacs, M. & Garrison, B. (1985). Hopelessness and eventual suicide: A 10 year prospective study of patients hospitalized with suicidal ideation. *American Journal of Psychiatry, 142*(5), 559–563.

Bernardo M. (2018). How to leave an abusive relationship.

Bel, R. J. (2014). Routledge Medical daily. *Jama Psychiatry*, 19 Dec.

Bem, S. L. (1974). The measure of psychological androgyny. *Journal of Consulting and Clinical Psychology, 42*(2), 155–162.

Bem, S. L. (1981). Gender schema theory: A cognitive account of sex typing. *Psychological Review, 88*(4), 354–364.

Benedeck, E. P., & Brown, C. F. (1999). No excuses: Televised pornography harms children. *Harvard Review of Psychiatry, 7*(4), 236–240.

Benson, H. (2000). *The relaxation response*. Harper Collins.

Bhatia, M. S., & Goyal, A. (2018). Anxiety disorders in children and adolescents: Need for early detection. *Journal of Postgraduate Medicine, 64*(2), 75–76.

Bhatnagar, A., Varshney, A., Sheoran, E., Dua, M., Nijhon, R., Jain, S., & Garg, V. (2012, August 22). Khap panchayat. https://www.slideshare.net/Mituldua/khap-panchayat

Bhattacharya, R. (2015, August 22). Men, not women leave their homes after marriage in these Indian communities. https://www.scoopwhoop.com/inothernews/matriarchal-communities-in-india/

Bhilwar, M., Upadhyay, R. M., Rajavel, S., Singh, S. K., Vasudevan, K., Chinnakali, P. (2015). Childhood experiences of physical, emotional and sexual abuse among college students in South India. *Journal of Tropical Pediatrics, 61*(5), 329–338.

Bierman, A., Fazio, E. L., & Milkie, M. A. (2006). A multifaceted approach to the mental health advantage of the married. *Journal of Family Issues, 27*, 554–582.

Biswas, S. (2016, April 12). *Why are India's housewives killing themselves?* BBC News. https://www.bbc.com/news/world-asia-india-35994601

Bouffard, L. A. (2010). Understanding men's perceptions of risks and rewards in a date rape scenario. *International Journal of Offender Therapy and Comparative Criminology, 55*(4), 626–645.

Bulman, R. J. (1992). *Shattered assumptions: Towards a new psychology of trauma.* Free Press.

Burgess, E. W., & Cottrell, L. (ed.). (1939). Role of emotional intelligence in marriage and adjustment. In *Predicting success and failure in marriage*. Prentice Hall.

Burr, W. R., Leigh, G. K., Day, R. D., & Constantine, J. (1979). Symbolic interaction and the family. In W. R. Burr, R. Hill, F. I. Nye, & I. Reiss (Eds.), *Contemporary theories about the family* (Vol. 2, pp. 42–111). Free Press.

Cahill, S. E. (1986). Language practices and self definition: The case of gender identity acquisition. *The Sociological Quarterly, 27*(3), 295–311.

Caroches, J., Deane, F. P., & Anderson, S. (2002). *Why marriage matters*. Institute for American Values.

Cambridge Dictionary. (2018). Cambridge University Press.

Carnes, P. (2001). The addiction cycle. https://www.researchgate.net/figure/The-addiction-cycle-Carnes-2001_fig1_247523538

Carnes, P. (2007, October 16). *Anorexia's childhood roots* (CBS News) [YouTube channel]. YouTube. https://www.youtube.com/watch?v=uKUSGOB-0V8

CBS News. (2013, May 7). Born bad? How to treat children who are predisposed to violence. https://www.youtube.com/watch?v=Q3GQ8hi4qi4

Chatterjee, I. (1999). *Gender, slavery and law in colonial India*. Oxford University Press.

Chaulagain, S., Soujanya P. U., Moras, S. M., Aranha, P. R., & Shetty, A. P. (2016). A study on knowledge regarding sibling rivalry in children among mothers in selected hospitals at Mangaluru. *Journal of Scientific and Innovative Research*, 5(4),122–124.

Cherickal, T. (2018, November 2). http://medium.com

Cherikal, (2018). How to deal effectively with children exposed to pornography on the internet?

Child Welfare Information Gateway. (2018). Preventing child abuse and neglect. https://www.childwelfare.gov/pubs/factsheets/preventingcan/

Childress, A. R. Mozley, P. D., & O'Brien, C. P. (1999). Limbic activation during cue induced cocaine craving. *The American Journal of Psychiatry*, 156(1), 11.

Chorpita, B. F., Taylor, A. A., Francis, S. E., Moffitt, C., & Austin, A. A. (2004). Efficacy of modular cognitive behavioral therapy for childhood anxiety disorders. *Behavior Therapy*, 35(2), 263–283.

Ciarrochi, J., Deane, F. P., & Anderson, S. (2002). Perceived emotional intelligence and marital adjustment. https://www.academia.edu/33123411/Perceived_Emotional_Intelligence_and_Marital_Adjustment_Examining_the_Mediating_Role_of_Personality_and_Social_Desirability

Clancy, C. (2019). The most common defense mechanisms of addiction. https://journeypureriver.com/defense-mechanisms-addiction/

Cochran, N H, Cochran, J. L., & Nordling, W. J. (2010). Child-centered play therapy: *A practical guide to developing therapeutic relationships with children*. Child centred play therapy. John Wiley and Sons.

Crome, S. A., & McCabe, M. P. (1995). The impact of rape on individual, interpersonal, and family functioning. *Journal of Family Studies*, 1(1). https://doi.org/10.5172/jfs.1.1.58

Crosby, A. E., Ortega, L., & Melanson, C. (2011). Self-directed violence surveillance: Uniform definitions and recommended data elements. National Center for Injury Prevention and Control. Division of Violence Prevention. https://www.cdc.gov/suicide/pdf/self-directed-violence-a.pdf

Cuber, J. F., & Harroff, P. B. (1966). The Cuber and Harroff's five types of marriage. https://www.bartleby.com/essay/The-Cuber-And-Harroffs-Five-Types-Of-PJGUFUMUG6

Curly Tales. (2020, May 27). *Kasturba hospital doctor shares experience on COVID-19* [YouTube channel]. YouTube. https://www.youtube.com/watch?v=LVrDYOpSWpA

Dalton Production. (2014, September 7). Theories of violence. https://www.youtube.com/watch?v=N3Jrmcz0CNE

Das, A. M. (2013, July 30). More than 80 percent of high school students exposed to porn, says study. https://www.newindianexpress.com/states/kerala/2013/jul/30/More-than-80-percent-of-high-school-students-exposed-to-porn-says-study-501873.html

Davenport, B. (2019). 10 signs of emotional abuse in a relationship (break the cycle of manipulation). https://www.youtube.com/watch?v=OZetpVv4lzs

Dhawan, A., Pattanayak, R. D. Chopra, A. Tikoo, V. K., & Kumar, R. (2017). Pattern and profile of children using substances in India: Insight and recommendations. *National Medical Journal of India*, 30(4), 224–229.

Dilli Aajtak. (2018, November 14). *Man commits suicide* [YouTube channel]. YouTube. https://www.youtube.com/watch?v=MdZ23P7B_DQ

Doidge, N. (2015). The brain's way of healing: Remarkable discoveries and recoveries from the frontiers of neuroplasticity. Viking Penguin.

Downey, A. (2017). Brain scans reveal how bad emotional abuse damages kids. *The New York Times*, November 2. https://nypost.com/2017/11/02/brain-scans-reveal-how-badly-emotional-abuse-damages-kids/

Durkheim, E. (1952). Suicide: A study in sociology (J. A. Spaulding and G. Simpson, trans.). Routledge and Kegan Paul (Original work published 1897).

Durkheim, E. (1974). Sociology and philosophy (D. F. Pcock, trans.). The Free Press.

Duckworth, K. (2015). Understanding mental disorders: Your guide to DSM-5. American Psychiatric Publishing.

Eagly, A. H. (1987). *Sex differences in social behavior: A social-role interpretation.* Lawrence Erlbaum Associates.

Elliott, J. M., Tong, C. K., & Tan, P. H. (1997). Attitudes of Singapore public to actions suggesting child abuse. *Child Abuse and Neglect*, 21(5), 445–464.

English, D., Graham, C., Newton, R. R., Lewis, T. L., Thompson, R., Kotch, J. B., & Weisbart, C. (2009). At-risk and maltreated children exposed to intimate partner aggression/violence: What the conflict looks like and its relationship to child outcomes. *Child Maltreatment*, 14(2), 157–171.

Erikson, H. (1968). *Identity, youth and crisis.* W. W. Norton and Company.

Eysenck, H. J. (1997). *Human addiction, personality and motivation.* John Wiley and Sons Ltd.

Federal Bureau of Investigation. (2013). Reporting rape in 2013. https://ucr.fbi.gov/recent-program-updates/reporting-rape-in-2013-revised

Fenichel, O. (1945). *The psychoanalytic theory of neurosis.* W.W. Norton and Company.

Feinauer, L. L., Callahan, E. H., & Gill H. (1996). Positive intimate relationships decrease depression in sexually abused women. *The American Journal of Family Therapy*, 24(2), 99–106.

Fernandez, E. (2010). Towards an integrative psychotherapy for maladaptive anger. In M. Potegal, C. Spielberger & S. Garhand (Eds), *International handbook of anger* (pp. 499–513). Springer.

Finkel, E. J., Larson, G. M., Carswell, K. L., & Hui, C. M. (2014). Marriage at the summit: Response to the commentaries. *Psychological Inquiry*, 25, 120–140.

Finkenauer, C., Kerkhof, P., Branje, S., Righetti, F. (2009). Living together apart: Perceived concealment as a signal of exclusion in marital relationships. *Personality and Social Psychology Bulletin*, 35(10), 1410–1422.

Fisher, B. L. (1982). Marriage and marital adjustment. https://www.researchgate.net/publication/273831376

FM Editorial. (2014). Cover story: Pornography and its devastating consequences on the youth & women in India. https://familymantra.com/2014/10/cover-story-pornography-and-its-devastating-consequences-on-the-youth-women-in-india/

Foret, M. M., Scult, M., Wilcher, M., Chudnofsky, R., Malloy, L., Hasheminejad, N., & Park, E. R. (2012). Integrating a relaxation response based curriculum into a public high school in Massachusetts. *Journal of Adolescence*, 35(2), 325–332.

Freud, S. (1923). The ego and the id. In S. Strachey & A. Freud (Ed.), *The standard edition of the complete psychological works of Sigmund Freud* (Vol 19, pp. 13–27). Hogarth Press and the Institute of Psychoanalysis.

Freud, S. (1957). Five lectures on psychoanalysis (1910, 1909). In S. Strachey & A. Freud (Ed.), *The standard edition of the complete psychological works of Sigmund Freud* (Vol 19, pp. 9–56). Hogarth Press and the Institute of Psychoanalysis.

Gaiger, A. (2016, February 14). Types of aggression. https://www.youtube.com/watch?v=ZOW4EosuhnI

Gallup. (2017). *State of the global workplace*. Gallup Press.

Ganguli, H. C. (2000). Epidemiological finding on prevalence of mental disorders in India. *The Indian Journal of Psychiatry*, 42(1), 14–20.

Geet, S., & Agashe, M. (1995). *Atmahatya va Echamaran* (Marathi). Nitin Prakashan.

Ginsberg, B. G. (2002). The power of filial relationship enhancement therapy as an intervention in child abuse and neglect. *International Journal of Play Therapy*, 11(1), 65–78.

Goldsmith, B., Beresford, M., & Thomson Reuters Foundation. (2018). India most dangerous country for women with sexual violence rife: Global poll. https://www.reuters.com/article/women-dangerous-poll-idINKBN1JM076

Gottman, J. M., Jacobson, N. E., Rushe, R. R., Shortt, J. W., Babcock, J., La Taillade, J. J., & Waltz, J. (1995). The relationship between heart rate reactivity, emotionally aggressive behaviour, and general violence in batterers. *Journal of Family Psychology, 9*(3), 227–279.

Hall, M., & Hall, J. (2011). The long-term effects of childhood sexual abuse: Counseling implications. https://www.counseling.org/docs/disaster-and-trauma_sexual-abuse/long-term-effects-of-childhood-sexual-abuse.pdf?sfvrsn=2

HarvardX. (2017, June 7). Direct, structural and cultural violence. https://www.youtube.com/watch?v=LW_rTeawAi0

Havighhurst, R. J. (1953). Havighurst's developmental task theory. https://practicalpie.com/havighursts-developmental-task-theory/

Havighurst, R. J., & DeHann, R. F. (1957). *Potentialities of women in the middle years.* Michigan State University Press.

Health, L. (2017, February 26). *Recognizing OCD* [YouTube channel]. YouTube.

Hendin, H. (1964). *Suicide and Scandinavia.* Grune and Stratton.

Hilberman, E., & Munson, K. (1978). Sixty battered women. *Victimology: An international Journal, 2*(3–4), 460–470.

Hindustan Times. (2018, February 9). How to report child sexual abuse in India. https://www.youtube.com/watch?v=o8irFN7ayII

Hines, M. (2011). Gender development and the human brain. *Annual Review of Neuroscience, 34,* 69–88. https://doi.org/10.1146/annurev-neuro-061010-113654

Horney, K. (1950). *Neurosis and human growth: The struggle towards self-realization.* W. W. Norton.

Hodal, K. (2018). Scientists confirm what women always knew: Men really are the weaker sex. *The Guardian.* https://www.theguardian.com/global-development/2018/jan/15/scientists-confirm-what-women-always-knew-men-really-are-the-weaker-sex

Howard, L. M. (2019). The domestic violence and abuse. National Institute for Health Research, WHO. https://www.rcpsych.ac.uk

Hurlock, E. B. (1979). *Developmental psychology* (5th ed.). Tata McGraw Hill Education.

Hyde, J. S. (1985). Half the human experience: The psychology of women (3rd ed.). D. C. Heath.

Hyde, J. S. (2005). The gender similarities hypothesis. *The American Psychologist, 60*(6), 581–592.

Huang, C. (2019). 10 signs of emotional abuse from parents. Psych2Go. https://www.youtube.com/watch?v=y7bKFMO0d-w

India Today. (2018, September 18). Telangana honour killing: Rs 1.13 crore to murder Dalit Christian son-in-law. https://www.indiatoday.in/india/story/telangana-honour-killing-rs-1-crore-murder-dalit-christian-1343611-2018-09-19

India Today. (2018). 8-month-old baby critical after being raped by cousin in Delhi. https://www.indiatoday.in/india/story/8-month-old-baby-critical-after-being-raped-by-cousin-in-delhi-1157100-2018-01-30

IndiaTV. (2014, November 19). Parents kill daughter in Delhi for inter-caste marriage. https://www.youtube.com/watch?v=By0595atO6Q

IndiaTV. (2018, June 2). *Man commits suicide in Punjab's Phagwara, records live video on Facebook* [YouTube channel]. YouTube. https://www.youtube.com/watch?v=U47Xgh41scE

Indian National Crime Record. (2012). *Crime in India*. National Crime Records Bureau.

Itimes.com. (2020). 5 cases of ragging in India that shocked the world! https://www.indiatimes.com/news/world/5-cases-of-ragging-in-india-that-shocked-the-world-278321.html

Jai Maharashtra News. (2015, December 17). Honour Killing: New married couple murder at Kasaba Bavada Kolhapur. https://www.youtube.com/watch?v=RdpkapWU-8s

Jaspreet Kaur. (2016, August 16). Honour killing. http://www.slideshare.net

Jecobs, J. (1971). *Adolescent suicide*. Wiley Interscience.

Jellinek, E. M. (1952). Phases of alcohol addiction. *Quarterly Journal of Studies on Alcohol, 13*(4), 673–684.

Johnson, S. A. (2007). *Physical abusers and sexual offender: Forensic and clinical strategies*. CRC Press.

Joiner, T. (2005). *Why people die by suicide*. Harvard University Press.

Jorgensen, S. R., & Gaudy, J. C. (1990). Self disclosure and satisfaction in marriage: The relation examined. *Family Relations, 29*(3), 281–287.

Joseph, K. (2019, December 24). Porn addiction in adolescents rising. *Deccan Herald*. https://www.deccanherald.com/metrolife/metrolife-lifestyle/porn-addiction-in-adolescents-rising-788369.html

Joseph, S., & Linley, P.A. (2005). Positive adjustment to threatening events: An organismic valuing theory of growth through adversity. *Review of General Psychology, 9*, 262–280.

Jung, C. G. (1933). *Modern man in search of a soul*. Kegan Paul, Trench, Trubner & Co.

Jung, C. G. (1954). The development of personality (R. F. C. Hull, trans.). Rouledge and Kegan Paul.

Kajal, K. (2020). The reasons why 63 Indian housewives killed themselves every day in 2018. https://scroll.in/article/9 j3545/the-reasons-why-63-indian-housewives-killed-themselves-every-day-in-2018

Kessler, B. L., & Bieschke, K. J. (1999.) A retrospective analysis of shame, dissociation, and adult victimization in survivors of childhood sexual abuse. *Journal of Counselling Psychology, 46*(3), 335–341.

Kelly, J. B., & Johnston, J. R. (2001). The alienated child: Reformulation of parental alienation syndrome. *Family Court Review, 39*(3), 249–266.

KLFY.com. (2018). Decade-plus sentence for man after 2nd child porn conviction. https://www.klfy.com/louisiana/decade-plus-sentence-for-man-after-2nd-child-porn-conviction/

Keller, M. A. (1979). Historical overview of alcohol and alcoholism. *Cancer Research, 39*, 2822–2829.

Kobler, A., & Stotland, E. (1964). *The end of hope: A social-clinical study of suicide.* Macmillan

Kohlberg, L. (1966). A cognitive-developmental analysis of children's sex-role concepts and attitudes. In E. E. Maccoby (Ed.), *The development of sex differences.* Stanford University Press.

Krahe, B. (2013). *The social psychology of aggression* (2nd ed.). Psychology Press.

Kristina, J. (2018). What is emotional abuse? The top emotional abuse warning signs. https://www.youtube.com/watch?v=W9QHncUU3IA

Kuhn, K. A., Ellen, B., Nigel, P. & Kevin, V. (2007). The pornography and erotica industries. In Binney, W & Brennan, L (Eds.), *Proceedings of the 2009 International Nonprofit and Social Marketing (INSM) Conference: Sustainable social enterprise* (pp. 1–9). Victoria University and Swinburne University of Technology.

Laurent, H. K., Kim, H. K., & Capaldi, D. M. (2008). Interaction and relationship development in stable young couples: Effects of positive engagement, psychological aggression, and withdrawal. *Journal of Adolescence, 31*(6), 815–835.

Lederer, W. J., & Jackson, D. D. (1990). *The mirages of marriage.* W. W. Norton.

Leenaars, A. A. (2010). Edwin S. Shneidman on suicide. *Suicidology Online, 1,* 5–18.

Levy, D. M. (1939). Trends in therapy. *American Journal of Orthopsychiatry, 9*(4), 713–736.

Lippa, R. A. (2010). Gender differences in personality and interest: When, where, and why? *Social and Personality Psychology Compass, 4*(11), 1098–1110.

Lisak, D., & Miller, P. (2002). Repeat rape and multiple offending among undetected rapists. *Violence and Victims, 17*(1),73–84.

Loganathan, S., & Murthy, R. S. (2011). Living with schizophrenia in India: Gender perspectives. *Transcultural Psychiatry Journal, 48*(5), 569–584.

Maddi, S. R., & Khoshaba, D. M. (2005). *Resilience at work: How to succeed no matter what life throws at you.* American Management Association.

Mann, J. J., Watenaux, C., Haas, G. L., & Malone, K. M. (1999). Toward a clinical model of suicidal behavior in psychiatric patients. *American Journal of Psychiatry, 156*(2),181–189.

Martin, C. L. (2000). Cognitive theories of gender development. In T. Eckes & H. M. Trautner (Eds.), *The developmental social psychology of gender* (pp. 91–121). Lawrence Erlbaum Associates Publishers.

Martin, L. L., Harris, G. T., Quinsey, V. L., & Rice, M. E. (eds.). (2003). *The causes of rape: Understanding individual differences in male propensity for sexual aggression.* American Psychological Association.

Maslow, A. H. (1943). *Motivation and personality.* Harper.

Mckibbin, W. F., Shackelford, T. K., Goetz, A. T., & Starratt, V. G. (2008). Why do men rape? An evolutionary psychological perspective Florida Atlantic University. *Review of General Psychology, 12*(1), 86–97.

Merdhekar, V., & Wadkar, A. J. (2012). Coping strategies and learned helplessness of employed and nonemployed educated married women. *Health Care for Women International*, 33(5), 495–508.

Miller, N. E. (1941). The frustration aggression hypothesis. *Psychological Review*, 48(4), 337–342.

Ministry of Women and Child Development. (2007). Government of India. http://www.wcd.nic.in/childabuse

Mitchell, M. R., & Potenza, M. N. (2014). Addictions and personality traits: Impulsivity, and related constructs. *Current Behavioral Neuroscience Reports*, 1(1), 1–12.

Medvarsity Online Limited. (2020, May 11). *The new normal—After lockdown* [YouTube channel]. YouTube. https://www.youtube.com/watch?v=7Itu32AyELg

MindChop. (2015, October 4). *5 most extreme cases of anorexia* [YouTube channel]. YouTube. https://www.youtube.com/watch?v=Ag7e3dnkTy4

Mojo Story. (2020, May 31). *Mumbai doctor dies after failing to get hospitalized in time* [YouTube channel]. YouTube. https://www.youtube.com/watch?v=sAtZh1tFq0E

Moreno, M. (2014). Molecular effects of traumatic stress. *Current Psychiatry Reports*, 19(11), 85.

Morton, K. (2014). 5 must know signs of emotional abuse. https://www.youtube.com/watch?v=A5fw-IT_phU

mynation.com. (2016). Enriching marriage and family life. Director General, Medical Service, Navy. http://www.mynation.com

Nair, D. (2014). Delhi child rape: Fired by porn and alcohol accused had sex with girl as she lay bleeding and unconscious. https://www.ibtimes.co.uk/rape-girl-delhi-bottle-candle-genitals-mutilated-460786

Nathawat, S. S., Mathur, A. (1993). Marital adjustment and subjective well-being in Indian-educated housewives and working women. *The Journal of Psychology*, 127, 353–358.

Napiorkowska, K. (2019, April 17). *Living with bipolar disorder* [YouTube channel]. YouTube. https://www.youtube.com/watch?v=AMsyfoLb9C0

Napiorkowska, K. (2016, June 20). *Living with OCD* [YouTube channel]. YouTube. https://www.youtube.com/watch?v=TD-xPiwtyHA

National Drug Use Survey. (2019). National Survey on Extent and Pattern of Substance Use in India' 2019. https://www.aiims.edu/en/national-drug-use-survey-2019.html

National Geographic. (2007, May 19). Multiple husbands. https://www.youtube.com/watch?v=d4yjrDSvze0

National Institute for the Clinical Application of Behavioral Medicine. (n.d.). How anger affects your brain and body. https://www.nicabm.com/how-anger-affects-the-brain-and-body-infographic/

National Institute of Justice. (2012, December 3). *The relationship between drugs and crime, Redonna Chandler (2 of 3)* [YouTube channel]. YouTube. https://www.youtube.com/watch?v=5lGEwdP9znY

NDTV. (2009, January 5). Homeless & addicted kids in Delhi [YouTube channel]. YouTube. https://www.youtube.com/watch?v=icVHU_U4YYI

NDTV. (2017, July 7). *I used smack, says Delhi's 8-year old. Another, 11, is an addict* [YouTube channel]. YouTube. https://www.youtube.com/watch?v=P3hmiVh-BBU

NDTV. (2018, September 27). For refusing sex, woman set on fire by husband in Maharashtra. https://www.ndtv.com/cities/beed-maharashtra-ayyub-pathan-kills-saira-pathan-by-setting-her-on-fire-she-refused-sex-1923348

NDTV. (2018, December 24). Telangana woman's body burnt, ashes thrown away for inter-caste marriage. https://www.ndtv.com/telangana-news/parents-alleg-edly-kill-daughter-for-marrying-man-outside-caste-in-telangana-1967090

NDTV. (2019, June 23). Over 12000 farmers committed suicide in 3 years: Maharashtra government [YouTube channel]. YouTube. https://www.youtube.com/watch?v=mPQB9TmVssU

Niaz, U., & Hassan, S. (2006). Culture and mental health of women in South-East Asia.

Official Journal of the World Psychiatric Association, 5(2), 118–120.

O'Connor, R. C. (2011). Towards an integrated motivational-volitional model of suicidal behaviour. 181–198. In: R. C. O'Connor, S. Platt, & J. Gordon (Eds.), *International handbook of suicide prevention: Research, policy and practice*. John Wiley & Sons.

Oddnaari. (2021). Pollachi sexual harassment case. https://www.youtube.com/watch?v=74qSx5rMpgE

OpIndia Staff. (2020). What happened to the juvenile rapist of the Nirbhaya gang-rape case: Here are the details. https://www.opindia.com/2020/03/nirbhaya-rape-case-juvenile-cook-sewing-machine-convicts-hanged/

Pandey G. N. (2013). Biological basis of suicide and suicidal behavior. *Bipolar Disorders, 15*(5), 524–541.

Pandey, M. (2017). What my interviews with convicted rapists in Delhi told me about male attitudes. https://thewire.in/law/interviewed-convicted-rapists-new-delhi-young-victim

Park, C. L., & Helgeson, V. S. (2006). Introduction to the special section growth following highly stressful life events, current status and future directions. *Journal of Consulting and Clinical Psychology, 74*(5), 791–796.

Parrott, D. J., & Gaincola, P. R. (2007). Addressing the 'criterion problem' in the assessment of aggressive behavior: Development of new taxonomic system. *Aggression and Violent Behavior, 12*(3), 280–299.

Pavlov, I. P. (1927). Conditioned reflexes: An investigation of the physiological activity of cerebral cortex. Oxford University Press.

PIB India. (2016). Komal: A film on child sexual abuse: CSA English. https://www.youtube.com/watch?v=5cBQtZRbRJU

Pretzel, P. W. (1972). *Understanding and counselling the suicidal person.* Abingdon Press.

Samachar Nama. (2017, May 19). *Demonic possession on an Indian girl* [YouTube channel]. YouTube. https://www.youtube.com/watch?v=SI38czy1N6U

Satyamev Jayate. (2012, May 13). Child Sexual Abuse. https://www.youtube.com/watch?v=Cw9lSkRBm3U

Saxena, S., Krug, E., & Chestnov, O. (2014). *Preventing suicide: A global imperative.* WHO.

Sbarra, D. A., Hasselmo, K., & Bourassa K. J. (2015). Divorce and health: Beyond individual differences. *Current Directions in Psychological Science, 24*(2). https://doi.org/10.1177/0963721414559125

Schmauder, C. (2015). The male brain on porn: Wheaton researcher speaks at Pitt. https://pittnews.com/article/66127/news/the-male-brain-on-porn-wheaton-researcher-speaks-at-pitt/

Seligman, M. E. P. (1975). *Helplessness: On depression, development, and death.* W. H. Freeman.

Sex Roles. (2012). *Encyclopedia of human behaviour* (2nd ed.). Academic Press.

Semel Institute Center for Neurobehavioral Genetics. (2012).

Sharma, H. (2018, August 1). Madhya Pradesh: Couple forced to drink urine for marrying against parents' wishes. https://www.indiatoday.in/india/madhya-pradesh/story/madhya-pradesh-alirajpur-couple-forced-to-drink-urine-for-marrying-against-parents-wishes-1302103-2018-08-01

Sharma, K. (2017, December 11). The reality behind the theory of killer game 'Blue Whale'. *The Times of India.* https://timesofindia.indiatimes.com/life-style/health-fitness/de-stress/the-reality-behind-the-theory-of-killer-game-blue-whale/articleshow/59881467.cms

Sharma, M. K., Rao, G. N., Benegal, V., Thenarassu, K., & Oommen, D. (2019). Use of pornography in India: Need to explore its implications. *The National Medical Journal of India, 32*(5), 282–284.

Sharma M. K., & Marimuthu, P. (2014). Prevalence and psychosocial factors of aggression among youth. *Indian Journal of Psychological Medicine, 36*(1), 48–53.

Sharma, N. (2018). 16-year-old girl gang-raped in private hospital's ICU. https://timesofindia.indiatimes.com/city/bareilly/16-year-old-girl-gang-raped-in-pvt-hosps-icu/articleshow/66492970.cms

Sharma, S. (2016). Substance use and criminality among juvenile under enquiry in New Delhi. *Indian Journal of Psychiatry, 58*(2), 178–182.

Sheth, H. (2020, April 14). India lockdown: Online child pornography consumption spikes by in India, says ICPF. https://www.thehindubusinessline.com/info-tech/india-lockdown-online-child-pornography-consumption-spikes-by-in-india-says-icpf/article31337221.ece

Shneidman, E. S. (1967). The NIMH Centre for studies of suicide prevention. *Bulletin of Suicidology, 1,* 2–7.

Shneidman, E. S. (1975). *Suicide and Life-threatening Behaviour, 5*(1). Wiley Online Library, onlinelibrary.wiley.com

Shneidman, E. S. and Farberow, N. L. (1957b). The logic of suicide. In clues of suicide by Shneidman E. S. and Farberow, N. L. (Eds), (pp. 31–40) McGraw Hill, New York.

Psych2Go. (2020, January 29). *The top 7 most common phobias* [YouTube cha. YouTube. https://www.youtube.com/watch?v=wVTvcxEWClg

Psycho Tools. (2020). Living with worry and anxiety amidst global uncerta https://www.psychologytools.com/assets/covid-19/guide_to_living_w worry_and_anxiety_amidst_global_uncertainty_en-us.pdf

PTI. (2019). BHEL's woman officer commits suicide over mental harassment senior, colleagues. https://www.indiatoday.in/india/story/hyderabad-bh woman-officer-commits-suicide-over-mental-harassment-by-senior-an colleagues-1610554-2019-10-18

punekarnews.in. (2021, March). Wife is not slave or property of husband, cannd be forced to live with him: Supreme Court. https://www.punekarnews.in wife-is-not-slave-or-property-of-husband-cannot-be-forced-to-live-with- him-supreme-court/

Rajkumar, R. P. (2020). COVID-19 and mental health: A review of the existing literature. *Asian Journal of Psychiatry*, *52*, 102066. https://doi.org/10.1016/j. ajp.2020.102066

Ratican, K. L. (1992). Sexual abuse survivor: Identifying symptoms and special treatment considerations. *Journal of Counselling and Development*, *71*(1), 33–38.

Real News of India. (2015, January 7). *Straight talk with a drug addict* [YouTube channel]. YouTube. https://www.youtube.com/watch?v=pvkGaa4IESY

Reddy, M. A., & Chandrashekhar, C. R. (1998). Prevalence of mental and behavioral disorders in India: A meta-analysis. *Indian Journal of Psychiatry*, *40*(2),149–157.

Redway, J. A. K., & Miville, M. L. (2013). Gender roles among African American women. In M. L. Miville (Ed.), *Multicultural gender roles: Applications for mental health and education* (pp. 65–95). John Wiley and Sons.

Reuters Staff. (2019). Statistics on rape in India and some well-known cases. https://www.reuters.com/article/us-india-rape-factbox-idUSKBN1YA0UV

Romeo, F. F. (2000). The educator's role in reporting the emotional abuse of children. *Journal of Instructional Psychology*, *27*(3), 183–186.

Roothman, B., Doret, K. K., & Marie, P. W. (2003). Gender differences in aspects of psychological well being. *South African Journal of Psychology*, *33*(4), 212–218.

Roy, L. D. (2020, April 7). Domestic violence cases across India swell since coronavirus lockdown. *Outlook*. https://www.outlookindia.com/website/ story/india-news-rise-in-domestic-violence-across-all-strata-of-society-in-the- coronavirus-lockdown-period/350249

Rudd, M. D. (2000). The suicide mode: A cognitive behavioral model of suicidal ity. *Suicide and Life-Threatening Behavior*, *30*(1), 18–33.

Sahni, U. (2020). COVID-19 in India: Education disrupted and lessons learned https://www.brookings.edu/blog/education-plus-development/2020/05/1 covid-19-in-india-education-disrupted-and-lessons-learned/#:~:text=In% India%2C%20320%20million%20students,embedded%20gender% and%20class%20divides.

Sheldon, W. H., Joiner, T. E., Pettit, J. W., & Williams, G. (2003). Reconciling humanistic ideals and scientific clinical practice. *Clinical Psychology*, *10*(3), 302–315.

Siam Paragon. (2020, May 11). *Welcome to the new normal innovative lifestyle* [YouTube channel]. YouTube. https://www.youtube.com/watch?v= yUFyoVEtVTg

Skinner, K. B. (2017). Seven levels of pornography addiction. https://www.scribd. com/document/339012121/Seven-Levels-of-Pornography-Addiction

Skinner, B. F. (1953). Science and human behaviour. Simon and Schuster.

Smoky Evening. (2019, October 24). *Bollywood celebrities and their shocking phobia* [YouTube channel]. YouTube. https://www.youtube.com/ watch?v=3b4jEXiKF2U

Stack, S., Wasserman, I., & Kern R. (2004). Adult social bonds and use of internet pornography. *Social Science Quarterly*, *85*(1), 75–88.

Stephanie Lyn Coaching. (2018). What you must do to leave an emotionally abusive relationship. https://www.youtube.com/watch?v=v0F_Dcg7BXM

Stephanie Lyn Coaching. (2018). Why you can't leave an abusive relationship/ trauma bonding. https://www.youtube.com/watch?v=EQAVLUSiddQ

Stevelos, J. (2010). Sexual abuse and obesity: What's the link? https://www.obesityaction.org/community/article-library/sexual-abuse-and-obesity-whats-the-link/

Study IQ Education. (2018, July 5). *Drug abuse in India—Current affairs 2018* [YouTube channel]. YouTube. https://www.youtube.com/watch?v= 17kUuuNnxc4

Sullivan, H. S. (1953). *The interpersonal theory of psychiatry*. W. W. Norton & Co.

Sutherland, S. (1947). Sutherland (1947): Theory of differential association. http://psychyogi.org/sutherland-1947-theory-of-differential-association/#:~:text=According%20to%20this%20theory%2C%20 the,and%20then%20'learning%20from%20others.&text=The%20most%20 important%20part%20of,persons%20close%20circle%20of%20friends.

Taylor, S. E., & Brown, J. D. (1988). Illusion and well-being: A social psychological perspective on mental health. *Psychological Bulletin*, *103*(2), 193–210.

Tandon, S., & Mehrotra, S. (2016). Post traumatic growth and its correlates in an Indian setting. *International Journal of Indian Psychology*, *4*(1). https://doi.org/10.25215/0401.014

Tedeschi, R. G., & Calhounin, L. G. (2006). Handbook of posttraumatic growth: Research and practice. Routledge, 291–310.

Tedeschi, R. G., & Calhounin, L. G. (1996). The post traumatic growth inventory: Measuring the positive legacy of trauma. *Journal of Traumatic Stress*, *9*, 455–471.

TEDx Talks. (2018). Why I stayed, why I left. TEDx University of Piraeus. https:// www.youtube.com/watch?v=5609_5FRjhY

TGF—The Guiding Factor. (2020, April 29). *Life after lockdown. The new normal: The restricted life* [YouTube channel]. YouTube. https://www.youtube.com/ watch?v=QTg7hHXlcQ0

The Better India. (2017). India is one of 36 countries where marital rape is not a crime. Here are the changes we need. https://www.thebetterindia.com/109672/marital-rape-an-unrecognized-evil/

The Guardian. (2018). Scientists confirm what women always knew: men really are the weaker sex. https://www.theguardian.com/global-development/2018/jan/15/scientists-confirm-what-women-always-knew-men-really-are-the-weaker-sex

The Hindu. (2017). Indian youth look modern, but inclined to conservatism and intolerance: Survey. https://www.thehindu.com/news/national/youth-modern-in-look-conservative-in-outlook-survey/article17819664.ece

The Hindu. (2019). Girl raped, set ablaze in U.P. https://www.thehindu.com/news/national/girl-raped-set-ablaze-in-up/article30308656.ece

The Indian Express. (2019). Mumbai: 13-year-old boy held for rape, murder of five-year-old cousin. https://indianexpress.com/article/cities/mumbai/mumbai-13-year-old-boy-held-for-rape-murder-of-five-year-old-cousin-6095163/

The Peacebuilding Practitioner. (2018). Analysis of violence for peacebuilders. https://www.youtube.com/watch?v=rPX3QHUyfxg

The Times of India. (2018, July 31). Bizarre! Man live streams suicide on Facebook, 2000 people watch, 29 share. https://timesofindia.indiatimes.com/videos/city/chandigarh/bizarre-man-live-streams-suicide-on-facebook-2000-people-watch-29-share/videoshow/65212877.cms

The Times of India. (2019). Haryana: Student stabs teacher for asking for homework copy. https://timesofindia.indiatimes.com/city/gurgaon/haryana-student-stabs-teacher-for-asking-for-homework-copy/articleshow/70127984.cms

The Quint. (2019). My parents never told cops about my rape. https://www.youtube.com/watch?v=TwkziNT2v28

The Quint. (2021). Badaun gang rape and murder sparks massive outrage; priest, two disciples booked. https://www.youtube.com/watch?v=HFA9rzx78rI

The United States Department of Justice. (2012). Attorney General Eric Holder announces revisions to the uniform crime report's definition of rape. https://www.justice.gov/opa/pr/attorney-general-eric-holder-announces-revisions-uniform-crime-report-s-definition-rape

TNIE Videos. (2020, April 23). *Lockdown tales: Kerala family used free time to dig a well at home in 17 days* [YouTube channel]. YouTube. https://www.youtube.com/watch?v=JhKsR6cV0_o

Trending 91. (2019, December 16). The real story of Laxmi Agarwal. https://www.youtube.com/watch?v=QebjSA0rgXg

Trivedi, S. (2019, December 16). Will consider my job done when Nirbhaya case convicts are hanged. *The Hindu.* https://www.thehindu.com/news/cities/Delhi/will-consider-my-job-done-when-nirbhaya-case-convicts-are-hanged/article30314878.ece

Union Health Ministry International Institute for Population Sciences. (2017). National Family Health Survey. Mumbai: Union Health Ministry International Institute for Population Sciences.

University of Pennsylvania. (2014, September 4). The biological roots of violence. https://www.youtube.com/watch?v=J-D2iWjUWiM

Update News. (2017). A woman interviewed 100 convicted rapists in India: This is what she learned. https://www.youtube.com/watch?v=HDnteYCTxeE

Walker, J., Archer, J., & Davies, M. (2005). Effects of male rape on psychological functioning. *British Journal of Clinical Psychology, 44*(3), 445–451. https://doi.org/10.1348/014466505X52750

Watson, J. B., & Rayner, R. (1920). Conditioned emotional reactions. *Journal of Experimental Psychology, 3*(1), 1–14.

West, D. J. (1965). *Murders followed by suicide.* Heinimann.

Wikipedia. (n.d.). Obesity in India. https://en.wikipedia.org/wiki/Obesity_in_India

Wikipedia. (2018). Wikipedia of divorce demography. https://en.m.wikipedia.org

Wikipedia. (2021). Gender role. https://en.wikipedia.org/wiki/Gender_role

WHO. (2018). Alcohol consumption in India doubled in 11 years: WHO report. https://www.livemint.com/Industry/0PBqBWHOYz8msKWSD6a84H/Alcohol-consumption-in-India-doubled-in-11-years-WHO-report.html

WHO. (2018). WHO's global status report on alcohol and health. https://www.who.int/publications-detail-redirect/9789241565639#:~:text=WHO›s%20Global%20status%20report%20on,doing%20to%20reduce%20this%20burden.

WHO. (2018). Youth violence. https://www.who.int/news-room/fact-sheets/detail/youth-violence

WHO. (2019, October 8). *Forty seconds to action.*

Wolman, B. B. (1977). *International encyclopedia of psychiatry, psychology, psychoanalysis, and neurology.* Van Nostrand Reinhold Co.

World Economic Forum. (2017). The global gender gap report. http://www3.weforum.org/docs/WEF_GGGR_2017.pdf

World Economic Forum. (2018). Here's what young Indians really want from life. https://www.weforum.org/agenda/2018/10/here-s-what-young-indians-really-want-from-life/

YouTube. (2016, June 16). YouTube Britain's worst paedophile Richard Huckle.

YouTube. (2018, May 19). Daisy Irani's shocking revelation: Abused at age 6.

YouTube. (2021, January 13). Marital rape ke khilaf India me kanun kyou nahi ban raha.

Zee News. (2013, December 13). Polyandry still practiced in Tibet's village. https://www.youtube.com/watch?v=11eGVWMVBTM

Zee News. (2019, December 26). DNA, crime statistics.

Zee News. (2019, December 4). DNA.

ABOUT THE AUTHOR

Alka Wadkar is a retired faculty from Department of Psychology, University of Pune. She has a rich experience of teaching, counselling, research, evaluation and extension activities.

Alka Wadkar has completed her MA and PhD in psychology and has been teaching postgraduate students since 1984. She had a bright career throughout her academic endeavour. She has received various prestigious awards and scholarships from primary education to PhD. She stood first in social sciences for her postgraduation in psychology. She has successfully guided 10 research students for PhD, 4 for MPhil and more than 100 students for MA and MEd.

Alka Wadkar is known as an effective teacher and orator. She is associated with training government officers, police officers, college teachers and education officers for more than 30 long years. She has delivered lectures for online refresher courses of psychology and management.

She has been associated with Symbiosis College for postgraduate teaching for last two years. She has been shouldering various responsibilities for the Indira Gandhi National Open University for last 12 years. She has been evaluating PhD theses of various universities for more than 25 years. She is involved in prestigious academic work of reviewing research papers for highly reputed foreign professional journal.

Alka Wadkar has authored 17 books and has received seven state-level awards. She is known for her socially relevant thought-provoking books, such as *Sexual Harassment of Women at Workplace*; *AIDS: A Psycho-social Perspective*, and *TV and Its Effects on Children*. All her books are based on scientific research and are for laypeople. She has also written six textbooks for different universities. She has been writing articles for radio, and daily, monthly and yearly publications for more than 35 years. She has published and presented more than 75 research papers in regional, national and international contexts. She has written articles for encyclopaedia and various state government publications. She has completed five research projects. Dr Wadkar has been actively involved in various government schemes, such as Sarva Shiksha Abhiyan, Anganwadi and the like, especially for the welfare of women and children. Dr Wadkar has been working for more than 30 years for the Government of India and the Government of Maharashtra on prestigious assignments related to highest examinations.

Wadkar has been involved in various institutes for differently abled children. She has been known for free counselling services for needy and differently abled individuals for years. She is also a trustee of a college of education.

INDEX